The Psychoanalytic Study of the Child

The Psychoanalytic Study of the Child

VOLUME I   1945

AN ANNUAL

INTERNATIONAL UNIVERSITIES PRESS

239 PARK AVE. SOUTH   NEW YORK, N. Y. 10003

Manufactured in the United States of America

The Psychoanalytic Study of the Child

VOLUME I   1945

MANAGING EDITORS

ANNA FREUD   HEINZ HARTMANN, M.D.   ERNST KRIS, PH.D.

CONTENTS

V. PROBLEMS OF GROUP LIFE

VI. SURVEYS AND COMMENTS

PREFACE

The contribution of psychoanalysis to the study of the child covers many areas. In therapy the range extends from child analysis to child guidance and group work; in theory, from the basic problems of genetic psychology to those concerned with the interrelation of culture and the upbringing of the child. While many psychiatric techniques and many concepts upon which psychologists and educators rely bear the imprint of psychoanalytic thought, contributions to this Annual center on psychoanalytic hypotheses. It is hoped that from this center contacts with neighboring fields will be established.

The Annual is an Anglo-American venture. We hope that in following volumes we may include contributions from other countries.

THE EDITORS

THE GENETIC APPROACH
IN PSYCHOANALYSIS

By HEINZ HARTMANN, M.D. and ERNST KRIS, Ph.D. (New York)

1. *Two Sets of Hypotheses*

The word "psychoanalysis" is commonly used to designate three things: a therapeutic technique, which we here call "psychoanalytic therapy", an observational method to which we here refer as "the psychoanalytic interview", and a body of hypotheses for which we here reserve the term "psychoanalysis". Two groups of hypotheses will be discussed: some dealing with dynamic and some dealing with genetic propositions. The former are concerned with the interaction and the conflicts of forces within the individual and with their reaction to the external world, at any given time or during brief time spans. The genetic propositions describe how any condition under observation has grown out of an individual's past, and extended throughout his total life span. Representative examples of dynamic propositions are those concerned with defense against danger and reaction to frustration. Genetic propositions state how these reactions come into being and are used in the course of an individual's life.

Psychiatrists, social workers and even social scientists base their findings frequently on a study of the past of the individual; however, in doing so, they need not have and frequently do not have genetic propositions in mind. The case record, that invaluable tool of modern medical and social exploration, or the psychiatric interview, may reveal that a conflict, a symptom or a pattern of behavior have occurred before. In using dynamic propositions the psychiatrist may reduce what appeared as a series of incomparable instances into a sequence of similar situations; when such regularity becomes perceivable, decisive progress will have been made. Thus we find the man who tends to drop his effort whenever in love or work an immediate competitor appears. This insight, however, is not gained with any genetic

11

proposition in mind. The finding establishes that an individual reacts similarly under similar conditions; in competition of a certain intensity he prefers retreat to continued pursuit of the goal in order to avoid what he experiences as fear and/or guilt.

If the investigator is guided by genetic propositions he will take such findings as a basis upon which to establish a causal relationship between the individual's retreat pattern in conflict situations and earlier experiences, in which the pattern was gradually formed. Experience in this context need not mean a single event but, more often, a constellation in an individual's early life that may have lasted for a stretch of time; no one isolated constellation need be meant, but rather the sequence of many that overlap in time and space. The expression "forming a pattern" does not only refer to a single trait, a symptom that is, as it were, attached to or superimposed upon the structure of the personality, but also to this structure itself. Investigators who follow the lead of genetic propositions will inquire when retreat from competition was "learned" or adopted as a solution; why, when the competitors were father or sibling, that conflict was solved by retreat, and what experiences had formed parts or earlier stages of the pattern long before the coincidence of situation and response was established. This pattern was learned through failure. The genetic propositions trace the way not only to earlier situations, in which similar behavior was displayed, but to situations in which different behavior was at least attempted: the attack against the rival and its failure in response to parental disapproval or to feelings of guilt.[1] And thus new areas open for the application of genetic propositions: when aggression was barred, why was it turned against the self and not against other objects or toward other activities?

The two types of propositions represent two aspects in the approach of psychoanalysis. The first is concerned with human behavior in a given situation; the second with the explanation of this behavior by an investigation of its origin. This investigaton regularly leads back to events that partly cannot be remembered, and tends to embrace periods of life when experiences could not be formulated in verbal symbols.

The forecast of human behavior that psychoanalysis can make is best, when based on both dynamic and genetic propositions. Generally

1. See in this connection the misapprehension of Lewin (1937) who assumed that in psychoanalysis behavior is merely traced back to similar earlier situations.
See bibliography for references.

speaking, one might say that the propositions concerned with psychological dynamics are more fully elaborated and more widely accepted. During the last decade they have gained some considerable influence upon the total field of medical therapy, partly through the studies in psychosomatic medicine, in which the dynamics of the "body" were correlated to those of the "mind". At the same time the verification of these propositions has acquired so independent a standing in experimental psychology that one tends to speak of "experimental psychoanalysis" as of a field of its own. Partly under the impression of this expansive activity in neighboring disciplines, some of the dynamic propositions of psychoanalysis are finding respectful consideration in practices of social control, in welfare, and in the social sciences. Briefly, they have deeply penetrated psychiatry and enlarged its scope and influence.

In many practices of child care and education genetic propositions have been hardly less influential. However, their influence in the practical fields up to the present has outweighed by far their importance in organized research. The academic study of child psychology and child development has not sufficiently taken notice of the genetic approach in psychoanalysis.[2] Psychoanalysts, on the other hand, have failed in many respects to take into account the data that child psychology has assembled; an omission that has led to many incongruities.

With this state of affairs in mind we here shall discuss two problems: first the relation of dynamic and genetic propositions of psychoanalysis, and second, the present stage of the development of the genetic propositions themselves.

2. Dynamic versus Genetic Propositions

The importance of the detailed and specific study of the actual situation in which human behavior occurs is not controversial; any attempt to apply any psychoanalytic hypothesis must start from here. Controversy begins when we wish to establish how much the understanding of the past, the genetically oriented investigation, can contribute to the understanding of the present. Clinical impressions and methodological considerations are both being brought forward in support of

2. For the different reaction of psychiatry and academic psychology to psychoanalysis see Herma, Kris and Shor.

the view that the genetic propositions are unduly stressed in psychoanalysis.

(a)   Genetic propositions and psychoanalytic technique.

Objections to the value of genetic propositions have been expressed by some clinicians since the early days of psychoanalysis. Thus C. G. Jung believed that Freud's ontogenetic propositions did not essentially contribute to an understanding of the actual conflict in which pathological behavior occurred; this claim led Jung to adopt the dichotomy that he has maintained for thirty years: he focuses his attention on the present situation of the individual and on the past of the race.   Others do not share his interest in the racial unconscious; however, they are inclined generally to stress that psychoanalysis is "too genetic" (Horney); less frequently do they object to one or the other of the genetic propositions.

A detailed discussion of such objections or a historical survey of the arguments used over a quarter of a century is not intended here.   Only one aspect of this controversy must be mentioned, since it concerns the data upon which, in clinical work, genetic interpretations have to be based.   Most of those who object to the importance of genetic propositions also object to the technique of psychoanalytic therapy.   This is true of authors as divergent from each other as Schultz-Hencke, Sullivan, Horney, or Thompson.   The controversy is best characterized if we relate it to the problem of "indication for psychoanalytic therapy" in general (Alexander).   Discussions center around three topics: that of contraindication of psychoanalytic therapy in certain types of cases; that of its modification in others; and that of its modifications in order to save time.   Modifications may then lead to substitution of less time-consuming therapies with comparable results; (where better results are expected by the use of other therapeutic techniques we would assume psychoanalytic therapy to be contraindicated).   The value of such investigations is uncontested and their urgency is great indeed.   In the course of these investigations, however, the tendency has developed to consider the technical procedures used in psychoanalytic therapy as random procedures.   The questions: "why should the patient lie on a couch"—or "why should the analyst refrain from guidance" are cases in point.   There would be indeed no reason for retaining either the paraphernalia of the interview situation or the elaborate technical prescriptions in handling interpretations, were we faced with accidental arrangements.   What today is being described as psychoanalytic therapy and its technique has grown out of many experiments in therapy, initiated by Freud and elaborated by others over many years. Some of the modifications suggested today have already been given a trial period and were rejected; others have been incorporated in what might be called "the standards". This development, starting out with Freud's road away from suggestive therapy, was largely due to the progress in psychoanalytic knowledge. To quote only one instance: the detailed discussions of techniques of interpretations, initiated in the twenties by W. Reich and continued by A. Freud, O. Fenichel, E. Glover and others, reflect the progress in understanding of the function of what Freud defines as ego: interpretation should start as close as possible to the experience of the patient—"from higher layers"—and elucidate the structure of "defenses" before they proceed to what stems from the id.[3]

These and similar rules aim essentially at obtaining the very data upon which genetic interpretations given to the patient have to be based: whatever traces of suggestive therapy survive in this procedure, whatever part cathartic discharges play—and their part is considerable—the ultimate goal is the capturing of the repressed. By the insight thus provided, the ego is given the strength to re-integrate; even the process of "re-living the past" during psychoanalytic therapy is part of that great venture in the acquisition of insight.

We formulate the following thesis: of all observational techniques dealing with adult individuals known at present the psychoanalytic interview is likely to lead to the most complete set of those data to which the genetic propositions refer. Insofar as it is assumed that genetic insight is a therapeutic asset, this thesis bears upon the problem of "indication"; the decision as to in which cases psychoanalytic therapy is not indicated, in which it should be modified, and in which it is the most promising or only possible therapy should be discussed with this point of view in mind. At the present stage of the discussion one frequently is tempted to believe that those who advocate changes in technique, e.g., the predominance of guidance in psychoanalytic therapy, are not aware of the consequences such changes will have upon the set of data to which they will be able to obtain access; and conversely those who do not appreciate the importance of genetic interpretations tend to change their technique.

3. For a recent summary of views on psychoanalytic technique see Fenichel.

(b)   Limitations of cross-sectional studies.

Discussions based on clinical impressions tend to leave many questions unsolved, and scientific decision in this area tends to be delayed, since the criteria upon which such decision has to be based lack decisiveness.   A greater clarity might be expected from academic psychologists, who in the last decade have reacted to the challenge of psychoanalysis.   As a first step, "objective verification" of psychoanalytic propositions has been attempted.   Sears recently surveyed the methods used and the results obtained.   The majority of these investigations test propositions established by psychoanalysts under controlled conditions, a procedure of considerable and manifold value. It establishes anew that the psychoanalytic interview is a source of valid scientific propositions, and reëstablishes unity in psychology by introducing "man and his conflict" into the reach of academic psychology.   By reformulating psychoanalytic findings into clear-cut propositions, work in this area is likely to force a greater logical sharpness upon psychoanalytic writing itself, which in turn may facilitate future scientific discourse.   At the present stage, the reformulation of psychoanalytic findings seems to have been most successful where concepts of learning theory were used.[4]   It is hardly necessary to stress other advantages of these experimental investigations: the rigor of the procedure which allows for quantification and the simplicity of the experimental situation facilitate demonstration of hypotheses to those who are unfamiliar with details in the general area of normal and abnormal behavior.

The limits of current experiments in the verification of psychoanalytic hypotheses become apparent when we realize that, at the present stage of investigations, the lack of experimental verification rarely, if ever, implies invalidation of propositions.   It proves rather that the ingenuity of the experimenters has not been able to master the translation from the area of life where the proposition was gained into that of the controlled situation where the experiment is performed.   Sears has made this point very clear, and his review of work in the field indicates the existing difficulties.   While it was comparatively easy to reproduce situations in which "displacement" and "substitution" operate, no comparable success has been achieved where other mechanisms of defenses are involved.   Thus experimental investigations in the area of repression tend to remain disappointing;

---

4. A survey of these reformulations initiated by Dollard and Miller was recently made by Mowrer and Kluckhohn.

repression, in Freud's definition, is a reaction to an experience which seriously affects the psycho-biological existence of the person; repression takes place in order to escape from danger or to avoid anxiety. All experimenters agree that danger cannot easily be induced in experimental setups.

The experiments select a limited number of factors and predictions are accurate only where these and no other factors operate.[5] Thus, the intensive studies of frustration and regression by Barker, Dembo and Lewin—a set of experiments in which the tools of research were sharpened with the greatest skill—do not permit us to generalize to what kind of frustrations and under what circumstances a child will respond with regression. Lewin and his collaborators investigated the reaction of children when suddenly deprived but still in view of highly desirable toys. When children visit department stores with their mothers, many of them are in an equally tantalizing situation. What will their reaction then be? It will depend on what meaning the "you can't have it" and the "it is too expensive" gains for the child by the way in which the mother puts it to him. This depends on a variety of factors: on the child's relation to the mother; on the mother's own relation to similar present and past experiences; and how, in the child's own previous development, tolerance for deprivation in general, and for certain specific deprivations has developed. These are the complexities with which the genetic and dynamic propositions of psychoanalysis grope. Only a consideration of both establishes favorable conditions for a successful prediction. The limitations of the experimental situation do not allow for a reproduction of this complexity. It deals with a limited time dimension and, however valuable in other areas, experimental investigation has produced hardly any verification where the genetic propositions are concerned.

The genetic approach in psychoanalysis does not deal only with anamnestic data, nor does it intend to show only "how the past is contained in the present". Genetic propositions describe why, in past situations of conflict, a specific solution was adopted; why the one was retained and the other dropped, and what causal relation exists between these solutions and later developments. Genetic propositions refer to the fact that in an adult's behavior, anxiety may be induced by paradoxically out-dated conditions and they explain

5. See for similar views, Bernfeld, Hartmann (1943) and for slightly different arguments, Rapaport.

why these conditions may still exercise influence. However, in speaking of the similarity of conditions eliciting anxiety we do not speak of an identity of situations. The man who retreats from competition in order to avoid murderous impulses against the man at the next desk, and a child who may experience similar impulses toward a newly born sibling do not live through the same situations. The various parts of the personality of the adult have undergone fundamental changes. Thus for instance, the appraisal of objective danger is clearly different with adult and child. In fact, the whole area to which a cross-sectional analysis of the adult's and the child's situation would refer is fundamentally different. But one part of the adult's personality behaves as if no change had occurred: it has, as psychoanalysts put it, not participated in the development. Briefly, the genetic propositions concerning fixation are in no way invalidated by Lewin's objections (1937).

The genetic propositions of psychoanalysis have grown out of empirical work. Not only did Freud draw attention to a large number of hitherto unknown facts concerning earliest childhood; but he soon was impressed by rules in the genetic relationship of psychological phenomena. The elements that constitute this relationship are "overdetermined", interdependent, and their complexity has in many instances not yet been sufficiently structured in a logical sense. The genetic propositions, however, made it possible to establish typical sequences in development and to trace individual behavior historically to its origins. As a consequence, psychoanalysis has adopted a preference to characterize psychological phenomena according to their position in the process of development. In the psychoanalytic study of personality, character traits are not grouped according to their similarity in a descriptive sense, but rather according to their common genetic roots. Examples in kind are the "oral" and "anal" characters. Here the procedure of psychoanalysis resembles that of biology in those cases where biological classification is based upon genetics (Hartmann, 1929).

Why have such classifications been adopted? What is the reason for the emphasis upon genetic propositions in this context? In order to simplify an extremely complex problem we start with an example: experience has shown that details of behavior that in a cross-sectional analysis appear indistinguishable may clearly be differentiated by genetic investigation. Conversely, details of behavior that in cross-sectional analysis appear different and are actually opposite may have grown out of the same root, and may justify the same prognosis. Pacifism may in one case be a reaction formation to the wish to attack and in the other an expression of fear of being attacked by a superior enemy. Extreme aggressiveness may be in one case the reaction to fear and its concealment, in the other, the direct expression of sadistic wishes. These are distinctions that the genetic methods permit us to establish. What appears to be similar behavior with the individuals when seen in the cross-section can be differentiated when we take account of its genesis. If we are able to indicate the position of such behavior in the longitudinal section what appeared as similar behavior gains in each individual case a very different meaning. It is here that we rely upon the genetic propositions especially when dealing with what has been called the central areas of personality; only the genetic propositions permit us to make perceivable the drives that a behavior detail represents, their direction, their intensity and their structural interconnection.

True, many elements of the past may actually be visible in behavior in a given field. But on the other hand, many elements of the past upon which the application of the genetic proposition has to be based are not contained as memories in "the field". We here refer to what psychoanalysis calls the repressed and to the unconscious parts of ego-defense. But they may appear in the field if a specific technique, that of the psychoanalytic interview, is being used. And every application of this method forcibly leads to a restructuring of the field.

The field theory as formulated by Lewin (who is inclined to speak of a method rather than a theory, 1943) has produced the sharpest and most logical formulation of the non-historical tendency in psychology (Brown, 1937). It nevertheless has much in common with psychoanalysis: the consideration of a large number of interdependent factors, the assumption that every event results out of a variety of factors (over-determination), are derived from psychoanalysis. One of the basic statements of the field theory, that "any behavior or any other change in a psychological field depends only upon the psychological field at that time", does not appear to be irreconcilable with psychoanalysis, and it seems possible that if the field theory or other cross-sectional approaches should develop new methods of investigation their scope may be considerably enlarged.[6] However, it seems essential

6. Thus Lewin in one of his latest papers seems to assume that those events of the past that are of immediate relevance for the present can be investigated as parts of the field and that such investigations may extend over "days and weeks" (1943). The analytic approach definitely postulates a reconstruction including the total life span.

not to overlook the pragmatic side: the field theory has as yet not suggested any definite answer to the question with which we are concerned in this paper: under what conditions is "testing the properties of a situation at a given time" the most productive and reliable method for the understanding of the dynamic and structural properties of psychological phenomena; and how far must such understanding be based upon what to field theorists may appear a detour via genetic investigation.

According to Lewin the postulates for an ideal topological investigation of the field will consider what is psycho-biologically relevant both in a phenotypical and genotypical sense (1935). No other observational method seems fit to establish this relevance except the psychoanalytic interview itself. It can reasonably be described as a field situation in which two people react to each other within conditions established by rules of procedure. The field situation is changed from day to day not only by changes in the experience of the patient in his daily life but also by the interpretation given by the analyst.

The patient whose mechanism of retreat from danger has been mentioned comes for analysis with no other complaint than that of lack of interest in his work. The analyst's first impression is that the lack of interest may not be genuine; a detail, the patient's affect when discussing events in his office supplies the cue. A first interpretation draws the patient's attention to the contradiction between lack of interest and intensity of emotional reaction. The structure of the field is changed since the patient has been stimulated to observe similar contradictions; for a time he has become allied to the analyst in observing under what conditions emotions of considerable intensity arise. From this first step a way leads to the insight that the first set of conditions is related to the second and that lack of interest occurs when continued participation might lead to a clash with competitors. In the course of the gradual elaboration of this pattern the following incident may take place: the patient's lack of interest may shift from his work to the treatment, which he may wish to discontinue. He has "suddenly" noticed other patients in the analyst's waiting room and reacts to this observation with a desire to retreat. At this point the field is restructured by a transference interpretation. He is told that the other patients have suddenly been noticed because he was predisposed to discover rivals and that this rivalry is related to the growing attachment to the analyst's person. The sequence attachment-rivalry-retreat is discussed as one that has shifted from professional life to the treatment room. When memory material supplies further cues a rivalry situation in childhood in relation to siblings and parents may emerge. This, as a rule, does not come about without the reexperiencing of repressed emotions. This in turn may lead to a reconstruction of the "original situation", in which, for example, the wish to attack was directed against sibling or parent, and in which attempts in this direction had been undertaken; the reconstruction may then include the dangers with which thought or action was fraught at the time, their suppression by the parents or by the patient's conscience and a large variety of other details. In many cases the reconstruction may then be supplemented by a recollection of a formerly repressed memory. Such reconstructions based upon traces in dream and fantasy life which supplement actual behavior may well be called predicting the past; predictions of this kind have by "objective verification" proved to be correct in astonishing details.[7]

Based on these and similar experiences the psychoanalytic interview itself has repeatedly been characterized as an experiment. But this experiment, however rich, is fraught with uncertainties. Observers who used the same observational method have not reached agreement on many points, especially on those referring to the genetic propositions. And thus the problem of objective verification of these propositions gains in importance; not only for those interested in integration of scientific approaches but for all those who do spade work in the field, for psychiatrists, social workers and educators.

3. The Present Stage of the Genetic Propositions

In the psychiatric and psychologic literature of the nineteenth century, concepts concerning dynamics played a limited part; Herbart's mechanistic dynamics reached Freud through the work of the neurologist Meynert, and his familiarity with the work of Lipps and with French psychiatrists redirected this influence. But from nowhere could Freud borrow models for an understanding of the ontogenetic development of man's psychological structure. Genetic thought came to him mainly through evolutionism; this accounts for the importance Freud was inclined to attribute to phylogenetic explanations; they play their part not only in his reconstructions of human history but also in explanations of concrete features of human behavior under clinical observation. However the recourse to the past of the race transmitted by the inheritance of acquired characteristics, inspiring as it is in Freud's presentation, does not find sufficient empirical support in our present knowledge of heredity. Moreover it seems that in most cases in which Freud introduces phylogenetic propositions, ontogenetic propositions could be carried one step farther. For instance, Freud argues that the intensity of the fear of castration experienced by the male child in our civilization is unaccountable if we consider it as a reaction to the actual threats to which the boy is being exposed in

7. For the theory of Reconstruction in Psychoanalysis, see Freud (1938); for an example of verification, see Bonaparte.

the phallic phase; only the memory of the race will explain it.[8]   To this we are inclined to reply with Freud's own arguments.   While in many cases the child in our civilization is no longer being threatened with castration, the intensity of the veiled aggression of the adult against the child may still produce the same effect.   One might say that there always is "castration" in the air.   Adults who restrict the little boy act according to patterns rooted in their own upbringing. However symbolic or distant from actual castration their threats might be, they are likely to be interpreted by the little boy in terms of his own experiences.   The tumescent penis with which he responds in erotic excitement, that strange phenomenon of a change in a part of his body that proves to be largely independent of his control, leads him to react not to the manifest content but rather to the latent meaning of the restriction with which his strivings for mother, sister, or girl-playmate meet.   And then, what he may have seen frequently before, the genitals of the little girl, acquire a new meaning as evidence and corroboration of that fear.   However, the intensity of fear is not only linked to his present experience, but also to similar experiences in his past.   The dreaded retaliation of the environment revives memories of similar anxieties when desires for other gratifications were predominant and when the supreme fear was not that of being castrated but that of not being loved.[9]   In other words: pregenital experience is one of the factors determining the reaction in the phallic phase. This simple formulation refers to a wealth of highly significant experiences which form the nucleus of early childhood; to the total attitude of the environment toward the child's anaclitic desires, when the need for protection is paramount, and toward the child's later erotic demands.

While phylogenetic speculation was suggested to Freud by theories current in the 1880's, his insight into the relevance of ontogenetic factors grew out of empirical material.   When, in the quest for the etiology of hysteria, clinical impressions led to the patient's childhood, Freud attempted to solve what appeared to him then as an unexplained difficulty; he made the assumption that one traumatic sexual experience, the seduction of the child by an adult, had been of decisive etiological importance (1896).   This assumption was soon dropped and replaced by descriptions of regular phases in the development of the child's instinctual needs.

8. See Freud, 1939, p. 124.

9. For a partly similar formulation, see Jones.

In establishing the sequence of oral, anal, and phallic phases of libidinal development, Freud did not distinguish between a biological process—maturation determined by constitution—and processes of development influenced by the environment. He simply presented the sequence and its consequences for the future life of man. It will remain an astonishing document in the history of science that from material so far removed from direct observation of the child as that of the analysis of adult neurotics, phenomena of high regularity in biological development could have been so accurately reconstructed. The genetic investigation then proceeded from the study of libidinal development to that of the inhibiting forces. In the course of these investigations one set of hypotheses has been elaborated in greater detail than others. More is known in psychoanalysis about the development of the superego than about that of the ego, in Freud's definition; thus the genetic propositions tend to be incomplete and in many cases unsatisfactory, where psychoanalytic ego psychology is concerned. The following discussion is aimed largely at this gap in our knowledge.

We start from Freud's greatest contribution to the psychology of the ego: the reformulation of the problem of anxiety in 1926. Anxiety is no longer traced to the transformation of libidinal energy into fear. What might be called a toxicological hypothesis was discarded. It was replaced by dynamic propositions that describe the function of the ego under the impact of perceived threats. Danger may come from within the organism itself when instinctual demands increase; such increase may become a threat to the very organization of the ego, or it may involve the individual in moral conflicts; but the increase in instinctual demands may also create conflict with the environment. The environment, on the other hand, may be the source of independent danger, when its impositions reduce indulgence. In each such case the function of the ego is related to what one might call a condition of imbalance in the total situation; anxiety of low intensity appears, as an emergency signal in order to stimulate action, and anxiety of high intensity appears in the adult mostly when the signal function has failed and the individual feels unable to restore balance either by attack or retreat of any kind; if this is the case, a traumatic situation, one of "no way out" and of helplessness, is experienced. Such situations have a tendency to revive the past. Past experiences with danger have been summarized by Freud as three main sets of situations: those in which the fear of the loss of the love-object arises, which finally leads to the fear of loss of love; those in which the fear of castration arises; and later those which lead to the fear of conscience—terms that refer to situations of high complexity and long duration.

In summarizing what is explicitly and implicitly contained in Freud's concept as far as genetic propositions are concerned, we suggest the following formulation. In the life of each individual crucial situations occur. They may be due predominantly to external events or they may be due predominantly to predispositions in the individual which then may invest insignificant situations with high significance. In order to assess the predispositions of an individual that meet those crucial situations, the data in every case would have to refer to his total past. For a considerable time the reference to the instinctual demands dominated the discussions of these predispositions and the functions of the ego were either incompletely described or the description was limited to that of mechanisms of defense at its disposal. Though at the present it is generally realized that the realm of the ego is wider, clinical and theoretical discussions are not conducted on the same level. While there is no hesitation to refer in clinical description to the capacities with which an individual is equipped in coping with pressures of many kinds at any stage of his development, this point of view is comparatively new in theoretical discussions.

If we turn to the ego as the psychic system that controls perception and motility, achieves solutions, and directs actions, we have to insist on distinctions that seemed irrelevant when Freud first formulated his genetic propositions. A number of functions of the ego related to the apparatus at its disposal develop largely outside of the reach of psychic conflict; Hartmann(1939) actually speaks of a sphere of the ego free from conflict. These functions gain for our discussion a specific importance since they exercise a considerable influence as independent factors; they determine together with other factors what mechanism of defense an individual adopts and with what results, or what substitute goals he adopts for his instinctual desires. However, this distinction between psychological processes predominantly dependent on biological maturation, and others predominantly dependent on influences of the environment, to which we here refer as "development", is not limited to ego psychology. The growth of the teeth and of the muscular sphincter control are according to Freud influential in determining the progress from one phase of libidinal development to the other; but these maturational sequences determine also the sequence of experiences that owe their special character to one or the other of the libidinal phases. Similarly, the maturation of the apparatus of motility or perception exercises influence on the progress of the general development of the ego—an area of problems which however has not yet been sufficiently clarified. Seen against this background, one of the most general findings of psychoanalysis which by now seems self-evident, gains a specific importance. This finding asserts that the importance of an actual experience through which a child lives, and the direction this experience may give to his life largely depend on the specific phase of the child's development. This is the reason why a superficial collection of anamnestic data concerning an individual's childhood is frequently misleading. The question is not that at some time in childhood a tonsillectomy was performed or that a child was left in hospital care, but under what conditions and when these events took place. The coincidence of hospitalization and the fear of loss of love, that of tonsillectomy and fear of castration, thus the coincidence of predisposition and experience, are the decisive points.[10]

Many of the child's experiences that are uncovered by psychoanalytic therapy are of such specific importance; i.e., many of them are traumatic. However, others of which the memory is recovered by the patient or which are reconstructed by the analyst do not concern experiences that in themselves necessarily had a decisive causal or formative effect, and yet such experiences are of considerable importance for genetic investigation: they are "signs", indicating important changes in the child's life and they impress us as symptoms of his general development. This again leads back to the two interacting chains of maturation and development.

Freud's insistence on this interaction has recently been misrepresented as "overemphasis on biology". In fact, however, Freud clearly stresses the existence of two aspects. He refers to the biological aspect when he states that in tracing an individual's life history we describe some processes that were bound to occur under alternative conditions and following alternative pathways. The other aspect, with far more momentous consequences, concerns the importance of the environment; the object of psychoanalytic observation is according to Freud not the individual in splendid isolation; it is part of a world. Psychoanalysis does not claim to explain human behavior only as a

---

10. A model of such coincidence in the regular normal development of the little girl and her discovery of the sex difference, is tentatively indicated by Rado. For similar theoretical views see Erikson.

result of drives and fantasies; human behavior is directed toward a world of men and things. The approach of psychoanalysis in many cases includes the structure of this world in its scope; and in this sense psychoanalysis is applied Social Science (Hartmann, 1944). Thus what we loosely call a child's "experience", is in psychoanalysis viewed both in relation to the child's biological growth and in its relation to the world around it, a distinction that proves its value, if applied over a long period of observation to the wealth of data psychoanalytic therapy brings to light.

We now define more closely the crucial situations in an individual's development: There are typical phases of conflict, either between drives with opposite goals or between drives and the ego structure, which regularly occur in both normal and abnormal development. They may be brought about mainly by maturation, when new demands or new tasks are brought into the individual's reach, or they may mainly be brought about by demands and influences of the environment, such as those regularly occurring in every human being's life. The crucial phases of maturation and of development actually coincide to a large extent; at which points they coincide, and at which lines cross each other, will to a considerable degree depend on cultural factors.

If we include these cultural factors it will become evident that however rich and manifold the data are on which psychoanalysis bases its views of the child's development, these data are on the whole not sufficient to allow for the full and detailed formulation of genetic propositions. In other words, it is essential to supplement the data supplied by the psychoanalytic interview with data established by other observational methods; there seems little doubt that in enlarging the set of data we shall approximate the postulate that the genetic propositions of psychoanalysis should be verified.

It might here briefly be recalled that up to 1909 the only data available were gained from the analyses of adults. In the second decade of this century unsystematic observations of children were interpreted as confirming what had been gathered from this source. In the third decade, with the systematic development of child analysis, new material was made available; it has deeply influenced psychoanalytic theory and technique and the more detailed propositions concerning defense mechanisms largely stem from this source. The next stage, the systematic observation of children by psychoanalytically trained observers, has not produced more than isolated sets of data.

Though we have learned a great deal an independent verification of the genetic propositions has only partly been achieved. Such verifications would have a different value from those concerning dynamic propositions. There, verification has largely confirmative value and serves, as we said, the purpose of scientific intercommunication. In the area of the genetic propositions, we are faced with problems of integration on a higher level. In many areas disagreement prevails. In certain cases psychoanalytic observation was able to falsify a genetic assumption; this we believe is true of the propositions concerning the trauma of birth as suggested by O. Rank. In other instances, a similar refutation has not been achieved. This is particularly true of propositions suggested by Melanie Klein, and though the uncertainty is partly due to a confusion of language it is also partly due to the limits of the observational methods used.[11]

One might have hoped for support in the experience and in the data made available by academic students of child development. Though the psychoanalyst is bound to find essential information in their work, and could be warned of many miscarriages in theoretical thinking by familiarity with it, it seems that the gaps in data to which we here refer, cannot be filled by what has been observed independently of a psychoanalytic orientation. It rather seems that only where the psychoanalytic hunch is directly linked to observation, new areas of problems are opened up.

As an example we refer to propositions suggested recently concerning the influence of earliest relationship with the mother upon survival and development of the child, by Ribble, Spitz and others. Similar investigations are lacking in other areas. We quote two examples: psychoanalytic hypotheses assert that isolated symptoms such as disturbances of concentration, eating difficulties, fears, and phobias or obsessional rituals are frequent with children between three and six. In other words, certain traits that are symptoms of neurosis in the adult are spread among young children who later become, or do not become "neurotics". A frequent formulation of this proposition states that the infantile neurosis is ubiquitous in our civilization. New data are required in order to determine under what conditions the infantile disturbance will develop to the adult neurosis (A. Freud, 1945).

11. For discussion of this controversy see Glover.

We are hardly in a better position where the changes of puberty are concerned; we are in many cases unable to predict both the extent and direction of these changes, a problem of decisive importance for child psychiatry; one which particularly suggests the importance of observation of a large number of cases, in various cultural settings.

Briefly, only the systematic observation of life histories from birth on can fill the gap. Such longitudinal research has been approximated with highly promising results by various groups, in relation to comparative studies, especially by anthropologists. It has been said that through the publications of Mead, Kardiner, Kluckhohn, Erikson, Gorer, and others,[12] we know more about the growing up in certain primitive civilizations than about the interrelation between the modes of childbearing and the formation of personality in our own civilization (Bateson, 1943). While this seems to be an exaggeration it is a healthy one which draws attention to the lack of data to which we here refer. If the longitudinal observation in our own civilization were to be systematized and the study of life histories were to be combined with that of the crucial situations in Freud's sense, many hunches might be formulated as propositions, and others might be discarded. This goal could best be achieved by the constant interaction of two observational methods, psychoanalysis and observation of life histories, which we here call the retrospective and prospective method. The method of retrospective research has been established by the technique of psychoanalytic therapy; the methods of prospective research have been elaborated by psychiatrists, psychologists, and anthropologists. The relationship of both observational methods is manifold: the retrospective method was in the past in a position to direct attention to new areas in the child's life, which have gradually been investigated by observers with various kinds of observational skills; there is no reason to assume that this function of pointing to the essential is exhausted. The retrospective method, however, can do more: it can establish interconnections between experiences that are bound to escape observers who have less intimate insight; it is here that child analysis may well be expected to play a part. There are, on the other hand, areas of problems in child development that have found little attention in psychoanalysis—or where the access remains unsatisfactory: examples of the former are those achievements of the ego that are independent of conflict; examples of the latter are the experiences of the pre-verbal stage of child

12. See Young and Linton for divergent summaries.

development.   Psychoanalysis is witness to the importance of this
sta⸱⸱e for the future; child observation, however, will have to tell the
tale of these eventful years.

BIBLIOGRAPHY

Alexander, F., 1944: "The Indication for Psychoanalytic Therapy", *Bulletin*,
    The New York Academy of Medicine, 20, pp. 319-332.
Alexander, F., 1944: "The Brief Psychotherapy Council and Its Outlook", in
    Psychosomatic Medicine, Procedings of the Second Brief Psychotherapy
    Council, Chicago, January 1944, pp. 1-4.
Barker, R. G., Dembo, T., and Lewin, K., 1941: "Frustration and Regression,
    an Experiment with Young Children", *Studies in Topological and Vector
    Psychology*, University of Iowa Studies in Child Welfare, XVIII, p. 1.
Bateson, G., 1944: "Cultural Determinants of Personality", *Personality and
    Its Behavior Disorders.*, ed. J. McV. Hunt, vol. II.
Bernfeld, S., 1934: "Die Gestalttheorie", *Imago*, XX, pp. 32-77.
Bonaparte, M., 1945: "The Analytical Discovery of a Primal Scene", *this
    Annual*, I.
Brown, J. F., 1937: "Psychoanalysis, Topological Psychology and Experimental
    Psychopathology", *Psychoanalytic Quarterly*, VI, pp. 227-237;
Brown, J. F., 1940: "Freud's Influence on American Psychology", *ibid*. IX,
    pp. 283-292.
Erikson, E. Homburger, 1940: "Studies in the Interpretation of Play, I, Clinical
    Observation of Play-disruption in Young Children", *Genetic Psychology
    Monographs*, XXII, pp. 557-671.
Fenichel, O., 1942: "Psychoanalytic Technique", *Psychoanalytic Quarterly*, XI.
Freud, A., 1937: *The Ego and the Mechanisms of Defence*.
Freud, A., 1945: "Indications for Child Analysis", *this Annual*, I.
Freud, S., 1896: "Etiology of Hysteria", *Collected Papers*, I.
Freud, S., 1936: *The Problem of Anxiety*.
Freud, S., 1938: "Constructions in Analysis", *International Journal of Psycho-
    Analysis*, XIX.
Freud, S., 1939: *Moses and Monotheism*.
Glover, E., "Examination of the Klein System of Child Psychology", *this An-
    nual*, I.
Hartman, H., 1929: über genetische Charakterologie, inbesondere über
    psychoanalytische", *Jahrbuch der Charakterologie*, VI, pp. 75-95.
Hartmann, H., 1939: "Ich-Psychologie und Anpassungsproblem", *Interna-
    tionale Zeitschrift für Psychoanalyse und Imago*, XXIV.
Hartmann, H., 1943: "Psychiatry: Its Relation to Psychological Schools of
    Thought", *Psychiatry and the War*, ed. Frank J. Sladen.
Hartmann, H., 1944: "Psychoanalysis and Sociology" in *Psychoanalysis Today*.
Herma, H., Kris, E., and Shor, J., 1954: "Freud's Theory of the Dream in
    American Textbooks", *Journal of Abnormal and Social Psychology*,
    XXXVIII, pp. 319-334.
Horney, K., 1939: *New Ways in Psychoanalysis*.

Jones, E., 1940: Review of *Moses and Monotheism, International Journal of Psycho-Analysis*, XXI, pp. 230-240.

Lewin, K., 1935: "Environmental Forces in Child Behavior and Development", *Handbook of Child Psychology*, ed. C. Murchison; Chapter XIV, (also Lewin, "A Dynamic Theory of Personality", Chapter III).

Lewin, K., 1937: "Psychoanalysis and Topological Psychology", *Bulletin of the Menninger Clinic*, I, 202-211.

Lewin, K., 1943: "Defining the Field at a Given Time", *Psychological Review*, L, pp. 292-310.

Linton, R., 1945: *Cultural Background of Personality*.

Mowrer, O. H., and Kluckhon, C., 1944: "Dynamic Theory of Personality", *Personality and Behavior Disorders*, ed. J. McV. Hunt, vol. I.

Rado, S., 1933: "The Fear of Castration in Women", *Psychoanalytic Quarterly*, II, pp. 425-475.

Rapaport, D., 1942: "Freudian Mechanisms and Frustration Experiments", *Psychoanalytic Quarterly*, XI, pp. 503-512.

Ribble, M., 1944: "Infantile Experience in Relation to Personality Development", *Personality and Behavior Disorders*, ed. J. McV. Hunt, vol. II.

Sears, R. R., 1943: "Survey of Objective Studies of Psychoanalytic Concepts", *Social Science Research Council, Bulletin LI*.

Sears, R. R., 1944: "Experimental Analyses of Psychoanalytic Phenomena", *Personality and the Behavior Disorders*, ed. J. McV. Hunt, vol. I.

Spitz, R., 1945: "Hospitalism", *this Annual*, I.

Young, K., 1944: *Social Psychology*, rev. ed. pp. 48-76.

THE BIOLOGICAL ECONOMY OF BIRTH

By PHYLLIS GREENACRE, M.D. (New York) [1]

I

It is the intention of this paper to ask a number of questions regarding the biological economy of birth, to bring together as much evidence as possible bearing on the answers, and to indicate certain lines of research emanating from them. In what way does the process of birth subserve the new individual, and through him the race? It is my belief that it exerts definite influences on the future psychic and physical patterns of the child, especially on these larger patterns of the distribution of energy and the intensity of drives rather than on the specific smaller patterns that characterize one neurosis or another. These influences are accomplished, I believe, mainly by the degree and shape of the organization of antenatal narcissism to meet postnatal needs, such organization resulting largely from the process of birth.

This paper concerns itself with normal birth—whatever that is. It is much easier to establish criteria for definitely abnormal births than to define normal birth. In fact some obstetricians will question whether human birth among civilized people is ever normal; and pregnancy has been defined by one as a disease of nine months' duration.

The lines of inquiry are as follows: the general implications of pain; the question of painful birth from the child's rather than from the mother's angle; an examination of the sensory-motor balance of stimulation and response possible in the infant just before, during and after birth; the possible relation of this sensory-motor ratio to patterns of normal tension potential established at birth; and finally the effect of such patterns on the primary narcissism of the infant and on the energy distribution.

1. From the New York Hospital and the Department of Psychiatry, Cornell University Medical College.

31

Physical pain is regarded as a signal to the individual that something is wrong with the body. Pain may differ greatly in quality, varying from the sharp, shooting character of neuritic pain to the dull ache associated generally with visceral disease. Cannon(1)[2] in his book *The Wisdom of the Body* states, "As a rule pain is associated with the action of injurious agents, a fact well illustrated in cuts, burns and bruises. There are, to be sure, instances of very serious damage being done to the body—for example in tuberculosis of the lungs—without any pain whatsoever; and there are instances, also of severe pain, as in neuralgia, without corresponding danger to the integrity of the organism. These are exceptions, however, and the rule holds that pain is a sign of harm and injury."

Pain occurs in varying combinations with pleasure as for example in the itch and especially in its paler relative the tickle. But in all these forms it is either a herald or a memory of danger and appears as one of the organism's self-protective devices. It resembles in this respect anxiety, the signal of hidden (future or inner) danger, and fear, the reaction to outer danger. Indeed in some states pain, anxiety, and fear are not readily distinguishable one from another, and in a larger sense all are varieties of pain, if we consider this as distress, the opposite of pleasure. The derivation of the word itself from the same root as is found in *penalty* indicates directly its relation to *wrongness* in some form.

It does not seem very important at this point to differentiate clearly between the general category of pain as distress, and the specific definition of pain as a sensory perception in the strictly neurological sense. It appears that pain in the perceptive sense is probably an evolutionary refinement accompanying the development of the nervous system and that in the lowly animals without developed nervous tissue there exist none the less indications of organismic distress. Indeed it may seem from the fact that "pain is a primitive sensory modality and the free nerve endings are the least differentiated of possible cutaneous receptors"(2) that the ability to feel pain in any degree in this perceptive sense is one of the most important landmarks in evolutionary development, and marks the inception of the differentiation of the nervous system.

The one situation in which pain seems conspicuously to appear as part of an ordinary physiological function is in childbirth. It seems best not to become involved here in the questions of the nature,

2. Numbers in parentheses refer to the bibliography at the end of the paper.

degree and inevitability of material pain. The obstetricians DeLee and Greenhill(3) consider that human birth is always painful and cannot be considered a normal physiological process for the mother. That the sensory perception of pain is readily influenced even by the factor of attention is a common experience and can be measured in the laboratory(4). Psychoanalysts(5, 6) have been impressed especially by the importance of unconscious attitudes of unwillingness and apprehension as contributors to the maternal pain of labor.

This inquiry is mostly concerned with the effect of normal birth, or of usual average abnormal birth, on the infant. While the birth of a baby may be likened to a loss of a part of the body by the mother, as is seen in so exaggerated and special a form in certain neurotic patients, this is hardly true in the same way from the infant's angle. Further, the special pain to the human mother caused by the birth of her baby seems due in some degree to the large size of the infant head, i.e., the pain of the mother may be in part the penalty for the large cerebral development of our species as represented by her off-spring. There is, too, the question of the pain or distress suffered by the infant in the process of being born. It does seem strange, however, that the head containing the most precious heritage, the well developed cerebrum, should be not only the cause of much of the stress of birth but especially that it is at the same time the very part of the infant most endangered during birth.

One might inquire why does Nature arrange for the infant to "lead with its head" in the struggle of being born. The head, being used in the majority of cases as the tool of dilatation of the cervix, is given a rhythmic pounding by the periodic uterine contractions. It is protected, to be sure, by the bag of waters during the first stage of labor, but even this protection is generally lost when the head is actually passing through the birth canal; and the effect of the pressure pounding is readily evident in the caput succedenum with which many infants are born or the molding where the pressure has been more severe and prolonged. It can readily be seen that it is a natural advantage for the baby to come head first in order to get its nose out quickly and its respiration stimulated. The dangers of breech presentation because of premature respiration are part of general knowledge. It is not the face of the infant, however, that generally presents at birth, but the top of the head, that portion exactly enclosing the cerebrum.

There is evidence that the trauma of birth may cause considerable damage to the infant(7, 8) and that blood is found in the cerebrospinal fluid of the newborn in a surprising number of instances even when there has been no clearly detectable clinical evidence of damage and sometimes when the birth itself has not been conspicuously long or hard. Looked at from a long biological range it might be expected that this organ, the cerebrum, would be the most protected part of the newborn rather than the most endangered. If the damage of ordinary birth were permanently and appreciably destructive to the cerebrum it would negate the development of that organ. The question then arises whether ordinary uncomplicated birth even with its considerable degree of trauma to the infant is not of some advantage, whether in some way this particular workout, rough as it is, serves as a good introduction to life, a bridge between the greater protected dependence of intra-uterine life and the incipient increasing extramural independence?

The question of the relation of birth to anxiety is one that I have discussed at some length in an earlier article dealing essentially with the possible effects of difficult abnormal births or poor antenatal or neonatal conditions in producing a state of excessive chronic tension or susceptibility to excitation, which I have characterized as a state of predisposition to anxiety(9). The rather tentative statements of that article were based on my clinical observations supplemented especially by laboratory experiments and observations of infants carried on by various investigators. Subsequent clinical experience has reinforced these impressions, but there has not yet been the opportunity to carry out the systematic clinical and experimental investigation necessary more thoroughly to validate or to discard the theory stated.

The problem of the relation of normal birth to anxiety was touched upon but not adequately dealt with in that paper. To recapitulate and re-define now: While anxiety as such cannot exist until there is some dawning ego sense and therefore some individual psychological content, the forerunner of anxiety exists in a condition of irritable responsiveness of the organism, at first appearing in a number of loosely organized reflex responses. The experience of birth is considered by Freud as a prototype of the anxiety reaction(10) but is conceived of as operating through the assimilation into the constitutional makeup (i.e., genetically) of all the births of the ancestors. Freud tended to discard the possibility that the individual birth was of any great importance in determining the strength of the later anxiety reaction. It appears to me, however, that there is little evidence that birth has changed in such a way as to have become less important or more incidental in the life of the organism and that it continues to be the period of organization and patterning of the somatic components of the anxiety response which have previously consisted of loosely constellated and relatively superficial defense movements. It marks also the time of the more definite participation of the respiratory and cardiovascular systems in the defense activities of the infant, these very components forming so characteristically the integral part of the commonest somatic pattern of anxiety responses later in life. I conceive of a situation in which the antenatal, natal and neonatal experiences have very slight or no true (differentiated) psychological content at the time of their occurrence, but do none the less leave some individual and unique somatic memory traces which amalgamate with later experiences and may thereby increase later psychological pressures. It is in fact extremely difficult to say exactly at what time the human organism develops from a biological to a psychobiological organization.

A general condition, omitted in my earlier paper but which I now believe to be important in the development of anxiety potentials in any human being, is the degree of tension existent, dependent on the sensory-motor balance, i.e., the ratio between the sensory stimulation and the capacity (development and opportunity) to effect some sort of motor discharge. Where there has been considerable disproportion between an increased sensory stimulation and a limited motor discharge over a period of time such tension may conceivably be incorporated into the working balance of the individual, and become temporarily or permanently a characteristic of his makeup. Where this is true, a sudden increase or decrease in the established tension level of the individual contributes to symptoms of anxiety. There is, however, in each individual a unique primary organization and level of tension that is determined, in some measure, by the birth experience, furnishing an important element in the patterning of the drive and energy distribution of that individual.

To examine the effect of the process of birth more specifically, one must inquire into the sensory motor state of the fetus, of the infant during the course of birth, and of the infant immediately after birth; and then consider the relations between these three states, which differ so very markedly. An imposing mass of literature dealing with the antenatal and neonatal states has grown up. The older investigators being largely morphologically oriented were concerned mostly with the presence or absence of various responses in the fetus and in the newborn infant. Later attention focussed more on the significance of such behavior responses.   Among all the investigations, the observations and experiments of Preyer, Minkowski, Langworthy and Windle stand out as most significant.

II

In antenatal life, the fetus is surrounded by a fluid medium which supports it and protects it against the fullest severity of external impacts.   That considerable stimulation may reach the fetus both from the outside and through unfavorable metabolic changes in the mother is definitely established.   By and large, however, in a relatively good pregnany the fetus appears to live a life of comparative ease, relaxation and passivity, even receiving its nutrition in an effortless fashion through the blood stream.   Thus its capacity for and rate of growth is enormous and will never again be approximated throughout its life.

When an attempt is made to examine the embryonic development of sensation and of motor activities, an interesting dilemma arises as to which capacity—to receive stimulus or to move—comes first, and it is easy to drift here into a kind of bio-philosophizing. Preyer(11) in his extraordinarily fine classical monograph on embryonic motility and sensitivity published as far back as 1885 concluded that the sensitivity of the embryo begins later than the motility, and describes early movements as both passive and irritative in type. The original passive movement of the fetus depends on the change of position of the mother, e.g., from standing to lying or in the movements of walking or even of breathing, as well as on such impacts of the maternal abdomen with external objects as might cause a change of position or dislocation of the embryo within the uterus. He notes that such passive movement merges over into clear reflex responsive movements, and that, for example, in the twisting of the umbilical cord which may occur quite early, it is not easy to determine whether this has been caused by the purely passive movement of the embryo or by some kind of irritative response to the movement of the mother.   Preyer seems in his statement about the late development of sensitivity to be considering this in its stricter sense of a function of differentiated nervous tissue, rather than in its more general biological sense of tissue irritability.   The more recent work (1939) of Hooker(12) indicates a response to tactile stimulation with a hair at a little after the eight-week embryonic stage, and he noticed spontaneous movement of a "total pattern" type at nine-and-a-half weeks, on which the local specific response to tactile stimulation could be super-imposed. Preyer (p. 40) deals with this problem in the following way, "I must agree with Griesinger and C. Wernicke, the latter of whom explains that the first movements of our body, the changes in the musculature, give rise to sensations, memory patterns of which remain in the cortex of the cerebrum. These memory pictures of *motion sensations,* motion pictures or ideas[3] of movement, persist alongside of the memory pictures of the sensations of senses." This is a particularly interesting statement, however, because it implies the possible participation of the cerebral cortex as a kind of repository of experience very early in fetal life, even though we know that its very presence is not essential for the existence of the infant even immediately after birth, as is so grimly demonstrated in the cases of monsters, who move, nurse and cry even with the complete absence of a cerebrum. Certainly it is known(13) that the "fetuses of three months have the gray substance arranged in what is essentially the permanent form."[4] While there is an ontogenetic indication of past changes in the cortex in response to varying needs in the course of phylogenesis, the functional relationship of the cortex to the experiences of the individual fetus remains as yet unclear and still assigned to the realm of speculation. According to some workers(16, 17) on the histological evidence of maturation in brains of newborn babies, there is no indication that at birth the cortex is functioning to any *appreciable degree as a mechanism for controlling behavior,* which appears rather to be mediated through the subcortical nuclei(18). This does not absolutely preclude the possibility, however, that the cortex might be a passive repository, as Preyer suggested.

Investigations carried on in recent years seem to substantiate Preyer's observations that the nervous mechanism for motor discharge functions before that for sensory perception. In the very earliest stages the cellular protoplasm has the property of irritable response which is later to be allocated to nervous tissue. During embryonic life, i.e., during the period before the body has taken on the specific form

3. One notes how hard it is to avoid the terminology really belonging to a later development. It is obvious from the context that Preyer does not mean *an idea* but only some sort of organic imprint which may later be a factor in an idea.

4. The description of the phenomenon of *neurobiotaxis* by Kappers(14) and Windle(15) gives one a glimpse of the possible participation of the cerebral cortex in the early embryonic life, and the realization that it is conceivable at least that it may be affected by the experience of the fetus. This phenomenon consists of the mass migration to new locations of nuclear cells, in response to special needs of the organism. This has been noted from one group to another among vertebrates, but more important for our purposes, is the fact that it has been observed in the development of individual embryos, and is thought to be a shift to an area closer to the source from which they receive most of their messages, i.e., it is an example of the economizing tendency of nature.

characteristic of its species, little movement occurs spontaneously but it may be elicited by stimulation of the embryo. These investigations in the human have been reported by Hooker as already mentioned. Such motion is at first a massive organismic response; later myogenic responses occur and finally reflex neuromotor responses are established. There are two trends of thought concerning the origin of these reflexes. One group of observers(18, 19, 20) has thought that reflexes developed by individuation from the mass or "total pattern" responses. The other school has believed that the early behavior consisted for the most part in a number of relatively simple reflex responses(21, 22). All this is concisely summarized in Windle's book, *The Physiology of the Fetus*(23).

It appears that the nerve endings which will later serve as receptors of pain, are the most primitive of all sensory nerve endings and mark the beginning development of the peripheral sensory system. Further, the fact that neuromotor functioning precedes neurosensory functioning even slightly would tend to establish a favorable situation for the fetus, i.e., that incoming stimuli would be effectively discharged without any degree of tension being established under ordinary conditions. Thus the passivity and protection of the fetus is furthered. This is stated in another way by Windle (p. 165): "The relative quiescences of the normal fetus in utero is somewhat surprising when one considers all of the activities of which the growing specimen is capable when removed from the uterus. The reasons seem to be twofold: lack of adequate stimulation and high thresholds in the fetal central nervous system."

The same differences of viewpoint as to relation between reflex behavior and "total pattern" response in the fetus are carried over to interpretations of the behavior of the newborn. As has already been mentioned, an anencephalic infant may survive birth for a short time with essential behavior carried on at a special reflex level. This does not indicate, however, that the normal newborn does necessarily function at this level. Irwin and Weiss(24) believe that the diffuse activity of the newborn is of a thalamic type of organization.[5] Although the fetus has been found by Minkowski(26) and Hooker to respond to tactile stimuli from a quite early period in its life many observers have noted the relative insensibility of the newborn to

5. This is of some interest inasmuch as it appears that certain types of head sensations or headaches occurring in states of chronic or severe anxiety later in life may be determined by the sensory patterns set up during birth and integrated at a thalamic level(25), with or without projections into the cortex. I shall present the clinical data in regard to this in a subsequent paper.

cutaneous stimulation. McGraw(27) remarks (p. 102), "When only a few hours or days old some infants exhibit no overt response to cutaneous irritation such as pinprick. It is impossible to know whether such absence of response should be attributed to an undeveloped sensory mechanism or to lack of connection between sensory and somatic centers, or between receptor centers and those mechanisms governing crying. Such infants usually do respond to deep pressure stimulation. In any event, this period of hypaesthesia is brief; by the end of the first week or ten days most infants respond to cutaneous irritation." Gesell(28) speaks of the newborn infant as being "quasi-dormant" and as showing an apparent "instability" in his reactions. Both authors emphasize the change that occurs at about four to six weeks, when the cortex begins definitely to take hold, as it were. Because of the organization of C. Bühler's(29) observations according to the supposed functional meaning of the behavior, it is difficult to get from her accounts a good composite picture of the newborn's activities. She mentions the extreme amount of sleeping or napping during the first day or two, the onset of hunger crying generally only on the second day, the twitching at the moment of falling asleep and the irregular twitchings which may occur at other times. In general she considers that "the sensitive and helpless bodies of newborn children encounter decidedly more situations from which to flee than to seek and probably also encounter much more displeasure than pleasure". One gets the impression that she found considerable individual differences in the behavior immediately after birth. Dewey(30) considers that it is practically impossible to investigate pain due to proprioceptive stimuli in the newborn; and sums up the literature up to 1935 with the statement that it is the general opinion that infants at birth do not react to these stimuli in ways that give evidence of much discomfort.[6] Canestrini(32) reported little reaction to pain stimuli, but like other authors found that the lips were the most sensitive. Koffka(33) states simply that the infant's pain sensitivity is subnormal. The Shermans(34) attempted a more extensive investigation of the reaction of the newborn to pain, and seemed to find that pain could be elicited in the first day if stimuli were repeated frequently enough, but that the reaction to the *first* pin prick was generally established only after the 76th hour. From all these observations it appears that

6. She quotes Carmichael(22) who accepts an earlier opinion of Genzmer(31) that the fetus has a poorly developed pain sense. This is based on the observations of the first post-natal day of a premature infant, who could be pricked until blood came without giving any response. This would seem to me hardly a reliable conclusion since it appears to ignore the trauma to an ill-prepared fetus of the impact both of birth and of external conditions.

there is some reduction of cutaneous sensitivity during the early neonatal period.

It is interesting that practically all of these investigators ignore the possible effect of birth in producing this change in the newborn. Dewey alone mentions that birth may give a spurt to the sensory development, referring especially to the special senses; but she does not seem to consider that sensory fatigue in some infants may be the cause of apparent regression of some functioning immediately after birth. Among the neurologists, Langworthy(35) makes the important observation that in the human infant birth serves as a great stimulus to the deposit of myelin in the nervous system. "In the first few weeks after birth, the optic and olfactory systems acquire myelin sheaths, and myelinated projection fibers from the thalamus extend to many areas of the cerebral cortex. The question arises as to the changes at birth that account for this increase in the deposit of myelin. Probably it is the *result of increased stimulation of the sensory organs.*" He believes that human sensory pathways are myelinated at the time when sensory endings receive adequate stimuli. It is not quite clear whether Langworthy considers such stimulation to occur during the course of birth or in the period soon after; probably both. This question of the state of functioning of the central nervous system, especially the possible participation of the cortex, will be again referred to later.

III

In the review of the literature on fetal and neonatal conditions, it is apparent that the great chiasma is that of birth. It is striking how little attention has been paid to the effect of this process on the development of the organism itself. It seems that serious scientific students following the development of the fetus, make meticulous inquiries into its life and activities right up to the time of birth; pick them up again with the infant after birth and start afresh, without daring to look at the effect of birth itself unless the damage has been so gross as unavoidably to rivet attention upon itself. Perhaps birth is inevitably too close to death in our feelings; perhaps the struggle of birth is at once too terrifying and too inspiring for us to regard it readily with scientific dispassion. Perhaps men have too much exclusion anxiety and women too much direct anxiety.

The fact remains that studies, even thought, concerning any of the subtler effects of birth on the newborn are very scant. Birth seems in the scientific world to be tacitly regarded almost as a rebirth or a reconception. This point can hardly be overemphasized, for among the hundreds of otherwise careful studies of the newborn as to its motor activities, its sensory responses, the state of its rudimentary psyche, and even in electroencephalographic studies immediately after birth, references as to the type of birth experience or its effect are conspicuously lacking.[7] Langworthy in his study of myelinization, already mentioned, makes the suggestion (p. 52), "Tracts in the nervous system become myelinated at the time when they become functional." Later he makes clear that the sensory tracts must function to some degree before myelinization, and that the increase in sensory stimuli, as for example during and immediately after birth, determines the further maturation including the myelinization of the nerve-fiber. Thus the myelinization in a premature infant exceeds that of an infant born at term of the same age, if age be considered from the time of conception; and preventing the opening of an eye at the proper time delays the process of medullation in the corresponding optic tract. Langworthy further states that conditioning reflexes may occur at subcortical levels. Windle(23, p. 163), too, states that "there can be a great deal of well organized activity in the brain before any nerve fibers become myelinated" and considers the possibility (p. 164) that with increasing fetal size, distances between points in the nervous system become greater and myelin may be laid down to compensate by increasing the conduction speed of the fibers. All this is important because it contributes to the idea stated sixty years ago by Preyer, that there may possibly be some traces of fetal experience deposited even at a cortical level but even more assuredly at a thalamic level. It seems further not only possible, but a reasonable expectation that birth itself may contribute to the patterning of the organic integration.

In the psychoanalytic field Rank made a contribution in his visionary theory in regard to the birth trauma, after which the subject was dropped. There have recently been a few articles attempting to penetrate into the intra-uterine psychology. While these may contain a nucleus of good observation, the specific interpretations appear as fantasies of patient and author, in which psychic constellations belong-

---

7. In this connection it is interestingly reported that Erasmus Darwin (grandfather of Charles) in a biological system of medicine published in 1796, under the title of *Zoonomia* describes fear as originating in each individual from the experiences at birth, a description which is said to have suggested Freud's concept of the organization of anxiety by birth. If one reads the original of Darwin, however, it is apparent that his conception was that fear was established by the on-rushing multiple stimuli of the world immediately after birth. He, too, could not, or at any rate did not, consider the process of birth. In fact, he gives little more than a paragraph to the business of birth itself, stating somewhat summarily that healthy women should not feel pain but that London ladies were spoiled by tight clothing and city air.

ing to considerably later periods of development are projected backward and make it appear as though the fetus lived a full and thoughtful life. The effect then is slightly wild and unconvincing.

Recently there has been some renewal of interest in the psychology of birth and the effects of different forms of birth experience on the offspring. Some very important work of this nature is being carried on in animal experiments by Windle and his co-workers, observing the effects of asphyxia and other deleterious conditions at birth.

Let us dare to look at the process of birth and its effects on the infant—or rather on transforming the fetus into the infant. In the majority of cases (approximately 96%) (3, p. 198), the child is born head first.[8] It is not clearly known whether there is any sort of forerunner of consciousness in utero; whether from the neurological angle, there is even slight relatively passive participation of the cortex in fetal life. All we can say is that it is not absolutely impossible. There are some workers who believe that there is a forerunner of consciousness, basing their conclusions on the periodic activities of the fetus which appear as though the fetus had times of something akin to sleep alternating with times of wakefulness.[9] I, myself, incline somewhat to this point of view not so much from these observations on the fetus about which I do not have the background for a discriminatingly critical attitude, but rather from observations on the newborn with which I am more familiar and especially from certain observations on psychoanalytic patients. Whatever the state of the fetal psyche, we do know that in the process of birth the fetal head is generally subjected to extreme pressure, sufficient to mold it and sometimes to produce hemorrhage, and that, likewise, too quick birth (precipitate or Caesarian) is also associated with increased tendency to cerebral hemorrhage. It would appear therefore, that even if there were some sort of fetal rudimentary consciousness, the process of birth would be in most instances, and perhaps always, a self-narcotizing or anaesthetizing experience to the infant—something akin to a

8. The distribution of presentations at birth is cephalic approximately 96-97%; breech between 3 and 4%; transverse generally less than ½%. Of the cephalic presentations approximately 94 of the 96% are vertex presentations. It is of special interest that pediatricians have made the general observation that there is a high degree of pathology (injuries to the neck, disorders of breathing, and many other disturbances) among babies born by breech presentation, but this subject has not been carefully studied. (Personal communication from Dr. Milton J. E. Senn.)

9. The anencephalic monster also has periods of "sleep" and "wakefulness" after birth, so that some degree of variation in consciousness must be conceded either at a spinal level or working through the total functioning of the organism. It would be a subject for investigation to determine the differences or similarities between this type of sleep and the sleep of the normal newborn.

pressure-concussion. It is necessary to concede, however, that there would be some threshold early in labor at which that rudimentary pre-consciousness would be lost. Further, one is confronted with the problem whether during birth the extreme sensory stimulation to the infant is such that it leaves some sort of central record, whether at cortical, thalamic or spinal level, or in combinations of these. These considerations cannot be dismissed lightly.

It seems likely that there is some sort of rudimentary consciousness or at least variations in degrees of unconsciousness, for in spite of the enormous sensory stimulation of birth and its probable self-narcotizing effect during birth, and the sensory fatigue immediately afterward, and in spite of the fact that the neonate may live at a spinal level (like an anencephalic monster) after birth until the cortex recovers, develops and participates in functioning, yet the newborn who has not been subjected to especially severe traumas of birth recovers more promptly from its immediate post-birth sluggishness and its variations between sleep and wakefulness soon become qualitatively different from those of the anencephalic. Its "recovery" generally occurs around the second or third day. Further, the recent electro-encephalographic studies of Smith(36) on the newborn extending through the first ten days of neonatal life indicate the presence of certain rhythmic waves that occur over the sensory-motor area during the sleeping periods of the infant but disappear on his awakening. It has been suggested that these waves are due to developing cortical function. Reasoning from Langworthy's and Windle's formulations (already quoted) this area may be dormant in the fetus although capable of some degree of activity if specifically stimulated. It seems probable that such stimulation does occur at some stage during birth and immediately afterward and thus promotes myelinization and increases efficiency and capacity of functioning.

The work of Stirnimann(37) on the reaction of the newborn to thermal stimulation is also of interest. Working on 50-100 babies, he found that they reacted to thermal stimuli as early as 10 minutes after birth, that the most sensitive area was the cheek and that throughout the first day of life this response to thermal stimulation was clearly greater when the infant was awake than when it was asleep. He concluded that some slight degree of consciousness participated in the response. Again, neither of these authors makes any attempt to correlate the findings with types of birth preceding. Perhaps the findings in themselves are not sufficiently intense or the observations made on a sufficient number of infants to warrant such attempt at correlation.

Another observation along this same line is that of Wagner(38) who studied the sleep of 40 newborns beginning 8 hours after birth and extending through the first 10 days. Using a polygraph, and classifying his records according to the depth of sleep, he noted great variations between infants and in the same infant at different times, but a general decrease in individual variability during the first 10 days. (As Gesell has remarked, the newborn is "unstable".) But especially he noted that yawning, sneezing and regurgitation were most likely to occur during complete waking and never occurred spontaneously during the three deepest stages of sleep. Even though these reactions may be provoked from the anencephalic monster it seems to me that these experimental findings, if confirmed, strongly suggest a general participation to some extent of nervous organization above a spinal level relatively soon after birth.

What do we see in this, in its effect on the rudimentary psyche, especially from a psychoanalytic point of view? We may concern ourselves at present with three general categories of inquiry: the effect on patterning of the sensory-motor tension level and its relation to anxiety; the effect on the organization of the narcissism of the fetus/infant; and the effect on the later sexuality of the individual especially in relation to masochism. While these are interrelated subjects, this paper will only attempt to touch upon the first two, leaving the subject of masochism for a further paper.

Birth seems to organize the anxiety pattern, setting in motion the genetically determined elements fused with those individually determined ones resulting from the special or unique birth experiences of the given infant. The commonest somatic elements are the cardio-respiratory ones and the ever present psychic element of later stages of development is the anxious attitude itself—the sense that something unpleasant or positively painful will happen. But there are a great variety of individual variations: one person feels his anxiety with creepy sensations in the skin, another in weakness in the legs, a third with headache, a fourth with diarrhea. One could go on to many more examples. From a careful scrutiny of reconstructed material from analytic patients, it seems that such patterning of the anxiety reaction always represents the genetic constitutional elements fused with birth experiences and further mediated through and increased by the traumata of the early years, with which we are so used to dealing in our analytic work. These traumata may in themselves be the predominantly determining experiences for later forms of anxious expression, but in any event never occur without some of the earlier elements. If the anxiety is extreme, these deeper elements always become more conspicuous. The psychic part of anxiety, the quality of anxious expectation, is generally considered to occur after the ego has developed somewhat. That anxious expectation occurs very early, however, in some rudimentary form can readily be directly observed in babies; e.g., a 7-months-old infant gasped and puckered its face with the appearance of frightened anticipation when a large inflated ball rolled silently toward it on the bed. In fact every new experience of the infant may have some tinge of this anxious reaction which is allayed when the experience is repeated or is related to some pleasantly tinged earlier experience. It is a further observation that this early anxious attitude varies greatly from infant to infant in the matter of what stimuli will provoke it. But the whole subject, and especially the questions of the time and stimulations of susceptibility to anxiety-like reactions in the first year require much more thorough systematic study.

While the establishment of the anxiety pattern is a protection against danger, the organization of the narcissism forms an instrument of positive attack, a propulsive aggressive drive. What is narcissism? Freud's deepening conception of it may be followed by consulting his early papers. In 1911, writing about the Schreber case(39), he described it as the stage between autoerotism and object love, "the individual . . . unifies his sexual instincts (which have hitherto been engaged in autoerotic activities) in order to obtain a love object, and he begins by taking himself, his own body and only subsequently proceeds to the choice of some person other than himself as his object." This description reminds one of the vivid slang taunt among adolescents, "I love myself, who do you love?" In 1914, Freud(40) wrote, "Narcissism in this sense would not be a perversion (referring to the original use of the word by Havelock Ellis in 1899 to refer to the specific perversion of self-admiration and love of one's own body) but the libidinal complement to the egoism of the instinct of self-preservation, a measure of which may justifiably be attributed to every living creature," and later in the same article he states, "We form a conception of an original libidinal cathexis of the ego, part of which cathexis is later yielded up to objects but which fundamentally persists and is related to the object cathexis much as the body of a protoplasmic animalcule is related to pseudopods it puts out," (p. 33), i.e., primary narcissism is partly given up to object love, but may be withdrawn again and appear in a secondary form. In his choice of this particular analogy, Freud approached a concept of the deepest and simplest form of narcissism, the biological. From a biological viewpoint, narcissism may be defined as the libidinal component of growth which may, how-

ever, become turned one way or another by the vicissitudes of experience at any time in the course of life. It is this fundamental biological
concept that I am especially considering.

What are the properties or characteristics of narcissism? How
does it act in times of stress and in times of plenty? Freud's own
simile of the animalcule is extremely helpful. I shall use it not just
as a simile but as the fundamental biological conception which it is.
In times of organismic distress, trauma, or deprivation, there is at first
an increase in the narcissism. It is the libidinal charge of the impulse
to conquer, to survive, to attack or to defend. In more elaborated forms
of life we see it operating in good and bad forms of attack and defense
—in humans in the increase in the wish for omnipotence, for magic,
for short-cuts to successful survival as well as in realistic ambition,
the drive to hard work, zestful interest, etc. In the ameba it appears as
part of the capacity of the organism to send out a pseudopod to engulf
its food. It would seem then to be somehow the force of the cellular
protoplasm flowing out through a lessened peripheral cellular tension,
some essence of the quality of life.

But what is the characteristic of fetal narcissism? Of the narcissism of the neonatal period of infancy? What does the process of
birth do in furnishing a bridge from the one to the other? Is birth a
chiasma, or is it a hiatus—a kind of blackout, very closely resembling
death? How much of its appearance as a hiatus is due fundamentally
to the scotoma even of the scientist? The process of human birth
actually does combine some of these opposites: it probably does involve
something of a blackout, an apparent almost complete interruption in
the life of the organism, but one through which a new arrangement of
organismic energy is effected. Perhaps the idea of birth as a rebirth
is not so fantastic after all, even though it may be used in quite
fantastic ways under stresses in our later life. In dreams and neurotic
symptoms, the symbolism of birth is always invested somewhat with
death, as for example in the impulses and phobias of jumping. Perhaps suicide always has lurking somewhere the hope of rebirth.

During fetal life under optimum conditions, the neuromotor
maturation preceding slightly the neurosensory, the piling up of
tension due to external stimuli is lessened. The libidinal charge, the
primary fetal narcissism, would appear to be distributed variously
throughout the fetal structure, its patterning determined almost entirely by the phylogenetic history of the species, i.e., any special accumu-
lations would accompany the maturation processes which were quicken-

ing at a given time.[10]   Probably even during a "good" pregnancy there is some slight infiltration of stimuli from the extramural world, with corresponding temporary effects upon the fetal narcissism, but these are generally negligible.

Birth itself is an enormous experience, with a sudden increase in the total sensory stimulation in the setting of limited opportunity for motor response, probably proceeding to some degree of sensory fatigue. There is in this way some sort of organismic tension established with a transformation of the relaxed, relatively sleepy narcissistic state of the fetus to a neonatal condition with a beginning propulsive psychic drive, the condition of primary infantile narcissism which has previously been considered.

It is apparent, however, that in the process of birth, the amount of stimulation is uneven.   Commonly there is an especially strong stimulation of the head, producing not only an effect upon the scalp and its underlying structures, but especially even a kind of cerebral massage.   Under good conditions this acts as a marked stimulation to the nervous system, but especially to the cortex, and according to Langworthy's work, there is thereby a stimulation of myelinization and a preparation for the development of cortical control which will begin to be apparent in a few weeks' time.   Under too severe birth conditions, it is obvious that the stimulation proceeds to a stage of destruction and gross damage.   In addition to this stimulation of the head, there is obviously a considerable stimulation of the entire body of the infant, with marked internal changes, and a toning up of the skin and muscular systems.   Here, indeed, in skin and muscles together with the mouth area (this latter probably largely genetically determined) is the first libidinal concentration.   Rado has referred to this as the "narcissistic rind of the ego"(41).

This birth stimulation probably produces a rudimentary erogenization of different body parts, at a level of development when erotism and aggression cannot be separated, but appear identical.   Under normal good birth conditions there is sufficient cerebral stimulation to make for good functioning, but not enough to make a vulnerable focus for the later castration anxiety.   In the study of psychotics, however, and of certain severe neurotic states, too great erotization of thinking with resultant overactivity and then blocking on a castration basis, is

10. It is obvious that such maturation processes may be affected by internal stimuli arising, e.g., from metabolic products received from the mother. Just how these may produce fetal distress and influence endogenously tensions of the organism, is extremely complicated, and embrace the field of fetal pathology. In a normal pregnancy they would presumably be minimal.

quite apparent. In a number of cases I have been able to recover sufficient material from adult dreams and from the interpretation of adult symptoms to give some idea of the special birth experiences of the given individual; and in the few cases in which it has been possible to check against objective birth records, subsequently obtained, my reconstructions have sometimes proved rather surprisingly correct.

These effects of birth may also be noted in regard to other body parts. For example a dry labor produces, among other things, a subsequent increase in skin erotization and seems the earliest determinant in certain instances, of a body-phallus identification. (I do not wish to imply, however, that this may not develop also in the absence of a dry labor if later conditions are such as generally to over-erotize the skin and kinaesthetic functions.) When a dry labor has occurred, the later special skin erotization and its corresponding narcissistic investment never disappears in the life of the individual but remains a part of his acquired "constitutional" equipment. It may be heightened by later experiences, to be sure, but is not lost.

Another example, which I have had the opportunity to study considerably in the course of analytic work, is the production of certain types of head sensations or headaches, which occur in states of marked anxiety. While these can be most easily studied in schizophrenic patients in whom they appear commonly, they may occur also if the anxiety is marked, in neurotic and even in severe reactive states. In my experience the type of head sensation may often be correlated quite definitely with the form of birth experience of the individual and appears under *any* conditions of very severe anxiety, but especially in later life situations in which the subject of birth is being stirred in the unconscious of the patient. M. Chadwick(42) has also made some valuable suggestions regarding the connections between birth experience and forms of headache, but has not presented much clinical material. It is a subject that requires a detailed presentation in order to be in the least convincing, and one that I hope to develop in a more careful study in a subsequent paper. Another special problem is suggested by Bak(43) who emphasizes the disturbed thermal orientation of the schizophrenic and relates this possibly to the thermal experiences, the too sudden cooling or near "freezing" of the baby immediately after delivery. He raises other interesting questions regarding the changes of libidinal cathexis of the skin determined at birth, and by the contrast between the antenatal and neonatal states. Jones(44) has hinted at similar questions in an earlier paper on "Cold, Disease, and Birth". This paper is only intended to lay the ground work for certain other studies, especially the one on masochism.

This paper obviously makes use of the concept of memory traces that exist in the organization of the individual,—organic memories determined by experiences from the very beginning of the life of the individual. Certain neurological aspects of this point of view were stated quite clearly by Preyer in the passage already quoted in which he in turn gave credit to Griesinger and Wernicke. In the psycho-analytic literature there are many references to conceptions of such memory traces as they appear in the behavior of the individual or of his organs, but the subject has not been very thoroughly presented. Ferenczi left a rather specific note (1932) on this subject, stressing that psychological events of the remote past may have left their hardly recoverable traces only in the "organophysical mimes of the individual". It should be further emphasized that such traces are generally amalgamated with and often almost concealed by the effects of later events. In the present paper the focus has been only on certain essentially normal patterning.

In summary, it seems that the general effect of birth is, by its enormous sensory stimulation, to organize and convert the fetal narcissism, producing or promoting a propulsive narcissistic drive over and above the type of more relaxed fetal maturation process that has been existent in utero. There is ordinarily a patterning of the aggressive-libidinization of certain body parts according to the areas of special stimulation. Specifically, birth stimulates the cerebrum to a degree promoting its development so that it may soon begin to take effective control of body affairs; it contributes to the organization of the anxiety pattern, thereby increasing the defense of the infant, and it leaves unique individual traces that are superimposed on the genetically determined anxiety and libidinal patterns of the given infant.

BIBLIOGRAPHY

1. Cannon, W. B., *The Wisdom of the Body*. W. W. Norton, New York, 1932, Chap. XIV, "Natural defenses of the organism", p. 229.
2. Morgan, C. T., *Physiological Psychology*. McGraw-Hill, New York & London. p. 265.
3. DeLee, J. B. and J. P. Greenhill, *Principles and Practice of Obstetrics*. 8th Edition. W. B. Saunders Co., Philadelphia, 1943. Introduction p. xiii.
4. Wolff, H. G. and H. Goodall, "The relation of attitude and suggestion to the perception of and reaction to pain", *Pain, Research Pub., Assoc. Nerv. & Ment. Dis.* Vol. XXIII, Williams & Wilkins, Baltimore, 1943, pp. 434-448. This article gives a concise statement of easily demonstrated variations in perception of pain under laboratory conditions.

5. Menninger, K., *Love Against Hate.* Harcourt Brace & Co., New York, 1942. pp. 97-98.
6. Jones, E. "Psychology and Childbirth", *Lancet,* Vol. 242, 1942. p. 695.
7. Ford, F. R., B. Crothers and M. C. Putnam. "Birth Injuries of the Central Nervous System", *Medicine Monographs,* Vol. XI, Williams & Wilkins, Baltimore, 1927. Section on Cerebral Birth Injuries. pp. 13-18.
8. Nevinny, H., "On Lesions of the Central Nervous System by Birth Injury", *Beilage zur Ztschr. f. Geburtshilfe u. Gynaekologie,* Vol. 114, 1936, Stuttgart.
9. Greenacre, P., "The Predisposition to Anxiety", Part I, *Psychoanalytic Quarterly,* Vol. X, 1941. pp. 66-94.
10. Freud, S., *The Problem of Anxiety.* W. W. Norton & Co., New York, 1936. pp. 96, 97, 102, 121-126.
11. Preyer, W., "Embryonic motility and sensitivity" (Trans. from *Specielle Physiologie des Embryo)", Monograph of the Society for Research in Child Development,* Nat. Res. Council. Washington D. C., 1937. pp. 42, 57.
12. Hooker, D., "Fetal Behavior", *Interrelations of mind and body. Research Pub.,* Assoc. Nerv. & Ment. Dis., Vol. XIX, Williams & Wilkins, Baltimore, 1939. pp. 237-243.
13. Arey, L. B., *Developmental Anatomy.* 4th Edition. W. B. Saunders Co., Philadelphia, 1942. p. 423.
14. Kappers, C. W. A., "Further Contributions on Neurobiotaxis", *Journal of Comparative Neurology,* Vol. 27, 1917. pp. 261-298.
15. Windle, W. F., "Neurofibrillar Development in Central Nervous System of Cat Embroyos", *Journal of Comparative Neurology,* Vol. 58, 1933. pp. 643-723.
16. de Crinis, M., "Die Entwicklung der Grosshirnrinde nach der Geburt in ihren Beziehungen zur intellecktuellen Ausreifung des Kindes", *Klinische Wochenschrift,* Vol. XL, 1932. pp. 1161-1165.
17. Conel, J. L. *The Postnatal Development of the Human Cerebral Cortex.* Vol. II, Harvard Univ. Press, Cambridge, Mass. pp. 39-41.
18. Angulo y Gonzales, A. W., "The Prenatal Development of Behavior in the Albino Rat", *Journal of Comparative Neurology,* Vol. 55, 1932. p. 395.
19. Hooker, D. "Early Fetal Activity in Mammals", *Yale Journal of Biology & Medicine,* Vol. 8, p. 579.
20. Coghill, G. E., *Anatomy and the Problem of Behavior.* Macmillan, New York, 1929.
21. Windle, W. F., J. E. O'Donnell, and E. E. Glasshagle, "The Early Development of Spontaneous and Reflex Behavior in Cat Embryos and Fetuses", *Physiology and Zoology,* Vol. 6, 1933. p. 521.
22. Carmichael, L., "Origin and Prenatal Growth of Behavior", *Handbook of Child Psychology,* edit. by Carl Murchison. 2nd Edition. Clark Univ. Press. Worcester, Mass., 1933. pp. 31, 159.
23. Windle, W. F., *Physiology of the Fetus.* W. B. Saunders Co. Philadelphia. 1940. p. 141.
24. Irwin, O. C. and A. P. Weiss, "A Note on Mass Activity in Newborn Infants", *Pedagogical Seminary,* Vol. 38. 1930. pp. 20-30.

25. Dusser de Barenne, J. G., "Central levels of sensory integration", *"Sensation: Its Mechanisms and Disturbances.* Assoc. Nerv. & Ment. Dis., Vol. XV, Williams & Wilkins, Baltimore. 1935. pp. 274-288.
26. Minkowski, M., "Neurobiologische Studien am menschlichen Fetus", *Abderhaldens Handb. d. biol. Arbeitsmethoden,* 1928. pp. 511-618.
27. McGraw, M., *Neuromuscular Motivation of the Human Infant.* Columbia Univ. Press. New York, 1943. pp. 7-10.
28. Gesell, A., H. Halvorson et al, *The First Five Years of Life.* Harper & Bros. New York, 1940. p. 18.
29. Bühler, C., *The First Year of Life.* John Day. New York, 1930. pp. 21, 22, 29, 30, 35, 39, 111, 119.
30. Dewey, E., *Behavior Development in Infants.* Columbia Univ. Press, New York, 1935. p. 85. This contains an excellent summary of literature from 1920-1934.
31. Genzmer, A., *Untersuchungen über die Sinneswahrnehmungen des neugeborenen Menschen.* Niemeyer, Halle, 1882. pp. 1-28.
32. Canestrini, S., *über das Sinnesleben des Neugeborenen,* Springer, Berlin, 1913. iv and 104 pp.
33. Koffka, K., *The Growth of the Mind.* 2nd Edition. Harcourt Brace, New York, 1931. pp. 133, 135.
34. Sherman, M. and I. C. Sherman, "Sensorimotor Responses in Infants", *Journal of Comparative Psychology,* Vol. 5, 1925. pp. 53-68.
35. Langworthy, O. R., "Development of behavior patterns and myelinization of the nervous system in the human fetus and infant", *Contributions to Embryology,* Carnegie Institute of Washington, D. C. Vol. XXIV, No. 139. 1933.
36. Smith, J. R., "The electroencephalogram during normal infancy and childhood; rhythm tendencies present in the neonate and their subsequent development", *Journal of Genetic Psychology,* Vol. 53, 1938. pp. 455-469 and 471-482.
37. Stirnimann, F., "Versuche über die Reaktionen neugeborener auf Wärme- und Kältereize", *Zeitschrift f. Kinder-Psychiatrie,* Vol. 5, 1939. pp. 143-150.
38. Wagner, I. F., "Curves of Sleep Depth in Newborn Infants", *Journal of Genetic Psychology,* Vol. 55, 1939. pp. 121-135.
39. Freud, S., "A Case of Paranoia", *Collected Papers,* III, Hogarth Press, London, 1934. p. 446.
40. Freud, S., "On Narcissism", *Collected Papers,* IV, Hogarth Press, London, 1934. pp. 30-59.
41. Rado S., "Fear of Castration in Women", *Psychoanalytic Quarterly.* Vol. II, 1933. p. 449, footnote.
42. Chadwick, M., *Difficulties in Child Development.* John Day, New York, 1928. p. 28.
43. Bak, R. C., "Regression of Ego Orientation and Libido in Schizophrenia", *International Journal of Psychoanalysis,* Vol. XX, Part I, 1939. pp. 1-8.
44. Jones, E., "Cold, Disease and Birth". *Collected Papers.* Chap. XXII. Baillière, Tindall and Cox, London, 1938. pp. 460-466.

HOSPITALISM

An Inquiry into the Genesis of Psychiatric Conditions in
Early Childhood[1]

By RENÉ A. SPITZ, M.D. (New York)

> "En la Casa de Ninos Expositos el nino se va
> poniendo triste y muchos de ellos mueren de
> tristeza."
> (1760, *from the diary of a Spanish bishop*.)

I. *The Problem*

The term *hospitalism* designates a vitiated condition of the body
due to long confinement in a hospital, or the morbid condition of the
atmosphere of a hospital. The term has been increasingly preempted
to specify the evil effect of institutional care on infants, placed in
institutions from an early age, particularly from the psychiatric point
of view.[2] This study is especially concerned with the effect of continuous institutional care of infants under one year of age, for reasons
other than sickness. The model of such institutions is the foundling
home.

Medical men and administrators have long been aware of the
shortcomings of such charitable institutions. At the beginning of
our century one of the great foundling homes in Germany had a
mortality rate of 71.5% in infants in the first year of life(1).[3] In
1915 Chapin(2) enumerated ten asylums in the larger cities of the
United States, mainly on the Eastern seaboard, in which the death rates
of infants admitted during their first year of life varied from 31.7%
to 75% by the end of their second year. In a discussion in the same

---

1. Preliminary report.

2. *Hospitalism* tends to be confused with *hospitalization*, the temporary confinement
of a seriously ill person to a hospital.

3. Numbers in parentheses refer to the bibliography at the end of the paper.

year before the American Pediatric Association(3), Dr. Knox of Baltimore stated that in the institutions of that city 90% of the infants died by the end of their first year. He believed that the remaining 10% probably were saved because they had been taken out of the institution in time. Dr. Shaw of Albany remarked in the same discussion that the mortality rate of Randalls Island Hospital was probably 100%.

Conditions have since greatly changed. At present the best American institutions, such as Bellevue Hospital, New York City, register a mortality rate of less than 10%(4), which compares favorably with the mortality rate of the rest of the country. While these and similar results were being achieved both here and in Europe, physicians and administrators were soon faced with a new problem: they discovered that institutionalized children practically without exception developed subsequent psychiatric disturbances and became asocial, delinquent, feeble-minded, psychotic, or problem children. Probably the high mortality rate in the preceding period had obscured this consequence. Now that the children survived, the other drawbacks of institutionalization became apparent. They led in this country to the widespread substitution of institutional care by foster home care.

The first investigation of the factors involved in the psychiatric consequences of institutional care of infants in their first year was made in 1933 in Austria by H. Durfee and K. Wolf(5). Further contributions to the problem were made by L. G. Lowrey(6), L. Bender and H. Yarnell(7), H. Bakwin (4), and W. Goldfarb(8-11). The results of all these investigations are roughly similar:

Bakwin found greatly increased susceptibility to infection in spite of high hygienic and nutritional standards. Durfee and Wolf found that children under three months show no demonstrable impairment in consequence of institutionalization; but that children who had been institutionalized for more than eight months during their first year show such severe psychiatric disturbances that they cannot be tested. Bender, Goldfarb and Lowrey found that after three years of institutionalization the changes effected are irreversible. Lowrey found that whereas the impairment of children hospitalized during their first year seems irremediable, that of children hospitalized in the second or third year can be corrected.

Two factors, both already stressed by Durfee and Wolf, are made responsible by most of the authors for the psychological injury suffered by these children.

First: Lack of stimulation. The worst offenders were the best equipped and most hygienic institutions, which succeeded in sterilizing the surroundings of the child from germs but which at the same time sterilized the child's psyche. Even the most destitute of homes offers more mental stimulation than the usual hospital ward.

Second: The presence or absence of the child's mother. Stimulation by the mother will always be more intensive than even that of the best trained nursery personnel(12). Those institutions in which the mothers were present had better results than those where only trained child nurses were employed. The presence of the mothers could compensate even for numerous other short-comings.

We believe that further study is needed to isolate clearly the various factors operative in the deterioration subsequent to prolonged care in institutions. The number of infants studied by Bakwin, Durfee-Wolf and Lowrey in single institutions is very small and Bender-Yarnell, and Goldfarb did not observe infants in the first twelve months of life. We are not questioning here whether institutions should be preferred to foster homes, a subject now hardly ever discussed—the decision can by implication be deduced from the results of the studies of the Iowa group in their extensive research on the "Nature Versus Nurture" controversy(13-18). It may seem surprising that in the course of this controversy no investigation has covered the field of the first year of life in institutions.[4] All Iowa investigators studied either children in foster homes or children over one year of age, using their findings for retrospective interpretations.[5] They did not have at their disposal a method of investigation that would permit the evaluation and quantification of development, mental or other-wise, during the first year of life. Their only instrument is the I.Q., which is unreliable(21), and not applicable during the first year. However, the baby tests worked out by Hetzer and Wolf(22) fill the gap, providing not only a quotient for intelligence but also quanti-fiable data for development as a whole, such as indication of Develop-mental Age and of a Developmental Quotient. They provide, further-more, quantifiable data on six distinct sectors of personality, namely: development of perception, body mastery, social relations, memory, relations to inanimate objects, and intelligence (which in the first

4. Woodworth(19) in discussing the results of the Child Welfare Research Station of the State University of Iowa makes the following critical remarks (p. 71): "The causes of the inferior showing of orphanage children are obviously open to debate. . . . It would seem that a survey and comparative study of institutional homes for children would be instructive. . . ."

5. Jones(20) takes exception to this method as follows: "It seems probable that we shall turn from retrospective surveys of conditions assumed to have had a prior influence, and shall prefer to deal with the current and cumulative effects of specific environmental factors. It may also be expected that our interest will shift to some extent from mass statistical studies . . . to investigations of the dynamics of the growth process in individuals."

year is limited to understanding of relations between and insight into the functions of objects).

With the help of these data ("dimensions"), a profile (personality curve) is constructed from which relevant conclusions can be drawn and with the help of which children can be compared with one another. Averages of development in any one sector or in all of them can be established for given environments. Finally, the relevant progresses of one and the same child in the several sectors of its personality can be followed up. The profiles present a cross-section of infantile development at any given moment; but they also can be combined into longitudinal curves of the developmental progress of the child's total personality as well as of the various sectors of the personality.

The aim of my research is to isolate and investigate the pathogenic factors responsible for the favorable or unfavorable outcome of infantile development. A psychiatric approach might seem desirable; however, infant psychiatry is a discipline not yet existent: its advancement is one of the aims of the present study.

II. *Material*[6]

With this purpose in mind a long-term study of 164 children was undertaken.[7] In view of the findings of previous investigations this study was largely limited to the first year of life, and confined to two institutions, in order to embrace the total population of both

6. It is interesting to note that independently of our approach to this problem (mapped out and begun in 1936) Woodworth(19) recommends a research program on extremely similar lines as being desirable for the better understanding of the problem of heredity and environment:

"Orphanages. Present belief based on a certain amount of evidence regards the orphanages as an unfavorable environment for the child but the causes are not well understood. Two general projects may be suggested.

(a) A survey of institutional homes for children with a view to discovering the variations in their equipment and personnel and in their treatment of the children, with some estimate of the results achieved.

(b) Experimental studies in selected orphanages which retain their children for a considerable time, with a view to testing out the effects of specific environmental factors. For example, the amount of contact of the child with adults could be increased for certain children for the purpose of seeing whether this factor is important in mental development. It is conceivable that an orphanage could be run so as to become a decidedly favorable environment for the growing child, but at present we do not know how this result could be accomplished."

7. I wish to thank K. Wolf, Ph.D., for her help in the experiments carried out in "Nursery" and in private homes, and for her collaboration in the statistical evaluation of the results.

(130 infants). Since the two institutions were situated in different countries of the Western hemisphere, a basis of comparison was established by investigating non-institutionalized children of the same age group in their parents' homes in both countries. A total of 34 of these were observed. We thus have four environments:

TABLE I.

Environment	Institution No. 1[1]	Corresponding private background[2]	Institution No. 2	Corresponding private background
Number of Children	69	11	61	23

III. *Procedure.*

In each case an anamnesis was made which whenever possible included data on the child's mother; and in each case the Hetzer-Wolf baby tests were administered. Problems cropping up in the course of our investigations for which the test situation did not provide answers were subjected to special experiments elaborated for the purpose. Such problems referred, for instance, to attitude and behavior in response to stimuli offered by inanimate objects, by social situations, etc. All observations of unusual or unexpected behavior of a child were carefully protocoled and studied.

A large number of tests, all the experiments and some of the special situations were filmed on 16/mm film. A total of 31,500 feet of film preserve the results of our investigation to-date. In the analysis of the movies the following method was applied: Behavior was filmed at sound speed, i.e., 24 frames per second. This makes it possible to slow action down during projection to nearly one-third of the original speed so that it can be studied in slow motion. A projector with additional handdrive also permits study of the films frame by frame, if necessary, to reverse action and to repeat projection of every detail as often as required. Simultaneously the written protocols of the experiments are studied and the two observations compared.

1. Institution No. 1 will from here on be called "Nursery"; institution No. 2, "Foundling Home".

2. The small number of children observed in this particular environment was justified by the fact that it has been previously studied extensively by other workers; our only aim was to correlate our results with theirs. However, during the course of one year each child was tested at least at regular monthly intervals.

IV. *Results.*

For the purpose of orientation we established the average of the Developmental Quotients for the first third of the first year of life for each of the environments investigated. We contrasted these averages with those for the last third of the first year. This comparison gives us a first hint of the significance of environmental influences for development.

Type of Environment	Cultural and Social Background	Developmental Quotients	
		Average of first four months	Average of last four months
Parental Home	Professional	133	131
	Village Population	107	108
Institution	"Nursery"	101.5	105
	"Foundling home"	124	72

TABLE II.

Children of the first category come from professional homes in a large city; their Developmental Quotient, high from the start, remains high in the course of development.

Children in the second category come from an isolated fishing village of 499 inhabitants, where conditions of nutrition, housing, hygienic and medical care are very poor indeed; their Developmental Quotient in the first four months is much lower and remains at a lower level than that of the previous category.

In the third category, "Nursery", the children were handicapped from birth by the circumstances of their origin, which will be discussed below. At the outset their Developmental Quotient is even somewhat lower than that of the village babies; in the course of their development they gain slightly.

In the fourth category, "Foundling Home", the children are of an unselected urban (Latin) background. Their Developmental Quotient on admission is below that of our best category but much higher than that of the other two. The picture changes completely by the end of the first year, when their Developmental Quotient sinks to the astonishingly low level of 72.

Thus the children in the first three environments were at the end of their first year on the whole well-developed and normal, whether they were raised in their progressive middle-class family homes (where obviously optimal circumstances prevailed and the children were well in advance of average development), or in an institution or a village home, where the development was not brilliant but still reached a perfectly normal and satisfactory average. The children in the fourth environment, though starting at almost as high a level as the best of the others, had spectacularly deteriorated.

The children in Foundling Home showed all the manifestations of hospitalism, both physical and mental. In spite of the fact that hygiene and precautions against contagion were impeccable, the children showed, from the third month on, extreme susceptibility to infection and illness of any kind. There was hardly a child in whose case history we did not find reference to otitis media, or morbilli, or varicella, or eczema, or intestinal disease of one kind or another. No figures could be elicited on general mortality; but during my stay an epidemic of measles swept the institution, with staggeringly high mortality figures, notwithstanding liberal administration of convalescent serum and globulins, as well as excellent hygienic conditions. Of a total of 88 children up to the age of 2½, 23 died. It is striking to compare the mortality among the 45 children up to 1½ years, to that of the 43 children ranging from 1½ to 2½ years: usually, the *incidence* of measles is low in the younger age group, but among those infected the mortality is higher than that in the older age group; since in the case of Foundling Home every child was infected, the question of incidence does not enter; however, contrary to expectation, the mortality was much higher in the older age group. In the younger group, 6 died, i.e., approximately 13%. In the older group, 17 died, i.e., close to 40%. The significance of these figures becomes apparent when we realize that the mortality from measles during the first year of life in the community in question, outside the institution, was less than ½%.

In view of the damage sustained in all personality sectors of the children during their stay in this institution we believe it licit to assume that their vitality (whatever that may be), their resistance to disease, was also progressively sapped. In the ward of the children ranging from 18 months to 2½ years only two of the twenty-six surviving children speak a couple of words. The same two are able to walk. A third child is beginning to walk. Hardly any of them can eat alone. Cleanliness habits have not been acquired and all are incontinent.

In sharp contrast to this is the picture offered by the oldest inmates in Nursery, ranging from 8 to 12 months. The problem here is not whether the children walk or talk by the end of the first year; the problem with these 10-month-olds is how to tame the healthy toddlers' curiosity and enterprise. They climb up the bars of the cots after the manner of South Sea Islanders climbing palms. Special measures to guard them from harm have had to be taken after one 10-month-old actually succeeded in diving right over the more than two-foot railing of the cot. They vocalize freely and some of them actually speak a word or two. And all of them understand the significance of simple social gestures. When released from their cots, all walk with support and a number walk without it.

What are the differences between the two institutions that result in the one turning out normally acceptable children and the other showing such appalling effects?

A.   *Similarities*:[8]

   1.   Background of the children.

Nursery is a penal institution in which delinquent girls are sequestered. When, as is often the case, they are pregnant on admission, they are delivered in a neighboring maternity hospital and after the lying-in period their children are cared for in Nursery from birth to the end of their first year. The background of these children provides for a markedly negative selection since the mothers are mostly delinquent minors as a result of social maladjustment or feeble-mindedness, or because they are psychically defective, psychopathic, or criminal. Psychic normalcy and adequate social adjustment is almost excluded.

The other institution is a foundling home pure and simple. A certain number of the children housed have a background not much better than that of the Nursery children; but a sufficiently relevant number come from socially well-adjusted, normal mothers whose only handicap is inability to support themselves and their children (which is no sign of maladjustment in women of Latin background). This is expressed in the average of the Developmental Quotients of the two institutions during the first 4 months, as shown in Table II.

---

8. Under this heading we enumerate not only actual similarities but also differences that are of no etiological significance for the deterioration in Foundling Home. These differences comprise two groups: differences of no importance whatever, and differences that actually favor the development of children in Foundling Home.

The background of the children in the two institutions does therefore not favor Nursery; on the contrary, it shows a very marked advantage for Foundling Home.

2. Housing Conditions.

Both institutions are situated outside the city, in large spacious gardens. In both hygienic conditions are carefully maintained. In both infants at birth and during the first 6 weeks are segregated from the older babies in a special newborns' ward, to which admittance is only permitted in a freshly sterilized smock after hands are washed. In both institutions infants are transferred from the newborns' ward after 2 or 3 months to the older babies' wards, where they are placed in individual cubicles which in Nursery are completely glass enclosed, in Foundling Home glass enclosed on three sides and open at the end. In Foundling Home the children remain in their cubicles up to 15 to 18 months; in Nursery they are transferred after the 6th month to rooms containing four to five cots each.

One-half of the children in Foundling Home are located in a dimly lighted part of the ward; the other half, in the full light of large windows facing southeast, with plenty of sun coming in. In Nursery, all the children have well-lighted cubicles. In both institutions the walls are painted in a light neutral color, giving a white impression in Nursery, a gray-green impression in Foundling Home. In both, the children are placed in white painted cots. Nursery is financially the far better provided one: we usually find here a small metal table with the paraphernalia of child care, as well as a chair, in each cubicle; whereas in Foundling Home it is the exception if a low stool is to be found in the cubicles, which usually contain nothing but the child's cot.

3. Food.

In both institutions adequate food is excellently prepared and varied according to the needs of the individual child at each age; bottles from which children are fed are sterilized. In both institutions a large percentage of the younger children are breast-fed. In Nursery this percentage is smaller, so that in most cases a formula is soon added, and in many cases weaning takes place early. In Foundling Home all children are breast-fed as a matter of principle as long as they are under 3 months unless disease makes a deviation from this rule necessary.

4. Clothing.

Clothing is practically the same in both institutions. The children have adequate pastel-colored dresses and blankets. The temperature in the rooms is appropriate. We have not seen any shivering child in either set-up.

5. Medical Care.

Foundling Home is visited by the head physician and the medical staff at least once a day, often twice, and during these rounds the chart of each child is inspected as well as the child itself. For special ailments a laryngologist and other specialists are available; they also make daily rounds. In Nursery no daily rounds are made, as they are not necessary. The physician sees the children when called.

Up to this point it appears that there is very little significant difference between the children of the two institutions. Foundling Home shows, if anything, a slight advantage over Nursery in the matter of selection of admitted children, of breast-feeding and of medical care. It is in the items that now follow that fundamental differences become visible.

B. *Differences*:

1. Toys.

In Nursery it is the exception when a child is without one or several toys. In Foundling Home my first impression was that not a single child had a toy. This impression was later corrected. In the course of time, possibly in reaction to our presence, more and more toys appeared, some of them quite intelligently fastened by a string above the baby's head so that he could reach it. By the time we left a large percentage of the children in Foundling Home had a toy.

2. Visual Radius.

In Nursery the corridor running between the cubicles, though rigorously white and without particular adornment, gives a friendly impression of warmth. This is probably because trees, landscape and sky are visible from both sides and because a bustling activity of mothers carrying their children, tending them, feeding them, playing with them, chatting with each other with babies in their arms, is usually present. The cubicles of the children are enclosed but the glass panes of the partitions reach low enough for every child to be able at any time to observe everything going on all around. He can see into the corridor as soon as he lifts himself on his elbows. He can look out of the windows, and can see babies in the other cubicles by just turning his head; witness the fact that whenever the experimenter plays with a baby in one of the cubicles the babies in the two adjoining cubicles look on fascinated, try to participate in the game, knock at the panes of the partition, and often begin to cry if no attention is paid to them. Most of the cots are provided with widely-spaced bars that are no obstacle to vision. After the age of 6 months, when the child is transferred to the wards of the older babies, the visual field is enriched as a number of babies are then together in the same room, and accordingly play with each other.

In Foundling Home the corridor into which the cubicles open, though full of light on one side at least, is bleak and deserted, except at feeding time when five to eight nurses file in and look after the children's needs. Most of the time nothing goes on to attract the babies' attention. A special routine of Foundling Home consists in hanging bed sheets over the foot and the side railing of each cot. The cot itself is approximately 18 inches high. The side railings are about 20 inches high; the foot and head railings are approximately 28 inches high. Thus, when bed sheets are hung over the railings, the child lying in the cot is effectively screened from the world. He is completely separated from the other cubicles, since the glass panes of the wooden partitions begin 6 to 8 inches higher than even the head railing of the cot. The result of this system is that each baby lies in solitary confinement up to the time when he is able to stand up in his bed, and that the only object he can see is the ceiling.

3.   Radius of Locomotion.

In Nursery the radius of locomotion is circumscribed by the space available in the cot, which up to about 10 months provides a fairly satisfactory range.

Theoretically the same would apply to Foundling Home. But in practice this is not the case for, probably owing to the lack of stimulation, the babies lie supine in their cots for many months and a hollow is worn into their mattresses. By the time they reach the age when they might turn from back to side (approximately the 7th month) this hollow confines their activity to such a degree that they are effectively prevented from turning in any direction. As a result we find most babies, even at 10 and 12 months, lying on their backs and playing with the only object at their disposal, their own hands and feet.

4. Personnel.

In Foundling Home there is a head nurse and five assistant nurses for a total of forty-five babies. These nurses have the *entire* care of the children on their hands, except for the babies so young that they are breast-fed. The latter are cared for to a certain extent by their own mothers or by wetnurses; but after a few months they are removed to the single cubicles of the general ward, where they share with at least seven other children the ministrations of *one* nurse. It is obvious that the amount of care one nurse can give to an individual child when she has eight children to manage is small indeed. These nurses are unusually motherly, baby-loving women; but of course the babies of Foundling Home nevertheless lack all human contact for most of the day.

Nursery is run by a head nurse and her three assistants, whose duties do not include the care of the children, but consist mainly in teaching the children's mothers in child care, and in supervising them. The children are fed, nursed and cared for by their own mothers or, in those cases where the mother is separated from her child for any reason, by the mother of another child, or by a pregnant girl who in this way acquires the necessary experience for the care of her own future baby. Thus in Nursery each child has the full-time care of his own mother, or at least that of the substitute which the very able head nurse tries to change about until she finds someone who really likes the child.

V. *Discussion.*

To say that every child in Nursery has a full-time mother is an understatement, from a psychological point of view. However modern a penal institution may be, and however constructive and permissive its reeducative policies, the deprivation it imposes upon delinquent girls is extensive. Their opportunities for an outlet for their interests, ambitions, activity, are very much impoverished. The former sexual satisfactions as well as the satisfactions of competitive activity in the sexual field, are suddenly stopped: regulations prohibit flashy dresses, vivid nail polish, or extravagant hair-do's. The kind of social life in which the girls could show off has vanished. This is especially traumatic as these girls become delinquent because they have not been able to sublimate their sexual drives, to find substitute gratifications, and therefore do not possess a pattern for relinquishing pleasure when frustrated. In addition, they do not have compensation in relations with family and friends, as formerly they had. These factors, combined with the loss of personal liberty, the deprivation of private property and the regimentation of the penal institution, all add up to a severe narcissistic trauma from the time of admission; and they continue to affect the narcissistic and libidinal sectors during the whole period of confinement.

Luckily there remain a few safety valves for their emotions: (1) the relationship with wardens, matrons and nurses; (2) with fellow prisoners; (3) with the child. In the relationship with the wardens, matrons and nurses, who obviously represent parent figures, much of the prisoner's aggression and resentment is bound. Much of it finds an outlet in the love and hate relationship to fellow prisoners, where all the phenomena of sibling rivalry are revived.

The child, however, becomes for them the representative of their sexuality, a product created by them, an object they own, which they can dress up and adorn, on which they can lavish their tenderness and pride, and of whose accomplishments, performance and appearance they can boast. This is manifested in the constant competition among them as to who has the better dressed, more advanced, more intelligent, better looking, the heavier, bigger, more active—in a word, the better baby.[9] For their own persons they have more or less given up the competition for love, but they are intensely jealous of the attention given to their children by the matrons, wardens, and fellow prisoners.

It would take an exacting experimenter to invent an experiment with conditions as diametrically opposed in regard to the mother-child relationship as they are in these two institutions. Nursery provides each child with a mother to the nth degree, a mother who gives the child everything a good mother does and, beyond that, everything else she has[10]. Foundling Home does not give the child a mother, nor even a substitute-mother, but only an eighth of a nurse.

9. The psychoanalytically oriented reader of course realizes that for these girls in prison the child has become a hardly disguised phallic substitute. However, for the purposes of this article I have carefully avoided any extensive psychoanalytic interpretation, be it ever so tempting, and limited myself as closely as possible to results of direct observations of behavior. At numerous other points it would be not only possible but natural to apply analytic concepts; that is reserved for future publication.

10. For the non-psychoanalytically oriented reader we note that this intense mother-child relationship is not equivalent to a relationship based on love of the child. The mere fact that the child is used as a phallic substitute implies what a large part unconscious hostility plays in the picture.

We are now in a position to approach more closely and with better understanding the results obtained by each of the two institutions. We have already cited a few: we mentioned that the Developmental Quotient of Nursery achieves a normal average of about 105 at the end of the first year, whereas that of the Foundling Home sinks to 72; and we mentioned the striking difference of the children in the two institutions at first sight. Let us first consider the point at which the developments in the two institutions deviate.

On admission the children of Foundling Home have a much better average than the children of Nursery; their hereditary equipment is better than that of the children of delinquent minors. But while Foundling Home shows a rapid fall of the developmental index, Nursery shows a steady rise. They cross between the 4th and 5th months, and from that point on the curve of the average Developmental Quotient of the Foundling Home drops downward with increasing rapidity, never again to rise (Curve I).

The point where the two curves cross is significant. The time when the children in Foundling Home are weaned is the beginning of the 4th month. The time lag of one month in the sinking of the index below normal is explained by the fact that the Quotient represents a cross-section including all sectors of development, and that attempts at compensation are made in some of the other sectors.

However, when we consider the sector of Body Mastery (Curve II) which according to Wolf[11] is most indicative for the mother-child relationship, we find that the curves of the children in Nursery cross the Body Mastery curve of the Foundling Home children between the 3rd and 4th month. The inference is obvious. As soon as the babies in Foundling Home are weaned the modest human contacts which they have had during nursing at the breast stop, and their development falls below normal.

One might be inclined to speculate as to whether the further deterioration of the children in Foundling Home is not due to other factors also, such as the perceptual and motor deprivations from which they suffer. It might be argued that the better achievement of the Nursery children is due to the fact that they were better provided for in regard to toys and other perceptual stimuli. We shall therefore analyze somewhat more closely the nature of deprivations in perceptual and locomotor stimulation.

11. K. Wolf, "Body Mastery of the Child as an index for the Emotional Relationship between Mother and Child" (in preparation).

First of all it should be kept in mind that the nature of the inanimate perceptual stimulus, whether it is a toy or any other object, has only a very minor importance for a child under 12 months. At this age the child is not yet capable of distinguishing the real purpose of an object. He is only able to use it in a manner adequate to his own functional needs(23). Our thesis is that perception is a function of libidinal cathexis and therefore the result of the intervention of an emotion of one kind or another.[12]. Emotions are provided for the

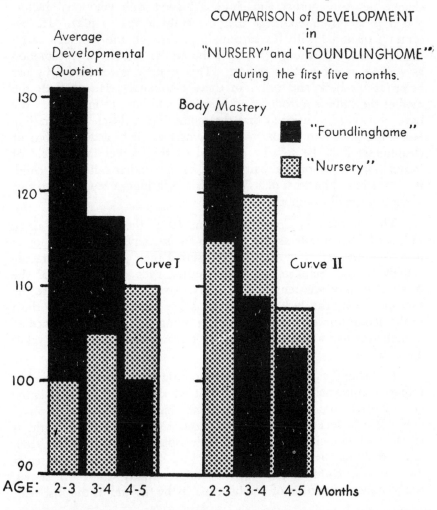

12. This is stating in psychoanalytic terms the conviction of most modern psychologists, beginning with Compayré(24) and shared by such familiar authorities in child psychology as Stern(25) and Bühler(26), and in animal psychology, Tolman(27).

child through the intervention of a human partner, i.e., by the mother
or her substitute. A progressive development of emotional interchange with the mother provides the child with perceptive experiences
of its environment. The child learns to grasp by nursing at the
mother's breast and by combining the emotional satisfaction of that
experience with tactile perceptions. He learns to distinguish animate
objects from inanimate ones by the spectacle provided by his mother's
face(28) in situations fraught with emotional satisfaction. The interchange between mother and child is loaded with emotional factors
and it is in this interchange that the child learns to play. He becomes acquainted with his surroundings through the mother's carrying him around; through her help he learns security in locomotion
as well as in every other respect. This security is reinforced by her
being at his beck and call. In these emotional relations with the
mother the child is introduced to learning, and later to imitation. We
have previously mentioned that the motherless children in Foundling
Home are unable to speak, to feed themselves, or to acquire habits of
cleanliness: it is the security provided by the mother in the field of
locomotion, the emotional bait offered by the mother calling her child,
that "teaches" him to walk. When this is lacking, even children two
to three years old cannot walk.

The children in Foundling Home have, theoretically, as much
radius of locomotion as the children in Nursery. They did not at
first have toys, but they could have exerted their grasping and tactile
activity on the blankets, on their clothes, even on the bars of the
cots. We have seen children in Nursery without toys; they are the
exception—but the lack of material is not enough to hamper them
in the acquisition of locomotor and grasping skills. The presence of
a mother or her substitute is sufficient to compensate for all the other
deprivations.

It is true that the children in Foundling Home are condemned to
solitary confinement in their cots. But we do not think that it is the
lack of perceptual stimulation in general that counts in their deprivation. We believe that they suffer because their perceptual world is
emptied of human partners, that their isolation cuts them off from
any stimulation by any persons who could signify mother-representa-
tives for the child at this age.[13] The result, as Curve III shows,
is a complete restriction of psychic capacity by the end of the first year.

13. This statement is to be developed further in a forthcoming article on "The
Beginning of the Social Relations of the Child".

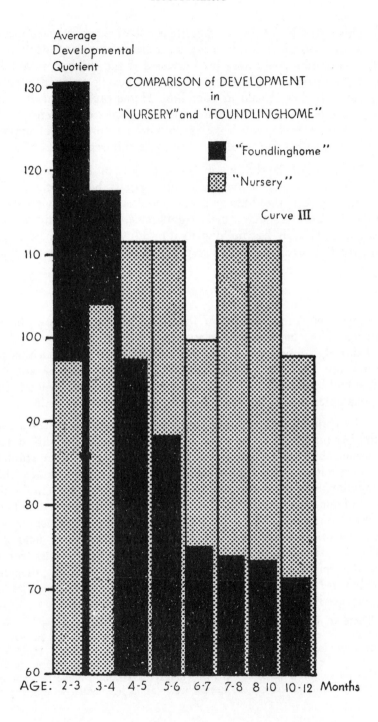

Average
Developmental
Quotient

COMPARISON of DEVELOPMENT
in
"NURSERY"and "FOUNDLINGHOME"

"Foundlinghome"

"Nursery"

Curve III

AGE: 2-3   3-4   4-5   5-6   6-7   7-8   8 10   10-12   Months

This restriction of psychic capacity is not a temporary phenomenon. It is, as can be seen from the curve, a progressive process. How much this deterioration could have been arrested if the children were taken out of the institution at the end of the first year is an open question. The fact that they remain in Foundling Home probably furthers this progressive process. By the end of the second year the Developmental Quotient sinks to 45, which corresponds to a mental age of approximately 10 months, and would qualify these children as imbeciles.

The curve of the children in Nursery does not deviate significantly from the normal. The curve sinks at two points, between the 6th and 7th, and between the 10th and 12th months. These deviations are within the normal range; their significance will be discussed in a separate article. It has nothing to do with the influence of institutions, for the curve of the village group is nearly identical.

VI. *Provisional Conclusions.*

The contrasting pictures of these two institutions show the significance of the mother-child relationship for the development of the child during the first year. Deprivations in other fields, such as perceptual and locomotor radius, can all be compensated by adequate mother-child relations. "Adequate" is not here a vague general term. The examples chosen represent the two extremes of the scale.

The children in Foundling Home do have a mother—for a time, in the beginning—but they must share her immediately with at least one other child, and from 3 months on, with seven other children. The quantitative factor here is evident. There is a point under which the mother-child relations cannot be restricted during the child's first year without inflicting irreparable damage. On the other hand, the exaggerated mother-child relationship in Nursery introduces a different quantitative factor. To anyone familiar with the field it is surprising that Nursery should achieve such excellent results, for we know that institutional care is destructive for children during their first year; but in Nursery the destructive factors have been compensated by the increased intensity of the mother-child relationship.

These findings should not be construed as a recommendation for overprotection of children. In principle the libidinal situation of Nursery is almost as undesirable as the other extreme in Foundling Home. Neither in the nursery of a penal institution nor in a foundling home for parentless children can the normal libidinal situation that obtains in a family home be expected. The two institutions have here been chosen as experimental set-ups for the purpose of examining variations in libidinal factors ranging from extreme frustration to extreme gratification. That the extreme frustration practised in Foundling Home has deplorable consequences has been shown; the extreme gratification in Nursery can be tolerated by the children housed there for two reasons:

(1) The mothers have the benefit of the intelligent guidance of the head nurse and her assistants, and the worst exaggerations are thus corrected.

(2) Children during their first year of life can stand the ill effects of such a situation much better than at a later age. In this respect Nursery has wisely limited the duration of the children's stay to the first twelve months. For children older than this we should consider a libidinal set-up such as that in Nursery very dangerous indeed.

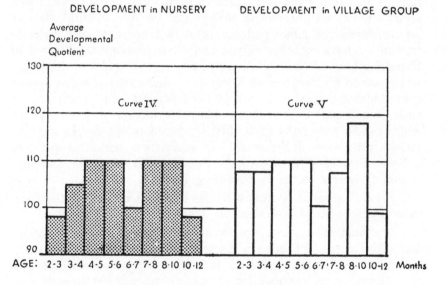

VII. *Further Problems.*

This is the first of a series of publications on the results of a research project on infancy that we are conducting. As such it is a preliminary report. It is not intended to show more than the most general outline of the results of early institutional care, giving at the same time a hint of the approach we use. The series of other problems on which this investigation has shed some light, as well as the formulation of those problems that could be recognized as such only in the course of the investigation, have not been touched upon in our present study and can only summarily be touched upon; they are headings, as it were, of the chapters of our future program of publication.

Apart from the severe developmental retardation, the most striking single factor observed in Foundling Home was the change in the
pattern of the reaction to strangers in the last third of the first
year(29). The usual behavior was replaced by something that could
vary from extreme friendliness to any human partner combined with
anxious avoidance of inanimate objects, to a generalized anxiety expressed in blood-curdling screams which could go on indefinitely. It
is evident that these deviant behavior patterns require a more thorough and extensive discussion than our present study would have permitted.

We also observed extraordinary deviations from the normal in the
time of appearance and disappearance of familiar developmental patterns; and certain phenomena unknown in the normal child, such as
bizarre stereotyped motor patterns distinctly reminiscent of the stereo-
typy in catatonic motility. These and other phenomena observed in
Foundling Home require an extensive discussion in order to determine
which are to be classified as maturation phenomena, (which appear
even under the most unfavorable circumstances, and which appear
with commensurate retardation when retardation is general); or
which can be considered as the first symptoms of the development of
serious psychiatric disturbances. In connection with this problem
a more thorough discussion of the rapidity with which the Developmental Quotients recede in Foundling Home is intended.

Another study is to deal with the problems created by the enormous over-protection practised in Nursery.

And finally the rationale of the one institutional routine as against
that of the other will have to be discussed in greater detail. This study
will offer the possibility of deciding how to compensate for unavoidable changes in the environment of children orphaned at an early age.
It will also shed some light on the social consequences of the progressive disruption of home life caused by the increase of female labor
and by the demands of war; we might state that we foresee in the
course of events a corresponding increase in asociality, in the number
of problem and delinquent children, of mental defectives, and of psychotics.

It will be necessary to take into consideration in our institutions,
in our charitable activities, in our social legislation, the overwhelming
and unique importance of adequate and satisfactory mother-child
relationship during the first year, if we want to decrease the unavoidable and irreparable psychiatric consequences deriving from neglect
during this period.

BIBLIOGRAPHY

1. Schlossman, A., "Zur Frage der Säuglingssterblichkeit", *Münchner Med. Wochenschrift*, 67, 1920.
2. Chapin, H. D., "Are Institutions for Infants Necessary?", *Journal of American Medical Association*, January, 1915.
3. Chapin, H. D., "A Plea for Accurate Statistics in Infants' Institutions", *Archives of Pediatrics*, October, 1915.
4. Bakwin, H., "Loneliness in Infants", *American Journal of Diseases of Children*, 63, 1942, pp. 30-40.
5. Durfee, H. and Wolf, K., "Anstaltspflege und Entwicklung im ersten Lebensjahr", *Zeitschrift fur Kinderforschung*, 42/3, 1933.
6. Lowrey, L. G., "Personality Distortion and Early Institutional Care", *American Journal of Orthopsychiatry*, X, 3, 1940, pp. 576-585.
7. Bender, L. and Yarnell, H., "An Observation Nursery: a Study of 250 Children in the Psychiatric Division of Bellevue Hospital", *American Journal of Psychiatry*, 97, 1941, pp. 1158-1174.
8. Goldfarb, W., "Infant Rearing as a Factor in Foster Home Placement", *American Journal of Orthopsychiatry*, XIV, 1944, pp. 162-167.
9. Goldfarb, W., "Effects of Early Institutional Care on Adolescent Personality: Rorschach Data", *American Journal of Orthopsychiatry*, XIV, 1944, pp. 441-447.
10. Goldfarb, W., "Effects of Early Institutional Care on Adolescent Personality", *Journal of Experimental Education*, 12, 1943, pp. 106-129.
11. Goldfarb, W. and Klopfer, B., "Rorschach Characteristics of Institutional Children", *Rorschach Research Exchange*, 8, 1944, pp. 92-100.
12. Ripin, R., "A Study of the Infant's Feeding Reactions During the First Six Months of Life", *Archives of Psychology*, 116, 1930, p. 38.
13. Skeels, H. M., "Mental Development of Children in Foster Homes", *Journal of Consulting Psychology*, 2, 1938, pp. 33-43.
14. Skeels, H. M., "Some Iowa Studies of the Mental Growth of Children in Relation to Differentials of the Environment: A Summary", *39th Yearbook, National Society for the Study of Education*, II, 1940, pp. 281-308.
15. Skeels, H. M., Updegraff, R., Wellman, B. L., and Williams, H. M., "A Study of Environmental Stimulation; an Orphanage Preschool Project", *University of Iowa Studies in Child Welfare*, 15, 4, 1938.
16. Skodak, M., "Children in Foster Homes", *University of Iowa Studies in Child Welfare*, 16, 1, 1939.
17. Stoddard, G. D., "Intellectual Development of the Child: an Answer to the Critics of the Iowa Studies", *School and Society*, 51, 1940, pp. 529-536.
18. Updegraff, R., "The Determination of a Reliable Intelligence Quotient for the Young Child", *Journal of Genetic Psychology*, 41, 1932, pp. 152-166.
19. Woodworth, R. S., "Heredity and Environment", *Bulletin* 47, Social Science Research Council, 1941.
20. Jones, H. E., "Personal Reactions of the Yearbook Committee", *39th Yearbook, National Society for the Study of Education*, I, 1940, pp. 454-456.

21. Simpson, B. R., "The Wandering I. Q.", *Journal of Psychology*, 7, 1939, pp. 351-367.
22. Hetzer, H. and Wolf, K., "Baby Tests", *Zeitschrift für Psychologie*, 107, 1928.
23. Bühler, Ch., *Kindheit und Jugend*, Leipzig, 1931, p. 67.
24. Compayré, G., *L'evolution intellectuelle et morale de l'enfant*, Paris, 1893.
25. Stern, Wm., *Psychology of Early Childhood*, London, 1930.
26. Bühler, K., *Die geistige Entwicklung des Kindes*, 4th ed., Jena, 1942, p. 106 and p. 116.
27. Tolman, E. C., *Purposive Behavior*, New York, 1932, p. 27 ff.
28. Gesell, A. and Ilg, F., *Feeding Behavior of Infants*, Phila., 1937, p. 21.
29. Gesell, A. and Thompson, H., *Infant Behavior, its Genesis and Growth*, New York, 1934, p. 208.

EXAMINATION OF THE KLEIN SYSTEM
OF CHILD PSYCHOLOGY[1]

By EDWARD GLOVER, M.D. (London)

INTRODUCTION

During the past twenty years the development of a specialized branch of child analysis has brought to a head a number of controversial issues the solution of which will influence analytic theory for some time to come. It was of course inevitable that clinical psychoanalysts should, sooner or later, begin to "specialize" in various branches of morbid psychology, thereby following the example of earlier colleagues who had "specialized" in different fields of applied psychoanalysis—anthropology, literature, folklore and the like. Indeed it is more than probable that as our knowledge of different varieties of mental disorder increases it will not be possible for the "general practitioner in psychoanalysis" to be equally competent in all branches of psychopathology. The apparent "all-round" ability he exhibits at present depends on the fact that our knowledge regarding the development of most psychopathological states, though accurate enough, is still rudimentary. Transference and other factors of technique apart, therapeutic results depend on the extent to which we apply sound analytic understanding; and we have just enough understanding of the main mental mechanisms common to all cases to produce some beneficial results. Up to the present, at any rate, there is no evidence that etiological fads or special systems of interpretation have any outstanding therapeutic virtue, still less that these isolated systems can be made the basis of a new metapsychology.

1. This paper is based on discussions conducted in the British Psychoanalytic Society during the last fifteen years. In addition to quoting from printed material extensive quotations are given from the mimeographed publication of the "Controversial Series of Discussions" organized by the British Psychoanalytic Society in 1943-44 and circulated among its members.

75

However that may be, it is interesting to note that the first sign of clinical specialization in psychoanalysis was the development of a branch of child analysis. This was followed by a clinically unjustified acquisition of prestige on the part of child analysts, and to this prestige factor[2] I attribute some of the chaos that has recently arisen in psycho-analytic circles in Britain. The present paper is intended to examine the views and theories put forward by the Klein Group of the British Psycho-Analytic Society.

THE DEVELOPMENT OF CHILD ANALYSIS

Up to the early 1920's child analysts in the real sense of the term (i.e., practitioners who devote their energies almost exclusively to the actual psychoanalysis of children up to the age of puberty) were few and far between. Psychoanalytically trained observers of children were common enough. Most practising psychoanalysts had been at one time or other at pains to collect observations of child behavior and to adduce these in confirmation of already established psychoanalytic findings. In short, child analysis was in the first instance a branch of applied psychoanalysis, a behavioristic study similar to the analytic study of the psychoses or of the behavior or ideologies of primitive races. Indeed as far as infancy is concerned it must remain an observational study, for until the child's mind has reached the stage of development at which it can apprehend the meaning of interpretations (even if these were made by dumb show) the psychic situation between the child and the analyst remains one of spontaneous or, at the most, of developed rapport only: no true "analytic situation" can exist.[3]

Nevertheless it is significant that some of the most important early advances in psychoanalysis arose from a psychic situation in which

2. A similar situation threatens to develop regarding the importance of the study of psychoses to psychoanalysis. The fact that the regressions, restitutive symptom-formations and disintegration products observed in the psychoses are of a primitive type tends to give the observer the impression that he is in specially close touch with unconscious mental processes, and encourages him in the belief that he may speak with special authority on psychoanalytic matters. Whereas the plain fact is that up to the present the study of psychoses remains for the largest part an observational field in which the essential techniques of psychoanalytic research are almost as limited as they are in the study of early infancy.

3. As a matter of fact even if Klein's entire system were sound, i.e., if the infant a few months after birth possessed a psychic apparatus already differentiated into ego and superego, capable of the elaborate and sophisticated system of unconscious and pre-conscious fantasy Klein describes, and, a priori capable of developing a classical transference neurosis, this would still not justify the assumption of a possible "analytic situation". Neither the transference nor its associated resistances could be analyzed until their meaning could be conveyed.

indirect observation was combined with vicarious interpretation. Freud's analysis of Little Hans resulted not only in a classical outline of the oedipus situation but in increased understanding of the dynamics of the unconscious mind and in particular of the role of anxiety and repression during that classical phase. As was only natural the work of the early child analysts (Hug-Hellmuth, Pfister, et al) reflected with some fidelity the existing state of psychoanalytic theory. So close was the correspondence, that it would not be unfair to say that the findings of the early child analysts were more corroborative than original in scope. They confirmed what psychoanalysis and analytic observation of adults had led Freud to infer regarding the unconscious mind of the child. And to a very considerable extent this has remained the case down to the present time. As Freud step by step expanded our knowledge of the structure and function of the unconscious mind, child analysts vied with analytical anthropologists and analytical psychiatrists to confirm his findings in their respective fields. This was at the same time a tribute to the amazing accuracy of Freud's observations and a step towards that corroboration that is necessary for the acceptance of analytic theories. But apart from filling in a few gaps here and there and from producing clinical illustrations from normal and abnormal children, all the more fascinating because they were observations made during actual analysis of children, it could not be said that child analysts had contributed much to the expansion of analytic theory.

Of course the lines of research were obvious enough. Freud had mapped out both positive and negative aspects of the oedipus situation, and had later outlined the structure of the mind at that phase. By his analysis of obsessional neurosis in particular he had been able to thrust deeply into the stage immediately preceding the oedipus phase. But between that pre-oedipus phase and the earliest phases of infantile psychic activity, which perforce were only understood in terms of hypothetical reconstruction, a gap remained only slenderly bridged by delineation of "stages in the development of the libido", by conceptions of the development of object relationships—"auto-erotism"—"narcissim"—"object-choice", and by etiological formulations regarding paranoia and melancholia. All these were expressed mainly in terms of libidinal development, although the use of phrases such as "oral-sadism", "anal-sadism", "ambivalence" and the like showed an understanding of the part played by impulses of aggression and attitudes of hate which were only later formulated by Freud with more precision. Not only was there a gap between hypothetical reconstructions of early mental function and clinical outlines of the mind at the oedipus phase; there were in existence no cross-sections of the mind during the pre-oedipus phases comparable with the cross-sections Freud had made for the three- to five-year-old children. Concepts of ego, superego and id, for example, were first mapped out in terms of the classical oedipus phase. Pre-oedipus regulator systems in the ego (concepts so essential to psychoanalytic psychology) were not described. Ferenczi, combining the concept of the anal-sadistic stage of the libido with that of the superego, had shot his bolt by describing "Sphincter-moral"; but although suggestive enough in theory and useful enough in practice this formulation was not sufficiently correlated with ego-structure(1).[4] The signposts to research could not be mistaken. Advances had to be made from two directions, from the clinical end where actual analyses could be effected and from the "reconstruction" end. It was a task that incidentally called for close correlation of effort in every branch of psychoanalysis. But above all it called for original work on the part of child analysts.

The dangers inherent in this situation were equally obvious. Hypothetical reconstructions of the mind in early infancy, however far they may be extended, can never meet and link up with clinical observations. They are of a different order. They can increase the plausibility of a clinical interpretation, and their own plausibility can be reinforced by clinical interpretations. But they cannot really dovetail with clinical facts. Attempts to merge them usually lead to the confusion that so often follows the blending of subjective fantasy with scientific fact.[5]

OUTLINE OF KLEINIAN THEORIES

Melanie Klein's theories fall into two phases. The first of these ended, for all practical purposes, with the appearance of her book, *The Psycho-Analysis of Children,* in 1932(2), and the second began with the publication of her paper on depression in 1934(3). The fact that there are two distinct phases of Kleinian theory is not sufficiently recognized. Some psychoanalysts who favored views put forward by Melanie Klein in her "first phase" have unthinkingly supported the theories produced in the second phase. They were evi-

4. Numbers in parentheses refer to bibliography at end of paper.
5. There are of course some exceptions to this rule. Freud himself provided one of the most distinguished exceptions to it. But he never confused hypotheses with facts. In less skilled hands the method results in absurdity.

dently under the misapprehension that the latter were mere logical extensions of earlier views. Admittedly there is some ideological continuity between the two phases, and it is not difficult to find in the earlier phase many of the confusions of thought and terminology that later on were developed into a heterodox brand of metapsychology. But the two phases are otherwise quite distinct. Klein's earlier theories constituted an attempt to fill in the gap I have described above: her later formulations, starting from the assumption of a "central depressive position", said to be characteristic of all mental development, are of a much more ambitious order. If accepted they would involve a complete recasting of our accepted ideas of mental development: if they are inaccurate, and that is the main contention of this paper, they represent a major deviation from psychoanalytic principles.

(a)   The First Phase.

Melanie Klein's book, *The Psycho-Analysis of Children,* was an expansion of two courses of lectures interspersed with a few chapters based on earlier papers on the subject. There is consequently a good deal of overlapping and repetition of argument, but the main outline is as follows:

From the middle of the first year onward the oral frustrations of the child together with increase of its oral sadism release oedipus impulses. The superego begins to develop at the same time. The immediate consequence of oral frustration is the desire to "incorporate" the father's penis. But this is accompanied by the theory that the mother "incorporates" and retains possession of the father's penis. The impulse is then aroused to destroy in various primitive ways the mother's body and its contents. In the case of the girl the impulse to destroy the mother's body gives rise to a danger situation equivalent to the castration anxiety of the boy, viz. fear of destruction of her own body. Incidentally, it is laid down that anxiety springs from aggression. As soon as the child's process of "incorporation" has begun, the incorporated object becomes the vehicle of defense against the destructive impulses in the organism. The child is afraid of being exterminated by its destructive impulses and projects them on an external object which it then tries to destroy by oral-sadistic means. And this in turn involves incorporating a "bad" object which acts as a severe superego. This primary defense by oral aggression soon extends to urethral and anal-sadistic systems. These all turn in the first place against the mother's breast, but later against other, sometimes corresponding, parts of the mother's body. These primary defenses continue unabated until the decline of the earlier anal-sadistic stage. Oral frustration also arouses an unconscious knowledge that the parents enjoy mutual sexual pleasures (at first thought of in oral terms), and the oral envy aroused makes the child wish to push into the mother's body and is at the same time responsible for its epistemophilic trends. These fantasied attacks are directed in particular at the orally incorporated penis of the father. The boy, for example, is ultimately afraid of the mother's body because it contains the father's penis, i.e. fear tends 'to be displaced from the penis to the body. The most anxiety-provoking situation is that where the mother's possession of the father's penis is regarded by the child as combination against him of both father and mother.

With the boy, oedipus conflict sets in with hatred of the father's penis in the mother's body and desire for genital union with the mother. The girl in her anxiety, turns from the mother (body) to the father (penis). In both, the impulses of hate bring about the oedipus situation and the formation of the superego. It is clearly laid down that the child's earliest identifications should be called a superego. This institution helps to overcome anxiety and sadism, but of course anxiety itself is partly responsible for the expansion of different erotogenic interests. The child's introjected objects (which are essentially organ-objects) exercise a fantastic severity, and therefore arouse intense anxiety. Indeed, in the early anal-sadistic phase the child is trying to "eject his superego", and not only his superego but his id. Up to the end of this phase we have all the fixation points for the psychoses. The processes of introjection and projection are reciprocal, and during these phases the ego deals with objects as the superego deals with the ego and as the ego deals with the superego and id. This introduces a confusion between the fantasied and the reality dangers of the object. The "real" object contributes a little but as a rule only a little to this anxiety situation. The child's original hate of the object is reinforced by hate of the superego and id.

Modification of these early anxieties and defenses is effected through the libido and through relations to real objects. Even the earliest turning from the mother's breast to the father's penis is a libidinal step forward from an anxiety situation, although not at first a very successful step. In the girl it is the precursor of the oedipus situation; in the boy it may, unless overcome by a second orientation to the mother, lead to a deep homosexual fixation on the father. What we call stages in the development of the libido really represent positions won by the libido in its struggle with destructive impulses. Moreover, suspicions regarding the external world evoked by projecting sadism on to it lead to a closer contact with real objects. These factors, following the process of ejecting the destructive superego, prepare the way for more successful introjection of "good" objects. The new introjections lead in turn to modification of the earliest anxiety phobias which are of a projective, paranoidal nature. In the later anal stage, when the superego begins to be "retained", anxiety develops into guilt, and obsessional features make their appearance. Ceremonials of object-restoration are a prominent feature at this stage, and are characterized by a belief in creative omnipotence which is necessary to counteract the belief in destructive (excretory) omnipotence. These obsessional symptoms are also a defense against early masturbatory systems, which themselves represent attempts to side-track sadistic oedipus content. To these "pathological" measures of defense are added the more "normal" mechanisms of play, and of curiosity (search for knowledge) which serve to allay fears in the outer world. An attempt is now made to approximate the superego to real objects, and to build up a realistic ego-ideal system. The development of the superego and of the libido cease at the onset of the latency period. In general, differences in the superego structure of the boy and girl relate to differences in the history of aggressive and libidinal development. The girl's oedipus phase is ushered in by oral desires for the father's penis which is thought to be in the mother's body. Her omnipotence then makes the girl believe that she has herself "incorporated" this penis. This reinforced incorporation tendency gives the girl a more powerful superego. Differences in the method of dealing with this "bad" introjected penis are responsible for differences in type observable amongst women. The girl's superego is also affected by ideas of sadistic omnipotence of excreta. And owing to the absence of a real penis she has more uncertainty about the inside of her body. In general, the girl's superego is more extensive than the boy's owing to the receptive nature of her impulses. The boy's primary omnipotence relates more to the possession of a real penis and less to the existence of an introjected father's penis. The girl introjects more than does the boy; she "needs" objects more, and is left ultimately with a more exalted superego. The boy in his original relation to the father's penis inside the mother's body concentrates more on destruction of the penis. In any case the stage of attack on the mother's body does not last so long as in the girl; moreover, the accompanying omnipotence is less excretory and more penile. Believing in the sadistic omnipotence of the penis, the boy concentrates on attacking the father's penis, and this leads to genital desires for the mother. When this penis-hate is displayed to the real penis of the father, typical castration anxiety develops.

Reviewing a book that sets out to describe in psychoanalytic terms the development of mind from the middle of the first year down to the latency period it is essential to keep the following questions clearly in mind: (a) to what extent has the author drawn on accepted Freudian findings; (b) to what extent are any new formulations either in the nature of hypothetical reconstructions or direct analytic interpretations of a given period of development; (c) how far are the new formulations either accurate or plausible. And these test questions raise a number of other issues, e.g., at what ages were the children under analytic observation; how far is the reconstruction concerned with fantasies alleged to exist in the child's unconscious, (and interpreted by the author) or on self-interpreting material; finally in the case of children of the age period three-to-five, by what criteria are the alleged stages of earlier development established, and in particular how does the author distinguish between, on the one hand, products of fixation and regression, and on the other, unconscious fantasies stimulated by the current psychological situation. Following these lines of approach it is possible to disentangle from a rather matted narrative the main outlines of early Kleinian theory.

At a first reading one is apt to become confused by the fact that although the author gives an adequate list of references to the work of Freud, Abraham, Ferenczi, Jones and others, it is not always easy to indicate the point at which she gives their ideas her own particular twist. For instance, she constantly lays stress on the view that early anxieties are reduced by exploitation of libidinal phases. Now this is not an original discovery. Neither is the companion view that sadism (or rather the impulses of aggression, destruction and mastery) is a determining factor in mental conflict. To Freud himself and later to Jones and Abraham is due the credit for first describing the fundamental conception of ambivalence in comprehensive terms. Indeed it was unfortunate that the author did not preserve the strict connotation of this term, for throughout her book, the term "sadism" becomes a catchword. Melanie Klein was evidently caught up in the swing of the analytic pendulum from purely libidinal etiologies and soon landed herself in theories that aggression causes anxiety and that anxiety can be credited with the calling out of different libidinal phases. Thus according to her, impulses of hate bring about the oedipus situation, and stages in the development of the libido really represent positions won by the libido in its struggle with destructive impulses. Possibly the author in formulating this sweeping hypothesis was biased by clinical observations made by Freud on homosexuality, in particular that an earlier ambivalence or rivalry can be covered by a later homosexual attachment. But the generalization she puts forward is not supported by direct analysis of a multiplicity of types of cases and in any event runs counter to all psycho-biological probability. Nevertheless the manner in which accepted Freudian views are interspersed with purely Kleinian hypotheses would lead the casual reader to imagine that the Kleinian conclusions arrived at are merely a logical extension of the more familiar Freudian premises. Throughout the book it is essential to distinguish clearly what is accepted Freudian teaching and what is specifically a Kleinian accretion to it.

A second pitfall for the unwary reader is the fact that the greater part of the author's description of mental development is purely hypothetical reconstruction. This merges gradually with views based on her clinical analysis of children beyond the age of three and four.[6] Of course it can be argued that the child analyst is just as entitled to draw conclusions regarding the first two years of life from the analysis of five-year-old children as the ordinary analyst is entitled to draw conclusions regarding the unconscious content of five-year-old children

6. From the age-table given by the author it appears that as far as the analysis of young children is concerned, her findings are based on the analysis of seven cases. The two youngest were 2¾ and 3¼ years respectively; the other five varied from 3¾ to 5 years (average 4½); all were diagnosed as severely neurotic: one exhibited psychotic traits. Of the others, five yere in the latency period (variation 6 to 9); two pre-pubertal (9½) and four pubertal (12 to 14); one adult case is included.

from the analysis of adults. This argument is not valid. Not only are conclusions drawn from adult cases based on observations of every variety of case but they can be confirmed by actual analysis of five-year-olds. The assumptions made about early infancy cannot be confirmed by direct analysis and must remain reconstructions to be judged by their plausibility. Naturally the same applies to what are alleged to be the unconscious fantasies of the young infant. Yet the merging of these alleged early fantasies with later fantasy systems (whether the latter are accurately analyzed or not) gives the former an air of objective description that is likely to lead the reader astray. This is best illustrated by the conclusions regarding the oedipus complex arrived at by the author. Melanie Klein holds that owing to oral frustration the oedipus complex is released at the middle of the first year. The sadism engendered by this frustration activates the oedipus situation. Now it has frequently been reported that infants from the age of six to eighteen months show *larval* genital reactions, and these observations have gained strength from the fact that genital excitation can be observed in small babies. These are interesting observations but they do not permit generalizations about the universality of an "oedipus complex" existing from the sixth month of life, and they certainly do not constitute proof that even in the cases described by Melanie Klein the sequence of events described by her is valid. The accepted theory of primacy of different libidinal components at different stages of development does not exclude the existence of genital elements at an early stage and, as Freud was ready to concede, there is no objection to calling all pregenital relations between the infant and its parent oedipus relations(4). But that is not Melanie Klein's point. She states specifically that fantasies concerning the father's penis (inside the mother) follow immediately on oral frustration, hence, that her "first year oedipus situation" is a true genital oedipus situation. Putting aside for the moment the question whether fantasies exist at this age, it will be seen that Melanie Klein while at some points accepting both explicitly and implicitly the concept of libidinal primacies, in effect undercuts the significance of later infantile genital primacy. No doubt the depth of true genital oedipus systems had previously been underestimated. Whether the author's conclusions are right or wrong, there can be no doubt that they led to a broader conception of the oedipus phase. The fact remains however that her own descriptions of the course of events are purely hypothetical and lack the clinical backing by which the classical Freudian views are supported. The Freudian view is that the oedipus situation results

from an infantile genital (phallic) primacy occurring at a phase when
the ego is definitely organized and about to undergo its final differentiation. I have every sympathy with the desire to trace genital elements in the primitive and unorganized ego: and in fact I have myself
postulated primitive genital (nuclear) formations in early infancy
but that is not the same thing as postulating an active oedipus situation. Moreover the Freudian position regarding the classical oedipus
situation is firmly based on analytic investigations. Melanie Klein's
theories as to the onset of the oedipus complex, the mechanisms that
activate it and the unconscious fantasies that precede the activation
remain purely hypothetical and incapable of direct confirmation. Indeed it is difficult to escape the conclusion that Melanie Klein's "discovery" of the first year oedipus complex was little more than a
"hunch" based on the conviction that as infants undoubtedly possess
some genital libido, there *must* be an oedipus situation at an early stage.

Concerning the early formation of the superego practically identical arguments are applicable. As I have pointed out earlier, the
question of "forerunners" of the superego, an institution which,
according to accepted Freudian theory, is specifically connected with
the disintegration of the oedipus situation, has long exercised the minds
of analytic investigators. But even in the field of hypothetical reconstruction, few attempts were made to describe the regulator systems
of the primitive ego. In the early days of superego controversy critics
used to take rather easily for granted that anything preceding the end
of the phallic phase should be regarded as belonging to the stage of a
"primitive ego" which was supposed partly to obey and partly to
project the urgencies of the id. But although I was among the first
to support Melanie Klein's view that true superego formation occurs
earlier than had previously been supposed, I expressed the opinion
that the earliest superego formations she outlined could be better
described as forerunners of the superego—that is to say as differentiations in the primitive ego brought about by the action of primitive
mechanisms during the earlier phases of reality-proving. In principle,
of course, any psychic imprint that is sufficiently permanent, and that
leads to the subdivision of instinctual energies within the ego (Freud's
"turning on the self") can be regarded as having superego characteristics in the sense that however rudimentary the formation may be, it
functions dynamically in the same way as the superego proper. And I
think it is probable that as the earlier components of infantile sexuality
lose their respective primacies and together with their associated
reactive (sadistic or aggressive) drives fall before the action of

repression, these primitive traces of ego-regulator systems become more organized and finally form substantial systems on which the superego proper is superimposed. Elsewhere I have put forward a "nuclear theory" of ego development which I believe meets many of the difficulties in reconstructing these earlier stages of ego development and differentiation. But these attempts belong mainly to the field of hypothetical reconstruction and are capable of clinical corroboration only insofar as the later pre-oedipus phases are concerned. Obviously, however early rudiments of superego systems may make their appearance, the lines of demarcation between the id, primitive ego nuclei and primitive superego nuclei can never be very clear. It may be that structural analogies are less useful in describing the early psyche than estimations of function in terms of energy, i.e., the quantities of unmodified instinct passing through a psychic system.

This, as I have said, is legitimate speculation. All we can say with certainty is that there is a good case for postulating earlier forms of superego. But it is one thing to outline hypothetical systems and quite another to affirm as Melanie Klein has done the actual existence of a superego based on the development of an oedipus situation at the sixth month of life. She maintains that the child, afraid of being exterminated by its destructive impulses, projects them on an external object which it then tries to destroy by oral-sadistic means and that this in turn involves "incorporating" a "bad" object that acts as a severe superego. The incorporated object becomes the vehicle of defense against the destructive impulses in the organism. The incorporated object is however an "organ-object", e.g., the father's penis existing in the mother; and apparently this organ-object, which when incorporated acts as a severe and destructive superego, can be "ejected". The description of later stages follows the same lines: a series of unconscious fantasies is postulated and extended in terms more appropriate to the description of mental mechanisms. By creating this confusion of terms it is easy for the author to adduce the postulated fantasies as a proof of the existence of the superego. Admittedly it is always hard to prevent anthropomorphism from creeping into psychological terminology, but the liberties Melanie Klein takes with metapsychological terms lead to the creation of a kind of slang in which it is no longer possible to distinguish between mechanisms, psychic imprints (nuclei or institutions) and unconscious presentations (including fantasies). The phrase "introjected penis", for example, is nothing more than a mixed metaphor. It is possible to maintain that the child unconsciously attributes psychic tension to the presence in its body of an imaginary penis or enemy. It can be maintained further that if the child unconsciously applies the mechanism of projection to the instinctual tension, he may then develop a new unconscious fantasy, namely, of ejecting the enemy from his body. But to talk of the child trying to eject the superego is manifestly absurd.

Most of the formulations contained in Klein's book depend on dogmatic assumptions regarding the psychic content of the first and second years of life, a period concerning which we know least. The book contains many generalizations that are extremely plausible, but it is interesting to note that the most plausible of them do not depend on the accuracy or otherwise of her postulated fantasies. Some are in the nature of reasonable reflections about mental development. Thus, it is certainly plausible that the superego of the classical oedipus phase has forerunners. And it is one of Melanie Klein's services to psychoanalysis that her insistence on the point focussed attention on a comparatively neglected problem. Again, quite apart from the question of precocious or delayed development of the classical oedipus complex, it is a reasonable assumption that earlier object relations with the parents constitute characteristic systems that are influenced by the primacy of certain unconscious mechanisms. Following Freud's views on the relation of the superego to the oedipus situation, I have pointed out that the structure of the ego is inevitably influenced by abandonment of the object cathexes characteristic of any given primacy, and it is extremely probable that each ego modification contributes to the mastering of the anxieties of the period(5). Again it is reasonable to suppose that since, in the later stages of development, libido can be exploited to counter anxieties (of whatever origin), similar exploitations occur in earlier stages, and it is likely that the interaction of these various factors influences the modification of both libidinal and aggressive impulses, and so ultimately influences the processes of fixation and regression. It is also clear that the formation of object imagines must be influenced by projection which therefore plays a reflexive part in the formation of introjections. Melanie Klein certainly deserves credit for having brought these and other reflections to bear on problems of early development. No doubt it was for this reason that her earlier formulations became popular.

Unfortunately the author was not content with these legitimate inferences from accepted Freudian theories. In her eagerness to give a theoretical basis to the fantasy systems she had postulated, she did not hesitate to develop theories that deviated from fundamental Freudian concepts. In some cases the deviation is quite apparent, as where she holds that libidinal positions or primacies are called out by struggles with the aggressive impulses. In others, the full implications of her views did not become clear until her "second stage" of theorizing was reached. Thus, having stated that the alternation of processes of projection and introjection introduces a confusion between the fantasied and the reality dangers of the object, she goes on to affirm that the "real" object contributes a little but as a rule only a little to this anxiety situation. It is instructive to compare this with Freud's categorical statement regarding the nature of anxiety in the last stage of infantile development, viz., "frightening *instinctual* situations can in the last resort be traced back to *external* situations of danger"; he adds that it is not the objective injury that is feared but a state of traumatic excitation "which cannot be dealt with in accordance with the norms of the pleasure principle"(5). By thus relating anxiety to a factor in *mental economy*, Freud not only gave a sound metapsychological basis to the theory of anxiety but cut the ground, once and for all, from all attempts either to interpret all mental development in terms of one stage of it or to interpret all mental disorders in terms of one etiological formula. Again Klein's view that the earliest identifications of the child should be called a superego is convenient enough for her own theoretical purposes but reduces our accepted ideas of ego-structure to inextricable confusion.

It remains to consider how this first phase of Kleinian theory was received in psychoanalytic literature. This can be summed up by saying that in Britain Kleinian theories became quite a vogue, in the continental countries they were either rejected outright or treated with considerable reserve, while in America they provoked no very definite reaction. The active support given in Britain came mostly from pupil-followers. There was however one important exception: Ernest Jones' papers on the "Phallic Phase" were based to a very considerable extent on Kleinian views regarding early development(6). At first no doubt a good deal of this support was due to dissatisfaction with the progress of psychoanalysis in mapping out early stages of development. This, together with the fact that Melanie Klein's views at first promised to extend our knowledge of these stages, made some analysts all the more ready to accept her formulations without too close scrutiny of their implications. There is still in my opinion a useful residue to be extracted from this early phase of Kleinian theory. Unfortunately this process of extraction did not take place.[1]

(b)   *The Second Phase.*

In her paper entitled "A Contribution to the Psychogenesis of Manic Depressive States"(3, 12) Melanie Klein stated that in her opinion "the infantile depressive position is the central position in the child's development".

1. My own reactions to the new system were as follows: From the time I first published some observations on the oral phase of the libido development (1924)(7), my main theoretical and clinical interests were devoted to attempted reconstructions of early stages of ego-development, and to the correlation of these stages with different forms of mental disorder. It had always appeared to me that until such correlations were made and distinctive etiological formulae established for different disorders, no important advances could be made in clinical psychoanalysis. When Melanie Klein first adumbrated her theories, I found them stimulating. As I have said, many of her reflections appeared to me to be sound inferences from the work of Freud, Abraham and Ferenczi. Possibly the fact that like Melanie Klein I had been a pupil of Abraham made me more readily responsive to her general line of thought, which both then and later was considerably influenced by Abraham's work. On the other hand, I was always dubious about the validity of her fantasy interpretations. For a time I set myself the task of trying to find a compromise between Kleinian and Freudian concepts. This resulted in a paper, "Grades of Ego-differentiation"(8). Summing up the situation, I expressed myself as follows: "I believe that when all due corrections have been made, the most important of Klein's findings will remain unchallenged, viz., the pre-phallic oedipus phase, and the pregenital phase of superego formation. Even granting this, we are no better off so far as the primitive phases of the Ego are concerned. Indeed the tendency of her work is one of Super-ego aggrandizement at the expense of the primitive Ego." And again: "There would appear to be a certain over-estimation of the Ego in the customary teaching and an under-estimation of the primitive Ego in Klein's teaching." My own main conclusion regarding the question of reality-proving was stated thus: "In the sense of organized reactive function we are entitled to say that a 'Real'-ego system exists from shortly after birth."
But as is so often the case, these unsolicited attempts at compromise ended by wringing concessions from their own sponsor rather than from the opposing parties. Not recognizing that Klein's primary observations were speculative rather than clinical, I assumed that they were clinically valid. If this should seem to represent a deplorable slipshodness on my part I would remind the reader that at that time (1924-29) most analysts inclined to accept papers published in analytic journals at their face value. For example, although in collaboration with James Glover I had examined and rejected Rank's birth-trauma theory of neurosogenesis, most analysts took Rank's theories on trust until Freud a few years later delivered the *coup de grace* in *Inhibitions, Symptoms and Anxiety*. In fact for some years both in public and in private discussions I lent considerable support to some of Melanie Klein's general conclusions, and referred freely to them in a number of clinical and theoretical papers.
But as time went on it was impossible to keep my misgivings from creeping into public comment on her work. This was at first very guardedly expressed in a paper called "The Therapeutic Effect of Inexact Interpretation" (1931)(9). By 1933 my misgivings took the form of explicit criticism; this was expressed in a review(10) of Melanie Klein's book, *The Psycho-Analysis of Children*. Even at this stage I paid tribute to the stimulus of her work in terms that were, I now recognize, unduly laudatory: nevertheless, the review contained practically all the criticisms that I have so far presented in this paper. But it was not until 1934 that, in a paper entitled "Some Aspects of Psycho-Analytical Research"(11), I came into open opposition, stating roundly that existing research activities in the British Psycho-Analytical Society were being "frozen" by the propagation of dogmatic views on matters concerning which a completely open mind was essential.

Starting with a brief re-statement of some of her earlier views, particularly concerning the phase of maximal sadism (which she believes to occur towards the end of the first year of life), the importance of introjection and projection of good or bad (part) objects and of the denial of psychic reality, she stated that a "depressive position" develops at the stage of passing from "part-object" to "whole-object" relations . . . "not till the object is loved *as a whole* can its loss be felt as a whole". At this point there is an increase in introjection processes in order that, among other reasons, the love-object may be preserved in safety inside oneself. There are, however, characteristic anxieties at this stage, in particular, "anxiety lest the object be destroyed in the process of introjection" and "as to the dangers which await the object inside". The situation that is "fundamental for the loss of the loved object" is when "the ego becomes fully identified with its good internalized objects and, at the same time, becomes aware of its own incapacity to protect and preserve them against the internalized persecuting objects and the id". The paranoid mechanisms of destroying objects (in particular "expulsion and projection") persist, although in a lesser degree, but lose value because of the dread of expelling the *good* object along with the bad. "The ego makes. greater use of introjection of the *good* object as a mechanism of defense. This is associated with another important mechanism, that of making reparation to the object." But "the ego cannot as yet believe enough in the benevolence of the object and in its own capacity to make restitution." Every access of hate or anxiety may temporarily abolish the differentiation between good and bad internal objects and this results in "loss of the loved object". The ego is "full of anxiety lest such objects should die". This represents a "disaster" caused by the child's sadism. In depression "the ego's hate of the id accounts even more for its unworthiness and despair than its reproaches against the object".

The paranoiac has also introjected a whole and real object, but has not been able to achieve a full identification with it. Sufferings associated with the depressive position may thrust him back on the paranoid position which can then be reinforced as a defense. The depressive state is genetically derived from the paranoid state. Another variety of defense is "manic" in type and is characterized by a sense of omnipotence, denial of psychic reality, and over-activity, all of which seek to deny the importance of the individual's good objects and to show contempt for them. The main aim of "manic defense" is to master and control all objects.

To sum up: The typical depressive fantasy might be crudely verbalized as follows—the good object is in pieces and cannot be put together again. In this connection although the child's relation to the father *imago* is referred to (particularly in connection with sadistic fantasies of parental coitus, hostility to and from the combined parents, and restitution fantasies concerning both parents), study of the clinical and theoretical contexts suggests that insofar as one object is referred to it is more often than not the mother *imago*. It is, however, specifically stated that "From the beginning the ego introjects objects 'good' and 'bad', for both of which its mother's breast is the prototype."

As has been noted, the publication of this paper marked the commencement of an entirely new orientation. The content of various papers soon indicated that a school of thought was growing, based exclusively on a new hypothesis of development. Thus, in the following year Joan Riviere suggested that the "manic defense" may motivate the "negative therapeutic reaction"(13). She accepted in their entirety Klein's ideas of the "depressive position" and of "manic defense". In a subsequent paper, "On the Genesis of Psychical Conflict in Earliest Infancy", she endeavored to establish a systematic metapsychological basis for the new views(14). Clinically, the most significant point in this paper was contained in a footnote where she committed herself to the explicit statement: *"We have reason to think since Melanie Klein's latest work on depressive states that all neuroses are different varieties of defense against this fundamental anxiety, each embodying mechanisms which become increasingly available to the organism as its development proceeds."* Readers who followed the history of Rank's deviation from psychoanalysis will not fail to note that by this time the Klein group had also committed itself to a monistic theory of neurosogenesis. The validity of Klein's views was also accepted without reservation in papers given to the British Society by Winnicott(15), Rickman(16, 17), Scott(18), Isaacs(19-21) and Rosenfeld(22), and in various contributions to discussions by Heimann and Matthew.

Criticisms for the most part were advanced by myself and by Melitta Schmideberg.[7] My main objections were as follows:

(a) that the building up of an "internalized-object-psychology" leads to confusion and obstruction instead of advancing existing concepts of early mental structure and function, e.g., confusion between "internalized-objects" and id-instincts, betwen "projection" and "expulsion", between an "object-imago", and "introjection", and a 'body-fantasy';[8] (b) that the "manic-defense" and "depressive position" are neither clinical syndromes nor defense mechanisms, but a compound of already established Freudian views with some inadequately substantiated theories; (c) that although the existence of depressive reactions, both symptomatic, and in the case of the child, developmental, is beyond dispute, there is no justification for postulating a "central position" of this sort; (d) that although the relations of clinical depression to clinical mania are also indisputable, it does not follow that there is a central and genetic sequence; that manic defense is an arbitrarily constructed concept including such mechanisms as denial (Freud and Abraham) which really belong to different phases or aspects of ego-development (cf. repression mechanisms); (e) that the "restitution" and "reparation" mechanisms associated with the "depressive position" are not organized until an obsessional phase that is clinically much later than that of depressive reactions; that some of the "mechanisms" de-

7. These criticisms were expressed on the first occasion that Klein's new paper was discussed (October 16, 1935)(23).

8. In his paper on "Introjection"(24), Foulkes endeavors to clear up the confusion arising out of various uses of this term. See also Knight(25).

scribed are not defense-mechanisms but fantasies, e.g. danger of injuring the object in the act of introjection; (f) that it has not yet been substantiated that analysts get better therapeutic results by basing their interpretations on the Klein hypotheses.

Melitta Schmideberg advanced similar criticisms, mainly:

(a) that Melanie Klein's description of fixed sequences of psychotic positions is based on three assumptions, viz., the predominance of aggressive impulses, the predominance of projection and introjection mechanisms and the lack of reality sense in the infant.   These assumptions have not, in Schmideberg's view, been adequately substantiated, and in any case the new theory involves a neglect of the importance of libido, of the effect of environmental factors in earliest infancy and of mechanisms like repression, isolation, conversion, sublimation, etc., which to some extent counteract projection and introjection; (b) that one should distinguish between the frequency of clinical depression and the supposed theoretical importance of the "depressive position"; (c) that a developmental etiology that leaves hysteria out of account and neglects schizophrenia cannot be regarded as satisfactory; (d) that dynamic aspects of psychic situations are neglected; (e) that some of the fantasies described are not primitive but of later origin, and in any case are frequently *distortions* of reality reactions and of more objective anxieties; (f) that it is not satisfactory to explain clinical disturbances, e.g. paranoia, by displacing the symptom backward into childhood and that there is no proof that the processes described actually take place in babyhood; (g) that interpretations on the Klein model, by their very inexactitude, can act as reassurances, covering more preconscious worries and anxieties, by deflecting affect and criticism and encouraging flight into unreality.

In all these discussions the issue of environmental factors in neurosogenesis entered. One of the main criticisms directed against the Klein system was its neglect of reality; to which it was replied that this lack of emphasis was more apparent than real. It was maintained by supporters of the method that not only did they study the interplay of environmental and endopsychic factors, but that the only way of understanding the importance of reality factors is to see them as refracted through the child's early anxiety situations and fantasies. In other words reality factors, whether occurring in childhood, in the current life-situation of the adult or in the transference, should not be assessed at face value but in terms of their "meaning" for the patient, which means is *a priori* an unconscious interpretation held to be made by the patient. To this line of argument Schmideberg replied (a) that the assumption of rigid sequences of positions cannot make proper allowance for environmental factors, in other words, environmental factors are regarded as merely of quantitative, not of qualitative importance; (b) that reality factors are assessed in a tendentious way, that in particular there is displayed a bias in favor of the parents; the parents' self-valuation is accepted at face value; every event is interpreted on the assumption that the patient is guilty about it, and this gradually induces guilt in the patient; (c) that the neglect of reality factors and the stress laid on the "good mother" implies an idealization of the mother-child relation and neglect of the ambivalence of both mother and child in more real levels.

The same author in a paper entitled "The Assessment of Environmental Factors"(26) stressed

(a) the genetic importance of more continuous factors (in contrast to "traumatic" ones), operating even in the average or favorable environment; (b) the role of specific environmental factors in the first months of life; (c) the emotional attitude of the attendants, so often in contrast to their professed "modern" ideas; (d) that events repeatedly affecting derivatives of primitive instincts may exercise as marked an influence as those affecting the primary instincts themselves. She insisted that environmental factors should not be regarded in isolation, but always in the interplay of unconscious factors and mechanisms.

In these discussions questions of evidence and of verification of hypotheses inevitably arose. These focused mainly on the assumptions made concerning mental processes in babyhood. These were considered in a series of "exchange" lectures between the British Society and the Vienna Society. Actually the exchange of views arose out of earler differences concerning infantile development, but in practice it was limited to a discussion of the new hypotheses. In a paper given before the British Society, on "The Problem of the Genesis of Psychical Conflict in Earliest Infancy"(27), Robert Waelder challenged the views of Klein and Riviere: this constituted the Vienna reply to Riviere's paper(14). Partly in reply to Waelder's criticism, Susan Isaacs, in the paper on "The Nature of Evidence Concerning Mental Life in the Earliest Years"(20), concluded (from behavioristic observations on babies and young children as well as from the analysis of older patients and children as young as two-and-half years) that pre-verbal fantasies already existed in the first months of life. She stressed the view that sometimes actual early experiences could be inferred in the course of later analysis, and supported her main argument in favor of drawing conclusions about babies from observations of older children by insisting on the principle of continuity. She also insisted that negative evidence should not be accepted as proof.

In the discussion Schmideberg objected to Isaacs' claims that negative evidence should be disallowed, and that there is no need to distinguish between analytic and behavioristic observations. She maintained that Isaacs did not distinguish sufficiently between observations and the conclusions drawn from them; and demanded that the principle of. continuity should be supplemented by that of development, adding that as we are not likely ever to have absolute certainty on what goes on in the mind of a baby under six months, we should avoid dogmatism.[9]

As a result of these and later discussions Klein and her followers produced a formal Kleinian metapsychology. Hence, although the issues under debate belong to what I have called the first and second phases of Kleinian theory, the metapsychological formulations deserve to be treated in a separate section.

THE NEW KLEINIAN METAPSYCHOLOGY

(a) *The Kleinian Concept of Fantasy.*

It may be said at once that even if the tendencies of Kleinian metapsychology had not already manifested themselves, it would not have been difficult to anticipate the form they would assume. If you believe that infants after a few months of life develop fantasies of internal objects which predicate the existence of a superego, if further you believe that these fantasies are of such vital importance that they exert an uninterrupted influence on progressive mental development, and that they determine the formation of a "central depressive position"; finally, if you believe that every variety of mental disorder can be traced back to this central position, you have certainly committed yourself to a quite novel metapsychology. You must prove that from the first all instinctual derivatives are what Freud would have called strongly cathected unconscious fantasy; further you must show that the mental apparatus possesses shortly after birth mechanisms that will preserve these apparently all powerful dynamic fantasies in a state of active cathexis throughout life; in other words, you must prove that the original Freudian unconscious system has at its core a central system or enclave as distinct from the rest of the unconscious as the Freudian unconscious is distinct from the Freudian preconscious; finally you must show that the continued existence of this

9. In the above summary I have drawn freely from the Appendix to "An Investigation of the Technique of Psycho-Analysis" by Glover and Brierley(28).

enclave is the primary factor in all pathogenesis. The first of these steps was boldly undertaken.[10]

In her paper on "The Nature and Function of Fantasy"(29; also 30, 31), Susan Isaacs took up the following position:

Admitting that the Kleinian definition of fantasy extended the connotation of the term as used by Freud, Isaacs stated categorically that "The primary content of all mental processes are unconscious fantasies . . . Such fantasies are the basis of all unconscious and conscious thought processes." All words stand for concepts but "the mind and mental process, thinking itself, are not in themselves abstract. As experience, as we experience them, they are immediate . . . Now in the infant experience and mental process must be primarily, perhaps at first entirely, affective, sensorial . . . At the first level of experience introjection is felt to be incorporation. At a later level it is imaged to be incorporation, later still it is felt to be getting something into the mind—that is to say, in the ego, that part of the self as experienced which remembers and imagines and has emotions." Hence: "When the child feels he has dismembered his mother, his mental life is split and disintegrated . . . The child experiences it as 'my-mother-inside-me-is-in-bits' . . . Fantasy is the mental corollary, the psychic representative of instinct, and there is no impulse, no instinctual urge which is not experienced as (unconscious) fantasy." Moreover: "Fantasy expresses the specific content of the urge (or the feeling, e.g., anxiety, fear, love and sorrow) which is dominating the child's mind at the moment; e.g., when he feels desires towards his mother, he experiences these as 'I want to suck the nipple, to stroke her face, to eat her up, to keep her within me, to bite the breast, to tear her to bits, to drown and burn her, to throw her out of me'—and so on and so forth." And not only feels " 'I want to' but 'I am doing this' ". "The capacity to hallucinate," in Susan Isaac's opinion "is either identical with fantasy or the precondition for it." The infant hallucinates "first, the nipple, then the breast, and later his mother, the whole person . . . hallucination does not stop at the mere picture but carries him on to what he is, in detail, going to do with the desired object which he imagines (fantasies) he has obtained . . . Thus we must assume that the introjection of the breast is bound up with the earliest forms of fantasy life." Here Isaacs quotes from Riviere(14) a slightly different version of the situation: ". . . from the very beginning of life . . . the psyche responds to the reality of its experiences by interpreting them—or rather, by misinterpreting them—in a subjective manner that increases its pleasure and preserves it from pain." Here Riviere forcibly links this "act of a subjective interpretation of experience" with Freud's use of the term "hallucination". "This act . . . which it carries out by means of the processes of introjection and projection, is called by Freud hallucination."

Subsequently Isaacs expands her definition still further: "Fantasies are in their simplest beginnings the content of implicit meaning, meaning latent in impulse, affect and sensation." This is repeated later in a confusing form.

---

10. In the Controversial Discussions of 1943-44 the views of her pupils were endorsed by Mrs. Klein.

"As we have seen the earliest rudimentary fantasy is bound up with sensory experience; it is an affective interpretation of bodily sensations, an expression of libidinal and aggressive impulses, operating under the pleasure-pain principle. Later on fantasy is inherent in sights and sounds, in touch and manipulation and perception of objects, as well as in gestures and vocal expression. At this stage it is still implicit fantasy."

After this statement of the Kleinian concept of fantasy Isaacs proceeds: "In the view I am here presenting, an essential feature of early mental development is the activity and intensity of early unconscious fantasies and their far-reaching and *uninterrupted* influence upon further progressive mental development."

Finally, on the nature of the evidence for these views, one of Isaacs statements deserves to be singled out: "When analytic experience leads us to reconstruct an internal situation or a particular relation to external reality, in the infant and young child, the behavioristic data can say whether or not such a reconstruction is possible or likely, at the given age."[11]

The foregoing abstract of the Isaacs paper cannot convey fully the confusion to which the author(s) has reduced Freud's basic psychological concepts: this was more clearly brought out in the sections of the paper in which Isaacs strove laboriously to show by quotation from Freud's writings either that Freud himself would have favored Kleinian conclusions or that these conclusions were merely natural extensions of Freudian concepts. Concerning these attempts the comment of Anna Freud(29) sums up the situation effectively: "To me it seems one of the most bewildering points about these new theories that existing analytic conceptions are explicitly retained and at the same time implicitly denied by the new formulations." To this I would add that Isaacs evidently found herself constantly hampered by existing Freudian concepts and that for the purposes of her own presentation she would have been well-advised to jettison them altogether and build up a separate psychological system with postulates of her own.[12]

To clarify the situation I have drawn up a list of the Freudian concepts, positions and definitions that are either confused, weakened or set aside by the Kleinian system.

In the first place Freud's distinctions between a memory-trace, an image, a "thing-presentation", an object-imago, a fantasy, an introjection and an identification are lost. They are all at one time or another subsumed under

11. It remains to add that in the course of the prolonged discussion of her paper Isaacs made one more significant statement regarding the nature of fantasy. She affirmed that " 'inner psychical reality' includes affects as well as fantasies but is otherwise indistinguishable".

12. I have expressed this conviction in the title I have given to this paper.

the Kleinian term "fantasy". Similarly the distinction between hallucinatory regression of instinct excitation to the sensory end of the psychic apparatus, a hallucinatory fantasy (clinically, hallucination) and fantasy (whether unconscious or preconscious) is lost. The concept of instinct derivatives is confused and in effect the fundamental distinction of affect from ideational presentation is lost. Distinctions between positive (tension or discharge) affects and reactive affects, in the long run, between gratification and frustration, are blurred; consequently the distinction between reality-ego-systems and fantasy-systems disappears. The relations between psychical reality, reality-proving and fantasy (in the Freudian sense) are obliterated. And both theoretically and practically (e.g. in Isaac's description of Kleinian stages of fantasy) the distinction between the unconscious, the preconscious and the conscious is blurred. Not only so the distinction between the id and the ego is flattened out. For although Freud agreed that the boundaries are hard to delimit, yet it is obvious that in her concept of "implicit meaning" and of its (somewhat contradictory) congener, "implicit fantasy", Isaacs is simply telling us what she (Isaacs) thinks the Primitive Ego would think if it (the Primitive Ego) could think and knew what was going on in the Id. In other words, what the Freudian would call Id-activity, the Kleinian calls implicit Ego (or Superego) fantasy.[13]

Anna Freud(29) pointed out also that the new definition of "unconscious fantasy" not only extended the reference of the term to include a number of early mental processes under a common connotation, but also "narrows it down from use for the unconscious only"; adding that no regard was paid to whether the mental processes are instinct-derivatives or not. Moreover she held that although Isaacs described unconscious fantasies as being partly subject to the primary process, she implicity rejected the action of other important

---

13. It would require several papers to trace all of these deviations from Freudian psychology to their roots, for although on occasion the deviation is directly stated or easily inferred, on others one has to follow the concept through a maze of exposition and definition watching carefully the exact meaning of the words employed. To give some examples: referring to the use by A. Freud of the phrase "the mother-image in the child's mind", Isaacs says, "Now I feel that this description of the 'mother-image in the child's mind' comes very close to Klein's postulate that the child introjects his mother"; and again "Anna Freud (to my mind) *implies* fantasies when she speaks of the 'mother-image in the child's mind' ". That is direct enough. On the other hand on the question of' instinct derivatives, i.e. affect and mental presentations (a distinction of supreme importance to the dynamics of mind), the reader may best appreciate the confusion Isaacs introduces by perusing the following summary of her views on the subject, viz:— unconscious fantasies are the primary content of all mental processes; in the infant experience and mental process must be primarily, perhaps at first entirely affective, sensorial: the child experiences his psychic reality in terms of his fantasy life; the "mental expression of instinctual needs" (a phrase used by Freud), *"is"*, says Isaacs, "unconscious fantasy"; fantasy is the mental corollary, the psychic representative of instinct; fantasy expresses the specific content of the urge (*or the feeling* anxiety, fear, love or sorrow); (yet) it soon becomes a means of defense against anxieties; fantasies are in their simplest beginnings implicit meaning, meaning latent in impulse, affect and sensation; (and finally) inner psychical reality includes affects as well as fantasies but is otherwise indistinguishable (from fantasy). Yet when Foulkes(32) taxed her with regarding fantasies as "primary motors", the reply given on behalf of the Klein group by Heimann(33) was, "unconscious fantasy is the mental representative of instinct: the conclusion being that unconscious fantasy is charged with instinctual energy",—indicating thereby either that the Klein group has forgotten about affect energy or that they believe affect-energy has no dynamic effect or that it is identical with the cathexis of a mental presentation!

factors in the primary process. She might well have asked why, if the secondary process applied also to primary unconscious fantasy, there was such an overpowering need to emphasize unconscious fantasy as the (apparently sole) expression of instinct and mental life. If anything emerges from the study of early Kleinian fantasies and of their exposition it is that the fantasies themselves combine characteristics of unconscious, preconscious and conscious mental systems.

When all is said, the most effective way of uncovering the poverty of the Isaacs (Klein) postulates is to outline again Freud's orderly series of concepts regarding the mental apparatus, concepts which we are invited to barter for the hypothetical benefits of hypothetical Kleinian "fantasies". Starting with the concept of a central mental apparatus dealing with instinctual excitation, governing the approaches to motility, and having a sensory receiver, Freud went on to describe the organization of memory traces in the various systems. These traces which form the groundwork of ego organization record a pleasure-pain series of experiences. And since, in contrast to the isolated stimulations of the external world, the stimulations of instinct are continuous, the earliest memory-trace systems are concerned primarily with various degrees of gratification or frustration of impulse. But since the ultimate aim of all instincts is gratification, the most important trace systems (which when cathected by psychic energy constitute memory images), are those that extend the "aim".[14] These images have as it were been burned into the mind through their respective association with psychic pain or pleasure. The realization of the aim thus comes to be the primary concern of the psychic apparatus. The pleasure principle is bound up with this dynamic aim. The function of memory together with memory images is however an adaptation function first and mainly developed in response to frustration. But so long as (what ultimately proves to be) the object of the instinct promotes the gratification of (what proves to be) the subject's aim (as in the case of the most important, infantile needs) this function remains larval. Nevertheless it is a potential reality function, which, after pleasure-pain experiences have led to the distinction of the self from the not-self, develops into a reality-proving ego-function. In other words when frustration becomes acute the cathecting of pleasure and pain image-associations develops reality value. The cathexis of images promoting activities that accelerate gratification and of images leading to avoidance of activities that increase

14. See also A. Freud(34): "What I mean to imply in my description of the child's narcissistic state, is a stage in which the aim of the instinct is of overwhelming importance, whereas the object is only dimly taken into account."

frustration, adds to the probability that instinct tension will be reduced. Summation of experiences of reduced tension leads ultimately to the development of reality-proving and this in turn promotes correlation between the subject, the aim and the object of any
given instinct. Not until this stage has been reached can we talk of
object-formation. Although therefore it is true that the pleasure
principle dominates psychic life in the early stages, the pleasure-pain
series of experience puts a premium on the development of reality-
proving. In this sense the baby, once the larval stages are passed,
has, relative to its conditions of life, just as good a sense of reality-
proving for any given instinct aim as any grown-up. The fact that the
mind is dominated by the pleasure principle does not mean that the
pleasure principle is invariably successful. At this stage therefore
there is no question of describing the cathexis of memory-trace-systems
as "meaning". Indeed even if an observer were asked to describe what
he thought about the baby's state of mind, he would have no need
to say more than that the baby, despite alternating states of experience
of pleasure (gratification) and pain (frustration), on the whole
pursues the main *aim* of all instincts, viz., gratification. But that
would of course be the observer's interpretation, not the baby's
"fantasy".

To the consideration of these "progressive" (development and
adaptation) aspects of mental activity Freud added some important
formulations regarding the "regressive" tendencies of the mental
apparatus. The relation of these regressive tendencies to prenatal
life has not been fully established(35), but of the postnatal factors
one of the most important is the peculiar nature of frustrations existing during sleep, a state that occupies by far the larger part of the
daily life of infants. This regressive tendency of the mental apparatus
must of course be distinguished clinically from the regression mechanisms occurring, for example, prior to symptom formation. It is
characterized by a backward flow of frustrated instinctual energy from
the motor to the sensory end of the psychic apparatus. The qualitative
aspects of this instinct tension have not been fully examined but we
may be sure that a certain amount of summation of different instinct
charges occurs, giving rise quantitatively to an acute damming-up of
energy. Anyhow the result is what is described as an attempt at hallucinatory gratification. The psychic relief secured (or sampled) in
this attempt varies in accordance with the depth of sleep and the
intensity of frustration but when previous pleasure experiences have
been intense or when previous frustrations have been acute, the hallu-

cinatory process is no doubt compensatory as well as being an unsuccessful attempt at adaptation. And it is of some relevance to the
discussion of early reality processes that this compensatory pleasure
is heightened when the hallucinatory regression frees energy once
more in the direction of motility, and some actions appropriate to the
hallucinatory activation of images occur—as in sucking movements
during sleep. But this is possibly only a marginal increase. The part
release of appropriate motility is in itself a proof of the reality nature
of the images cathected in the regression to the sensory end of the
apparatus. The hallucinatory process is an attempt at gratification
initiated by frustration but arrested at the imaginal level and so
doomed to failure.

Now there is nothing here to justify the Kleinian equation of
memory-images, unconscious fantasies, introjections and "internal objects". There is no question of using the term "fantasy" for such
psychic events. There is an essential distinction between on the one
hand image-presentations, whether associated with reality gratification
or with the attempts at hallucinatory gratification (i.e. regression to
the sensory end) and on the other hand any variety of fantasy either
conscious or unconscious. Fantasy in the sense in which it is used
by Freud is a much later, more complicated, and from the point of
view of reality a more revolutionary development. Possibly the
confusion arose in the Klein system because of slipshod thinking regarding the clinical hallucinations observed in the psychoses. The fact
that a schizophrenic may behave as if his fantasies are real is no proof
of the existence of these fantasies in the first months of life(26, 32).
The ruling psychic concept is not "fantasy", it is the concept of
"imaginal presentations" (based on the organization of memory
traces) and of their cathexis. Development in the direction of reality
thinking and of fantasy can then be traced in an orderly series and
correlations made that are appropriate to their respective exciting
causes. Not only is the behavioristic study of sucklings in favor of
Freud's system, but the whole weight of biological evidence of survival is against the Kleinian assumption. As I have pointed out,
when the infant's hallucinations of sucking obtain some expression
in motility, the actions are appropriate not to a Kleinian fantasy but to
the reality of sucking. It is a sound assumption therefore that during
this sensorial regression the instinct has retained a realistic aim. In
this respect the infant is neither a fool nor a fantast.

Moreover, if Isaac's view that reality thinking is a derivative of
primary fantasy thinking were correct, our existing conception of the

function, timing and psychic locality of unconscious defense mechanisms would have to be completely recast. It would imply, for example, that ego-syntonic as well as ego-dystonic presentations are subject to repression and that in some way or another, ego-syntonic impulses contrive to escape this censorship. It is to my mind unthinkable that presentations of instinct, in particular those advancing the aim of preservation, which are capable of conscious gratification without interference from unconscious defense mechanisms (*bewusstseinsfähig*), should begin to be distinguished at some later date from an original fantasy nexus. Again the whole weight of biological evidence of survival is against the assumption. By abolishing the distinction between cathected memory-traces and fantasies Isaacs abolishes the economic function of repression, and thereby obliterates the distinction between the dynamic unconscious and the preconscious.

To sum up: the history of reality thinking and fantasy thinking is a long and complicated one. The former can be traced from its final conceptual form through the processes of "word-presentations" and "thing-presentations" back to the earliest formation of memory traces. Its development is influenced by the pleasure-pain series, the operation of reality-proving and the expansion of the reality principle. On the other hand the beginnings of fantasy are determined by three factors; the failure of the hallucinatory process, the development of object formation and the action of repression. The existence of fantasy implies the psychic capacity to form correlations between the subject, aim and object of an instinct. Purely narcissistic organization comes to an end with the failure of the hallucinatory technique. Fantasy in the Freudian sense is a frustration product which should be set off not so much against reality-thinking as against reality-action. Without the mechanism of repression, effective unconscious cathexis of fantasy could not be maintained. Despite all the involved discussion of instinct derivatives and of the relation between "psychic-reality" and so-called "external-reality" there is no difficulty in either the statement or the comprehension of these ideas that has not already been met in Freud's basic formulations.

But it is high time to return to the list of Kleinian deviations from Freudian theory. To continue: The biological progression of an instinct-series (the Freudian development of the libido) with its psychological implications of fixation points and of a regressive series is sacrificed for the sake of Kleinian oro-phallic ego[15] and/or superego of the first year, which constitute(s) according to her an independent, dynamic and (except presumably to Kleinian therapeutists) immutable system. Friedlander(29) summed up the situation as follows:

"We see that the Freudian conception of regression is of course intimately bound up with Freud's conception of libidinal development up to the genital phase. This conception is based on the biological tendency of the instincts to develop. Contrariwise in Klein's view . . . The so-called early fantasies which we can only perceive as being inborn or universally formed in the first months of life and which already contain oral, anal-sadistic and phallic impulses as well as guilt-feelings and defense mechanisms, are thought to be of primary importance insofar as the further development occurs as a flight from too great a fear or too great a guilt-feeling aroused by these fantasies . . . Naturally therefore, the conception of regression has no place in this theory. The whole of the libido remains fixated to these early fantasies throughout life . . . The important fact which emerges from these ideas is not, in my opinion, that Klein lays less stress on a mechanism on which Freudians lay more stress. The importance of the depreciation of the mechanism of regression, which Isaacs admits as such, is the fact that it is the result of giving up Freud's conception of the biological development of the libido."

Following this line of thought it is possible to outline clearly one of the clinical bones of contention between the Kleinian and the Freudian Groups, viz., the importance of the classical oedipus situation. Freudians hold that the Klein Group depreciate the importance of the classical oedipus situation, both clinically and theoretically. To which the Kleinians reply that they do not—that on the contrary they emphasize how important it is by discovering the oedipus complex in the sixth month of life. But their assumption of a primary active core in the *Ucs* (Id) based on the persisting cathexis of unconscious fantasies at this period—a core which, according to Isaacs, retains its power to influence all later progressive mental development, commits her to a depreciation of the specific significance of the classical oedipus situation. Her views on the dynamic significance of "early fantasy" and her views on regression may still allow her to plead that the classical oedipus phase has a secondary significance. Yes, but a significance shorn of dynamic importance. Freud's view was that whatever the pregenital phases of infancy contribute, the oedipus phase, as described by him, is of primary significance in the dynamic, economic and structual aspects of the term.

15. I have coined the term in order to emphasize one of the descriptive features of the Klein system. It is worth noting that although Klein talks of the factors of anal and urethral erotism, she neglects the all-important factors of e.g. gastro-intestinal and skin erotism in ego differentiation.

Indeed we may conveniently close the provisional list of deviations by considering the economic and topographic implications of the Kleinian theory of fantasy. These turn on the relation of the pleasure-principle to stages of auto-erotism and narcissism, and to the beginnings of object-relationship. This issue was stated succinctly by A. Freud(34) as follows:

> "One of the outstanding differences between Freudian and Kleinian theory is that Klein sees in the first months of life evidence of a wide range of differentiated object-relations, partly libidinal and partly aggressive. Freudian theory on the other hand allows at this period only for the crudest rudiments of object-relationship and sees life governed by the desire for instinct gratification in which perception of the object is only slowly achieved." Again, "The assumption of early object-fantasies in Klein's theories is bound up with the theoretical substitution of a very early stage of rich and varied object-relationship, for the early phases of narcissism and auto-erotism as described by Freud." And again, "I consider that there is a narcissistic and auto-erotic phase of several months duration which precedes what we call object-relationship in its proper sense, even though the beginnings of object-relation are slowly built up during this initial stage. According to Isaacs' descriptions, the newborn infant, already in the first six months loves, hates, desires, attacks, wishes to destroy and to dismember his mother . . . According to my own conception of this same period, the infant is at this time exclusively concerned with his own well-being . . . I believe that the psychic processes (during the child's narcissistic state) are governed by the urge for satisfaction, that is, by the aim of the instinct and not by fantasies of its object . . . It is . . . in agreement with the Freudian conception of a narcissistic beginning of life to conceive of auto-erotism as an intrinsic source of pleasure, independent of relations to the object."

Lantos(29) puts the position in the following way: referring to the primitive reactions, actions and play of the child she wrote:

> "We believe that the bodily functions, the functioning of the sensory apparatus, are pleasurable in themselves. So is mental development with its gradual acquisition of knowledge and understanding . . . they are all the same insofar as they are pleasures in themselves, that is to say: pleasures without meaning . . . Thumb-sucking, masturbation, hair-pulling and other habits are at that age still auto-erotic . . . We do not believe that masturbation makes him (the infant) feel, 'I shall bring my mother back' . . . The difference (between Freudian and Kleinian views) is not that we are building on different facts (behavioristic observations) but that we are interpreting the same facts differently."

In the introductory part of this paper I pointed out that for some time a gap existed between psychoanalytic formulations concerning mental life at the latest pre-oedipus stage, and hypothetical reconstructions of the primitive ego: also that the tendency of most analysts then was to regard developments occurring prior to the immediately pre-oedipus stage as belonging to the primitive phase. On various occasions I maintained that the application of the terms autoerotism and narcissism to these comparatively advanced stages was no longer justified. In this respect I held that the terms had to some extent outworn their usefulness. In particular I found the concept of a unified stage of late narcissism an obstacle to understanding, and when I developed the "nuclear theory of ego-formation" I became convinced that only in the earliest stages of infantile development could either term be used with advantage and then only provided one kept in mind the scattered forms of early ego-organization. But this issue is not at present in dispute. Existing controversies, as A. Freud pointed out, turn on the Kleinian definition of the term fantasy, the date of fantasy, and the content of fantasy. And so we come back once more to the dispute over "meaning" and "implicit meaning". I would only add a few considerations appropriate to the discussion of auto-erotism and narcissism in the first year of life. In the first place the concept of auto-erotism is bound up with the polymorphous nature of infantile sexuality.[16] It takes cognizance of the fact that whereas certain components of sexuality are (whether the infant knows it or not) anaclitic in nature in the sense that their complete gratification requires the support and collusion of (what the observer knows to be) an external object; other components are comparatively independent of external objects. Some of the most important erotisms, e.g., skin and muscle erotism, are of this nature. And it is precisely the autonomic function of many of the early erotisms that promotes a narcissistic organization of the early ego (in my view, early ego-nuclei). In the early stages even those libidinal gratifications that involve the collusion of (what the observer knows to be) an external object are, *qua* experiences, of an "auto-erotic" character. They can have an object reference only when (a) the object has been distinguished from the subject; (b) the object imago has been cathected with instinctual energy. "Meaning" whether attached to reality presentations or later to fantasy presentations is a product of frustration which implies the capacity to correlate the affective derivatives of instinct with both subject and object. Without frustration there would be no more "meaning" in extra-uterine life than there is in intra-uterine life. After sleep, and reality gratification of hunger needs, auto-erotism affords the closest approximation to a frustration-free existence—

16. The polymorphous structure of early ego-nuclei seems to me entirely congruous with concepts of "components" of sexuality.

although admittedly it involves expenditure of both psychic and physical effort. Later, no doubt, auto-erotisms acquire meaning in both realistic and fantastic senses of the term but it is significant that auto-erotic libidinal components that escape the processes of sublimation are by comparison with object impulses singularly ineducable. In short, however desirable it may be to extend our knowledge of early object relations there is no advantage to be gained by presuming, as Klein does, organized and unified ego patterns at a time when, according to the overwhelming weight of clinical evidence and of theoretical probability only a scattered and uncorrelated series of organizations of memory traces can be presumed.

(b)   *Introjection and Projection.*

The next stage in the development of Kleinian metapsychology consisted in applying to the description of mental mechanisms the Kleinian concepts described in the previous section, together with some of the assumptions laid down as axiomatic during the first phase of Kleinian theory. It is obvious for example, that if there is no difference betwen an image, an imago, a fantasy, a meaning, an introjection, an "internal object" and a superego (that can for example, be "ejected") and if all this primary mental activity is thought of in terms of oral experience, it will not be long before mental mechanisms are equated with bodily processes. This is in fact what happened. Speaking on behalf of the Klein Group, Heimann(36; also see 37, 38) began with the following statement:

"I shall use the terms *introject and project* when referring to the mental mechanisms which are modeled on and correspond to the bodily experiences of taking in and expelling respectively." (The baby) "devotes an intense attention to his surroundings (to the objects around him) . . . the modification of his mental apparatus through this function of attention and of his 'tasting' the stimuli comes about by his taking in with his mouth and hands and eyes and ears every object which attracts his attention. His first attempts to make acquaintance with any new thing are expressed in efforts to take hold of it and suck it or taste it. As he does so he actually introjects it; in his experience he incorporates it, sucks it in, eats it up . . . The earliest relation to an object is effected by means of introjecting it . . . the most fundamental vital processes of any living organism consist of intake and discharge . . . the mechanism of taking in and expelling, or if we think of their psychic correlates, introjecting and projecting, are vital processes of the first magnitude . . . In the Ucs the oral significance of loss and gift are maintained, so that under circumstances in which this fundamental pattern becomes reactivated all acquiring means devouring, all giving means spitting and defecating, with the result that guilt and anxiety arise along with these activities . . . The earliest introjections establish a protective and a persecuting agency within the mind ('good' and bad' breast) . . . The early introjections represent the early stages of the later genital superego . . . The introjected breast is the object of the infant's auto-erotic wishes and experiences . . . The narcissistic condition is bound up with a libidinal cathexis of internal objects . . . We should not draw a sharp line between auto-erotism and narcissism . . . Hallucinatory gratification may be considered as the supreme instance of auto-erotic activity . . . (it) is based on the relation to a 'good' inner breast, which the infant rediscovers in a part of his own body . . . (it) is stronger when its object is a part i.e. the nipple, than when it is a whole person: for the nipple was really 'inside' the infant, completely enclosed by the lips, the gum and the tongue . . . The first roots of the superego are to be found in the introjected 'good' and 'bad' breast, to which are added the 'good' and 'bad' parents and the 'good' and 'bad' penis."

Having quoted passages from *Beyond the Pleasure Principle* in which Freud, discussing the protective functions of cell structure, refers to the differentiated outer layer of the living vesicle whose protective function against outer stimuli is almost more important than its receptive function, Heimann goes on to say "what Freud describes in these and other passages is that the ego, or surface part of the id, comes into being and functions by means of both *taking things*[17] into itself and conversely rejecting them from itself". Now in fact Freud was not then considering "taking things" into the ego; he was discussing the biological function of a protective layer (the concept of the Reizschutz) and he went on to point out that in more highly developed organisms the *sense organs* constitute such a protective "layer". Freud never suggested, as Heimann does implicitly and explicitly, that the mouth is a rudimentary thought-organ taking precedence over the central nervous system. The fact is that Heimann, following Klein, converts analogies into literal identities. "Taking in things" and "rejecting" them are, as Heimann's later argument indicates, regarded as *identical* with introjection, which (see Isaacs) is identical with "experience", "psychic-reality feeling" and "meaning" of actually taking the nipple into the mouth or spitting out of the mouth. But Heimann goes on: "Thus the mechanism of taking in[18] *recurs* in the operation of attention. Then comes a slight change. The function of keeping out dangerous *stimuli* "is akin to the function of discharge and expulsion". Apparently dissatisfied with the use of "akin" she adds, "However it *is*[19] an expulsion insofar as the *decision*

17. My italics throughout this passage.
18. Note that this is now a mechanism.
19. Only the word "is" is underlined in the original: the other italics are intended to draw the reader's attention to two facts (a) that even when elaborating a biological analogy Heimann falls into confusion between biological and psychic function: (b) that the resultant confused ideology is anthropomorphised and expressed in terms of consciousness.

not to *let in* the dangerous stimuli presupposes that a small sample of it has been taken in, *decided upon* as being *bad,* and *expelled;* and the *whole* from which the sample was *taken, kept out* in consequence of the *judgment* to which the sample was subjected."

The conclusions do not follow from the argument: rather is the argument an *apologium* for the conclusions. The conclusions themselves are nothing more than postulates. It is clear that Kleinian views on introjection and projection merely paraphrase in pseudo-metapsychological terminology the fantasies alleged to exist in the oro-phallic phase described by Klein in her *Psycho-Analysis of Children,* fantasies that were never more than unsubstantiated assumptions. But the tendency is much more significant than this fact would indicate. Brierley(37) remarked that to limit ourselves to understanding the subjective meaning of our unconscious pre-conceptions about mental processes and to equate these with the processes themselves would be comparable to limiting our knowledge of the outer world to perceptional knowledge. She might as well have said quite frankly that this equation is the basis of mysticism.

For the same reason it is instructive to read the passages in Heimann's paper where she seeks to fortify Kleinian theories by an appeal to the Freudian concept of the death-instinct. Having discussed the concepts of life-instincts and death-instincts at some length, Heimann reaches a very remarkable conclusion. "Here," she says, "we have to face the fact that the aims of the instincts to which the organism is subject are in opposition to one another; in other words, that we deal with an organism which is by its very nature in a condition of conflict." Lest the use of the term "organism" confuse the issue, the following quotations make clear that Heimann is thinking of *psychic* conflict: "One conceives of the human mind as being by its very nature compelled to manipulate constantly between two fundamentally opposed instincts. . . . And since the instincts are inborn, we have to conclude that some form of conflict exists from the beginning of life." Now it is hardly necessary to take this point seriously. As Friedlander(37) put it, "This misconception leads at once to a further psychoanalytical impossibility, namely, to the fight of two instincts without intervention of what we call the mind." And again: "The further result of this misconception is the theory (advanced by Heimann) that the life-instinct employs a defense mechanism, namely, projection, against the death-instinct. In Freudian theory defense mechanisms are employed by the ego against the instincts." Indeed in her own reply Heimann(38) herself provided the complete refutation of her own remarkable theory. She stated that she uses the term death-instinct when discussing theoretical matters but that when dealing with clinical considerations she uses the term "destructive instinct". But what else is the concept of "conflict" but a clinical concept?

Foulkes(32),[20] discussing the Isaacs-Klein concept of fantasy, re-marked, "It looks as if we were back at the religious and spiritual level with an independent soul having energies of its own from another world. This is particularly true when these fantasies have attained the dignity of 'inner objects'." In Heimann's paper we can trace the outlines of a new religious biology. The ultimately moral values "good" and "bad" can be followed back to early fantasies of "good" and "bad" introjected breasts, and, via the function of taking in the good and expelling the bad, to a "conflict" between the life and the death instincts which exists before any psychic organization is de-veloped. Whatever else this may mean, it certainly represents a pro-jection into biological science of moral values.

In my opinion the Klein system has broken through the limitations of metapsychology to postulate a bio-religious system which depends on faith rather than on science.

(c) *The Concept of Regression.*

In the first two papers on the Controversial Series, discussion was essentially non-clinical. But when it comes to a discussion of the concept of regression it is increasingly easy to confuse the meta-psychological with the clinical aspects of the subject, and consequently increasingly important to distinguish between them. No such dis-tinction was effected by the Klein protagonists. In their joint paper on "Regression"(42), Heimann and Isaacs continued to assume that Kleinian fantasy systems existing from the sixth month of life were not in dispute, although in fact these fantasies were the original cause of the Controversy. Discussing the data regarding fixation the authors maintained that the relation of libidinal wishes to im-pulses of aggression "can be directly noted"; anxiety and the earliest defenses against it "can be seen"; the child's relations to his objects together with his fantasies "can be studied"; early processes of symbol-formation, etc., "can be watched", and so forth. The casual reader might not realize that in fact there are no such direct notes, views,

20. The subject had already been considered exhaustively in a paper by Schmideberg (39); see also her papers(40-42).

studies and observations. There are only interpretations of the infant's behavior or utterances from which hypothetical reconstructions are arrived at. Nevertheless it is impossible to discuss regression without entering on the clinical field and it is equally impossible to modify the Freudian concept of regression without altering the Freudian theory of neurosogenesis(43).

Starting with the relation of anxiety to fixation, Heimann and Isaacs stated:

"When stirred too intensely (by whatever situation) anxiety contributes to a fixation of the libido at that point . . . A fixation is thus partly to be understood as a defense against anxiety." If, however, anxiety is not overpowering it "acts as a spur to libidinal development . . . Anxiety itself, however, . . . arises from aggression . . . It is the destructive impulses of the child in the oral and anal phases which are, through the anxiety they stir up, the prime causes of the fixation of the libido." Frustration initiates aggression "not only by a simple 'damming-up' of the libido but also by evoking hate and aggression and consequent anxiety". This cannot be understood "without appreciating the part played by fantasies . . . fantasies of the destruction of the desired object by devouring, expelling, poisoning, burning, etc., etc., with ensuing dread of total loss of the source of life and love, the 'good' object, as well as the dread of retaliation, persecution and threat to the subject's own body from the destroyed and dangerous 'bad' object . . . The primal oral and anal anxieties give rise to the homosexual fixation and to the regression to paranoia." Under non-traumatic conditions they can influence development favorably. Thus "These oral fantasies and aims have remained uninterruptedly active in the unconscious mind exerting a favorable influence and promoting genitality . . . Bound up with these fantasies, moreover, are the reparative tendencies . . . In our view the part played by internal objects and the superego is an essential part in the regressive process." Discussing Freud's theory of the life and death-instincts, the authors remark: "The question now arises whether regression is not the outcome of a failure of the libido to master the destructive impulses and anxiety aroused by frustration." Agreeing that Freud's view of inhibition was bound up with excessive erogenicity of the organ concerned, Heimann and Isaacs say, "We venture to think that it is precisely this, the fantasy of violence, derived from the admixture of destructiveness which causes anxiety and guilt and enforces—by the intervention of the superego—an inhibition of that activity."

Regarding the relation of the libido to destructiveness, the authors take the view that analysts in the past put too exclusive emphasis on the role of the libido in regression because the libido was the first instinct energy to be studied. Whereas the truth is that libidinal regression was emphasized because of the *nature* of the libido. It is a commonplace that despite their adhesiveness, libidinal impulses are by comparison with other instincts remarkably labile. It is this lability that, together with the prolonged history of modification of

different phases of sexuality, prepares the way for subsequent regression; in other words the reversal of this process is the main feature
of regression. The sexual impulses can change their aims as well as
their objects. Aggressive impulses may change objects but modify
their aims to a comparatively small degree. It is true that certain
varieties of "fused" impulse appear to behave as if the sadistic component had a specific aim but it should not be forgotten that the libido
acts as the pilot impulse both in the fusion and in the sadism. Both
biologically and psychologically regarded, it is in the highest degree
improbable that regression operates primarily through the aggressive
series. This is supported by the constant reactive function preserved
by aggressive impulses. If aggressive impulses possessed the same
lability of aim as the libidinal impulses, not only would their general
biological function as reactive instincts be dangerously impaired but
their particular function in the service of libidinal drives would be
jeopardized. Even so, a clinical distinction should be drawn between
recognized fusions such as anal-sadism and instinct drives in which
the destructive or libidinal aims respectively dominate.

If arguments concerning regression are to be based on the study
of instincts which, clinically regarded, represent an important fusion,
the question of the *specific* influence of aggressive and of libidinal
components respectively must obviously be begged. Despite their
emphasis on aggression factors the authors are careful to emphasize
the element of fusion with libido. By so doing they provide themselves with a convenient avenue of escape should their favored thesis
become inconvenient. Anxiety, they say, arises from (is a primary
reaction to) aggression. This statement is then carefully hedged:
"It is evoked by the aggressive components in the pregenital stages of
development" (whether these are independent components or fused
components is left to the imagination). Anyhow they go on to say
that further anxiety can be evoked by libidinal frustration and consequent further anxiety and hate. Incidentally, it seems curious that
libidinal energies, which, according to the authors, have such effective
power that they can neutralize the alleged all-important forces of
aggression, which are (again according to the authors) the primary
stimulus to anxiety, cannot apparently give rise to primary anxiety
when frustrated. It is true the authors go on to say that regression
is due "*not only*" to libidinal frustration "*but also*" to hate, aggression
and consequent anxiety. But in view of the persistent emphasis on
aggression and the death-instincts, this reservation does not seem to
have much practical value.

But after all the pragmatic test of a metapsychological theory is its application to *clinical* psychoanalysis.   And in the clinical sense, this paper on "Regression" is more subversive of Freudian teaching than the two preceding papers.   Its tendency is to ascribe a predominating influence in mental development to destructive and defensive systems; i.e. to negative reactive factors; for the authors have apparently little interest in the constructive force lent by the instincts of mastery when these are placed at the service of object-libido.   The theory that fixation is a reaction to aggression is merely a special illustration of this main Kleinian viewpoint which ascribes to the destructive instincts some of the characteristics and tendencies Freud ascribed to the libido.   For if fixation can be regarded as a reaction to (result of) aggression and if regression itself works backwards through a developmental aggression series, it follows that progression must be attributed to the same factors. Indeed from the very beginnings of Kleinian theory its author has held this view.   The oedipus (i.e. libidinal) complex of the sixth month is, according to Klein, *released* by oral *sadism*.   But what then becomes of the psycho-biological theory of the life instincts?   What has happened to Freud's libido theory of neurosogenesis?

The answer is that the Kleinians have developed an entirely *new theory* of neurosogenesis. In terms of this new theory, the classical oedipus factor in neurosogenesis *must* be regarded as secondary or even tertiary.   It is not enough to say that the Kleinians have simply displaced backward to early stages the situations Freud placed at the age period of three to five.   They certainly have done so in the case of the fantasy-systems of reparation, which Freud placed in a late (obsessional) pregenital phase and which Klein now places in the center of an alleged depressive position occurring in the first months of life.   But they have done more; they have, as Riviere explicitly and implicitly maintained, based all psychopathology on oro-phallic sadistic fantasies and introjections alleged to occur after the first few months.   In the process the Freudian conception of regression has, as Friedlander put it, "vanished into thin air" (43; see also Hoffer, ibid., for a comparison of the clinical systems of Freud and Klein).

(d)   *The "Depressive Position"*.

By comparison with her earlier papers on ego development and with her original papers on the depressive position Klein's paper on "The Emotional Life and Ego-development of the Infant, with Special Reference to the Depressive Position" (44) is much more subdued in tone. She is at pains to find in the work of Freud and Abraham on anxiety, guilt, object-formation, etc., quotations that she holds prove that her own views on fantasy, aggression, internal objects, etc., are extensions of their lines of thought. She includes also a lengthy discussion of the affective states which she assumes exist in the infant and reviews the significance of early feeding difficulties, in terms which imply that behavioristic data all prove the accuracy of her metapsychological assumptions. To these points I shall return. In the meantime it is necessary to summarize the passages in her description of the depressive position (which, it will be remembered was one of the main points of controversy) that amplify or clarify earlier statements of this particular hypothesis.

Starting with "the strong and emotional relation to the mother *as a person* (my italics), which can be clearly observed from at least the beginning of the second month" she proceeds to say of genital impulses:

"I think it possible that even from the beginning they influence, however dimly, the relation to objects . . . We can assume that love towards the mother in some form exists from the beginning of life . . . It is obviously *still more fundamental* that, when he becomes separated from his mother at birth, the infant who was at one with her feels her to be his first and main love object . . . One may assume that from the beginning the mother exists as a whole object in the child's mind but in vague outline as it were . . ." Turning then to the infant's feelings of anxiety and guilt which, she believes, originate from sadistic impulses and fantasies, she goes on to describe the infant's mental fear of loss of the love object: "But the ego experiences it as a psychic reality that the loved object has been devoured, or is in danger of being devoured and therefore the loss of the love object is the immediate consequence of these cannibalistic desires." And "the infantile depressive position arises when the infant perceives and introjects the mother as a whole person (between three and five months). The fear lest she should be destroyed by his cannibalistic desires and fantasies gives rise to guilt . . . However the assumption seems justified that the seeds of depressive feelings, insofar as the experience of birth gives rise to a feeling of loss, are there from the beginning of life . . . My experience showed me that depressive feelings arise in infants, and that these feelings originate in early introjective processes." To repeat: "The infant experiences feelings akin to mourning and those feelings arise from his fear of destroying and so losing his loved and indispensable object (as an external as well as an introjected object) through his cannibalistic desires and through his greed . . . Defenses against greed are possibly the earliest of all . . . I suggest that the depressive position in infancy is a universal phenomenon." Standing, crawling and walking "help the infant to overcome the depressive position . . . The coordination of functions and movements is bound up with a defense mechanism which I take to be one of the fundamental processes in early development, namely, the manic defense. This defense is closely linked with the depressive position and implies a control over the internal world."

The first point that strikes the reader is the baffling nature of the presentation. This is due not solely to endless repetitions and paraphrasings but also to the fact that the author cannot tell a developmental story straight. Take, for example, her views on object-formation. These are complicated by the fact that the author has to run two theories simultaneously: on the one hand, the theory that shortly after birth the infant can "love" the mother as a "person" or a "whole" object; and on the other, that primitive object-formations are "part-objects" or "organ-objects" capable of immediate introjection, as witness, the introjection of "good" and "bad" breasts. What exactly constitutes the instinctual reference of the "whole" object is not clear. Klein thinks it may be an oral (breast) reference or a genital reference, the genital interests of the infant operating from birth through oral (breast) relations, and so giving rise to "love" of the whole. The depressive position involving the formation of a "whole" object already starts at the third month and the attachment to a whole object at the beginning of the second month. But, says Klein, rudiments of "whole" love also exist from birth. So there is no reason why the depressive position should not start from birth. And that, I really believe, is what Klein is driving at, for she links the depressive reaction of the infant to the birth trauma. Anyhow we soon get into difficulties with the Kleinian "psychic-reality" system, for apparently although the infant applies "psychic" reality to the breast situation (i.e., it interprets, or according to Riviere, misinterprets, the situation in terms of feeling-fantasies), the infant seems to react to the whole object in a manner that is extremely reminiscent of an adult's reaction to external reality. And this means in turn that secondary processes involving reality perceptions and conscious reactions are more readily applied to the "whole" object (the person) than to the "part"-object (the breast). Whereas I should have said that if there is anything in the Klein fantasy theory the exact reverse should be the case.

For all practical Kleinian purposes, cannibalistic means oral-sadistic, aggressive impulses, despite Abraham's patent definition of them in terms of the libido. Indeed it is interesting to note that whereas in the early Klein papers the early ego is an oro-phallic ego, in the present paper, despite a few cursory references to genital libido, it is clearly an oral ego. The cannibalistic-sadistic fantasies are throughout concerned with the breast and its introjections. The real truth of the matter is that Klein made three cardinal blunders in these attempts at hypothetical reconstruction: first, to lay exclusive emphasis on an oro-phallic ego, subsequently scaling this down to an oral ego; second, and despite reference in earlier papers to anal components, to exclude in effect all other libidinal components; and third, to compress all her theories of development into the concept of a unified ego. If the whole object is formed at the beginning of the second month and can be introjected as such, the primitive ego must have a unified and organized structure, for the unity of the ego is bound up with the existence of "whole" objects. True, Klein talks about rudimentary phases of object-formation, but at the same time she believes that from birth onwards rudimentary whole objects exist. Had she been ready to accept the nuclear theory of ego-development she might have avoided in part the bundle of contradictions with which she has saddled her own metapsychology.

The same confusion between rudimentary and complex psychic manifestations occurs in her description of the affects alleged to be experienced by the infant. In an early paper on the nature of affects I have indicated the necessity of closer differentiation of affects, in particular the distinction between primary affects and later fused affects, between affects that are characteristic of different states of instinct excitation (tension and discharge affects) and reactive affects that are secondary to traumatic states of tension. The later fusion of affects goes hand in hand with the development of more complicated forms of object relationship. By a sweeping simplification which is at the same time merely a sweeping assertion, Klein postulates "love" feelings for a "whole" object practically from the beginning of life. Similarly with feelings of loss, grief, and depression, the two- to three-months-old infant is saddled with affects of a sophisticated nature that presuppose complicated object-formations. And despite frequent references to early anxieties and to hypothetical guilt-feelings, the total result of the Klein formulations on infantile affect is to weaken rather than to strengthen the basic concept of an anxiety response to danger situations of over-excitation. This weakening of Freud's concept of anxiety is increased by the concentration of Kleinian interest on oral impulses to the neglect of other instinctual components that are capable of evoking anxiety responses.

Nevertheless the parts of Klein's paper where she deals with infantile affects and with affective interpretation of the behavior of sucklings are in one sense the most illuminating of all. The author evidently regards them as important pieces of evidence in support of her theories. Whereas in fact they merely go to show that Klein cannot imagine the infant's feelings in any psychic situation without injecting into them not only her own knowledge as an observer but her own emotional bias. Thus speaking of the infant's reaction when his smile is not responded to, she says "The smile disappears, the light fades from his eyes, and something akin to sorrow and anxiety creeps into his expression." Or again referring to situations where the mother leaves the room, "a fleeting expression of sadness came into the child's eyes". And again referring to the return of the mother, "Her very presence and signs of love reestablish the infant's belief in her as an unharmed and loving mother. This implies that his trust in his good internal and external objects increases and his fear of persecution by bad objects decreases." Some years ago Schmideberg criticized the tendentious nature of the Klein interpretations both of the infant's reactions and of environmental influences, and certainly if we were to string together the interpretations of the infantile situation given in this paper, we would be entitled to assume that infancy is a state in which loving mothers do nothing but love their babies while babies alternate between loving their mothers and being very sad and depressed because they have destroyed the mothers not merely in the real world, but in their own bodies and in their own minds. Now this is more than a gross over-idealization of the mother's behavior. It is a process of mother-justification which can be simply expressed in this formula: "If babies are sad, and fundamentally they are sad, it is their own fault: the real mother is good." It is a welcome change to have some evidence brought regarding the method and tendency of interpretation on which the Klein theories are based, but behavioristic interpretations have to include an objective assessment of the actual (ambivalent) behavior of the mother during the infancy of the child.

However absurd the results of these behavioristic studies may have been they served one useful purpose. One of A. Freud's criticisms of the fantasy concept was that it involved the operation in the unconscious mind of "secondary processes". To which I added that the fantasies as described were evidently derived from unconscious, preconscious and conscious mental systems. This view is strongly supported by the content of the last Klein paper. Hypothetical interpretations of infantile fantasy and mechanisms are interwoven with behavioristic descriptions of the infant's reactions to external objects and of the development of reality estimations. Once this interweaving is unravelled the different methods of approach stand out clearly each with a different relation to consciousness. Even so, on many occasions it is left uncertain whether the alleged feelings of the infant are conscious or unconscious. At any rate, it is interesting to note that with every step toward behavioristic corroboration of Klein theory, the previous (Isaacs-Klein) concept of "psychic-reality" is weakened, since in some of the behavioristic studies the infant's feelings are regarded as reality estimates, whereas according to the "psychic-reality" hypothesis they ought to be fantasy misinterpretations. Indeed some of Klein's behavioristic descriptions sound as if the infant itself had, unwittingly, repudiated the Kleinian view that reality thinking is derived from an earlier phase of pure fantasy thinking.

CONCLUSIONS

It is true that there have been fallow periods in the development of psychoanalysis, that its expansion was almost exclusively the work of Freud himself. But that does not imply the existence of a "closed" system. On the contrary, Freud's own development of psychoanalytic theories indicated an unusual capacity on his part to modify or extend where the clinical evidence demanded modification or extension. It if often and loosely thought that because Freud, for example, made important changes in his views on traumatic experiences or on the relation of the libido to anxiety, his basic formulations on the mental apparatus were equally subject to major modifications. Freud clung with tenacity to his basic formulations regarding mind and was justified by events. He measured deviations from psychoanalysis by the degree to which their sponsors abandoned fundamental principles. It is no more true to say that Freud was ready to abandon his basic conceptions than to say that because cardiologists may change their clinical assessments or theories of heart disease, they are ready to abandon their belief in the circulation of the blood.

When the Klein group are taxed with major deviations from Freudian theory they select quotations from Freud's writings that appear to lend support to their views. Freud's only explicit reference to the controversy occurs in a paper on "Female Sexuality" (4, p. 295): referring to a paper by Fenichel on the pregenital antecedents of the oedipus complex, Freud said:

"He (Fenichel) . . . protests against Melanie Klein's displacement backwards of the Oedipus complex, whose beginnings she assigns to the commencement of the second year of life. This view of the date of origin of the complex, which in addition necessitates modification of our view of all the rest of the child's sexual development, is in fact not in accordance with what we learn from the analyses of adults and is especially incompatible with my findings as to the long duration of the girl's pre-Oedipal attachment to her mother. This contradiction may be softened by the reflection that we are not as yet able to distinguish in this field between what is rigidly fixed by biological laws and what is subject to change or shifting under the influence of accidental experience. We have long recognized that seduction may have the effect of hastening and stimulating to maturity the sexual development of children, and it is quite possible that other factors operate in the same way: such, for instance, as the child's age when brothers or sisters are born or when it discovers the difference between the sexes, or, again, its direct observation of sexual intercourse, its parents' behavior in evoking or repelling its love, and so forth."

It will be observed that the date in question is the beginning of the second year. Later Klein specified the sixth month of life. It is not clear from her last paper how much earlier the Klein version of the oedipus complex appears but the depressive position is said to originate at the third month of life, relations to whole objects at the second month, and genital elements from birth: so the reader is free to draw his own conclusion on the matter.

I do not intend to recapitulate here the list of Kleinian deviations I have set out in this review. They can be summed up as follows: first, by their definitions of fantasy the Klein Group have reduced to complete confusion the basic Freudian concepts of the mental apparatus and have opened the door to a mystical interpretation of life immediately after birth; second, in their outline of the development of instincts, mental mechanisms and ego structure, they have departed from the Freudian theory of the libido and have undermined the basic distinctions between unconscious, preconscious and conscious systems; third, by their theories of the "uninterrupted influence" of the concepts of fixation and regression, they have abandoned the Freudian theory of neurosogenesis. If ever there was a "closed" system it is surely the Kleinian theory of a central depressive position developed between the third and fifth month of life. Not only does it run in direct contradiction to Freudian theories of neurosogenesis but if accepted, it would arrest all possibility of correlating the normal and abnormal manifestations of adult life with stages of development in infancy. It subverts all our concepts of progressive mental development from the unorganized to the organized.

But it is perhaps more interesting to consider what manner of deviation the Klein system constitutes. As regards neurosogenesis it resembles most closely the Rank "Birth Trauma" deviation. Instead of Rank's birth trauma we have offered to us a "love trauma" of the third month which is as fateful for subsequent development as Rank thought the birth trauma to be. I imagine, however, that the Klein system is not simply an attempt to find new explanations for the clinical data of psychoanalysis but that it owes its existence also to some urge towards a new *Weltanschauung,* together with a natural desire to bridge the gap in our reconstruction of life between the intra-uterine and the extra-uterine state. In my opinion the concept of a three-months-old love trauma due to the infant's imagined greedy destruction of a real loving mother whom it really loves is a variant of the doctrine of Original Sin.[21]

BIBLIOGRAPHY[22]

1. Ferenczi, S., *Further Contributions to the Theory and Technique of Psychoanalysis,* London, 1926, p. 267.
2. Klein, M., *The Psycho-Analysis of Children,* London, 1932.
3. Klein, M., "A Contribution to the Psychogenesis of Manic Depressive States", *International Journal of Psycho-Analysis,* XVI, 1935, pp. 145-174.
4. Freud, S., "Female Sexuality", *Internat. J. Psa.,* XIII, 1932, pp. 281-297.
5. Freud, S., *New Introductory Lectures,* 1933, pp. 124, 129.
6. Jones, E., "The Phallic Phase", *Internat. J. Psa.,* XIII, 1932.
7. Glover, E., "Significance of Mouth in Psychoanalysis", *British Journal of Medical Psychology,* IV, 1924, pp. 134-155.
8. Glover, E., "Grades of Ego-Differentiation", *Internat. J. Psa.,* XI, 1930.
9. Glover, E., "Therapeutic Effects of Inexact Interpretation", *Internat. J. Psa.,* XII, 1931, pp. 397-411.
10. Glover, E., Review: *Psycho-Analysis of Children, Internat. J. Psa.,* XIV, 1933, pp. 119-129.
11. Glover, E., "Some Aspects of Psychoanalytic Research", paper read Oct. 3, 1934.
12. Klein, M., "Mourning and its Relation to Manic Depressive States", paper read Oct. 16, 1938.
13. Riviere, J., "A Contribution to the Analysis of the Negative Therapeutic Reaction", *Internat. J. Psa.,* XVII, 1936, pp. 304-320.
14. Riviere, J., "On the Genesis of Psychical Conflict in Earliest Infancy", *Internat. J. Psa.,* XVII, 1936, pp. 395-422.

21. It has been argued that all this is a storm in a tea-cup, that even if the Klein system constitutes a major deviation from Freudian theory, this does not matter very much. In the long run, it is said, scientific method and thinking will prevail. If the election of members of psychoanalytic Groups (which up to the present in Britain is the equivalent of an official Diploma to practise Psychoanalysis) followed the lines adopted by societies for the promotion of natural science, there might be something in this argument. But it does not. The transferences and counter-transferences developing during training analysis tend to give rise in the candidate to an emotional conviction of the soundness of the training analyst's theories. This means that many candidates trained at the present time will for the next twenty-five years practise and themselves propagate the Kleinian precepts.

22. Unpublished papers quoted were read to the British Psychoanalytic Society.

15. Winnicott, D. W., "Manic Defense", paper read Dec. 4, 1935.
16. Rickman, J., "A Study of Quaker Beliefs", paper read June 3, 1935.
17. Rickman, J., "The Nature of Ugliness", paper read Jan. 20, 1937.
18. Scott, W. C. M., "Psychoanalysis of a Manic Depressive Patient in an Institution", paper read June 2, 1937.
19. Isaacs, S., "An Acute Psychotic Anxiety Occurring in a Boy of Four Years", paper read Feb. 2, 1938.
20. Isaacs, S., "The Nature of the Evidence Concerning Mental Life in the Earliest Years", paper read April 6, 1938.
21. Isaacs, S., "Temper Tantrums in Early Childhood and Their Relation to Internal Objects", paper read Dec. 7, 1938.
22. Rosenfeld, E., "Psychoanalytic Approach in a Case of Psychosis", paper read May 4, 1938.
23. Glover, E. and Schmideberg, M., Discussion, British Psychoanalytic Society, Oct. 16, 1935.
24. Foulkes, S. H., "Introjection", *Internat. J. Psa.*, XVIII, 1937, pp. 269-293.
25. Knight, R., "Introjection, Projection and Identification", *Psychoanalytic Quarterly*, IX, 1940, pp. 334-341.
26. Schmideberg, M., "Assessment of Environmental Factors", paper read Feb., 1936.
27. Waelder, R., "The Problem of the Genesis of Psychical Conflict in Earliest Infancy", *Internat. J. Psa.*, XVIII, 1937, pp. 406-473.
28. Glover, E. and Brierley, M., *An Investigation of the Technique of Psycho-Analysis*, Appendix, London, 1940.
All dates following refer to the meetings organized by the British Psychoanalytic Society for the Controversial Series of Discussions, 1943-44:
29. Discussion, anuary 27, 1943.
30. Discussion, February 17, 1943.
31. Discussion, May 19, 1943.
32. Discussion, February 7, 1943.
33. Discussion, March 17, 1943.
34. Discussion, April 7, 1943.
35. Discussion, April 17, 1943. See also H. Hoffer.
36. Heimann, P., "Some Aspects of the Role of Introjection and Projection in Early Development", Discussions, October 20 and November 17, 1943. Controversial Series II.
37. Discussion, October 20, 1943.
38. Discussion, November 17, 1943.
39. Schmideberg, M., " 'Introjected Objects': an issue of Terminology or a Clinical Problem?" December 3, 1941.
40. Schmideberg, M., "Proof and Error in Psychoanalytic Conclusions", November 6, 1940.
41. Schmideberg, M., "The Relative Validity of 'Pre-conscious' and 'Deep' Interpretations", March 19, 1941.
42. Controversial Series III. Discussions, January and February, 1944.
43. Discussion, January, 1944. See K. Friedlander and W. Hoffer.
44. Klein, M., "Emotional Life and Ego-development of the Infant, with Special Reference to the Depressive Position", Controversial Series IV. Discussion, March, 1944.

NOTES ON THE ANALYTIC DISCOVERY
OF A PRIMAL SCENE

By MARIE BONAPARTE (Paris)

A forty-two-year-old woman is undergoing analysis. In the fourth week of her analysis the patient one night dreams that she is in a small cot on the grassy slopes of a park, near a lake, looking intently at a married couple whom she knows lying quite near in their bed. The analyst asserts that she must have seen sexual scenes in her childhood, that the dream must derive from an unconscious reminiscence of what she saw. She must not only have *heard* those scenes in the dark, as is so often the case with children, but she must have *seen* them in full daylight. The patient did not at first accept this interpretation of her dream, she even reacted violently against it, but the analyst persisted in his assertion. The patient's mother had died when the little girl was born but she had had a wet nurse, and the analyst suggested that she must have observed scenes between that nurse and some sexual partner.

I shall now report the first memory of the childhood of this patient.

She is sitting very low, on a small chair or a small box, in her nurse's room. The nurse is standing in front of the looking-glass of the chimney, in which the fire burns; the child is looking at her intently. The nurse is smearing her own black hair with pomade. The pomade, in a little white pot, is on the marble of the chimney; that pomade is black. The child finds that disgusting. The nurse has a long yellowish face and looks like a horse.

Rumors had been going about in the household, rumors which the patient had heard, that her nurse had had a lover, the master of her father's horses. The screen-memory confirmed these rumors. For the nurse had in no way had a face resembling that of a horse: on the contrary, an old photograph showed her with a sound and pleasant face. So the horsy look of the woman must have expressed some real function of hers; she had been ridden as a horse by some

119

horseman. The identity of her partner was betrayed by the woman's presumed looks. And the yellow tinge of the face itself must have been some reminder of the yellowness of horse's teeth.

The fire expresses the fire of sexual love in accordance with its general significance. The chimney is also a very general symbol of the cloaca. And the black pomade—which in fact the nurse used— manifests the anal character of the cloaca, at a time when the child did not yet distinguish between anus and vagina. No doubt the hair itself of the nurse is displaced from the lower to the higher part of the body. Here occurs a condensation of pubic hair and hair on the head.

The nurse remained with the little girl from the day of her birth until after her third year. So this screen-memory may refer to the early months of the child's fourth year. But the visual memories lying beneath it cannot have been posterior to the child's second year, as the lovers must have feared to perform sexual acts in full daylight when the child, having begun to speak, might have given them away.

When the little girl at about seven had learnt to write fluently, she began writing little books in which she gave free play to her imagination in wild fantastic stories. The little books she discovered among her father's papers after his death, shortly before going into ana- lysis. Their contents seemed at first sight mad, full of extravagant sadistic symbols.

They were in English, though the little girl was French. The English language, which she had begun to learn when she was four, and in which she wrote the fantastic stories she invented, was no doubt used by her as a "secret" language in which to express her unconscious "secrets". At the time when she was writing these mysterious books, she also was keeping a journal of her everyday activities, this one written in French. Of these latter writings she never lost the memory. But the "secret" English books she did not remember having written, though they were unmistakably in her own hand. And even when the analysis had discovered their for- bidden secret meaning, the memory of having written them never came back.

These stories were symbolic presentations of what the child had seen in her early years. They expressed those sexual scenes in a transposed language, in which many of the usual symbols of mankind stood for repressed unconscious memories.

Even the titles of some of the stories are suggestive of what lies beneath them: *"The mouth pencil"*—*"The rabbit without skin"*—*"The waiting drop"*—*"Spitting man"*—*"The velvet tear"*—*"The bursting woman"*—*"The bursting stomach"*—and so on.

In order to exemplify the way in which the unconscious memories were worked out, I shall report one of the most characteristic of the little stories invented by the child:

"The smoking Deadimannishfon goat (explication of the goat)

"Kami and Kama were two brothers ther father in daying left only a goth to them they agry to gother that they woud cut the goat in two. in the night they went with a handle in the stable of the goth and they cut er in two they said that they would take ther part of goat in the morning and in the morning when they went in the stable the goat was stikend again and she was complete. and as they had cutten the goat with a knife that they had cutten bad smelling rockfort there were bad smelling rokfort that grew on the goat. they woud make get rid of that to the goat and they made her smok nervously in a pipe. and as she was not accouted to smoke she vomit and they they saw on the ground the rockfort and his roots.

"in the night the goat went up the stairs and she spit at the face of Kami and Kama then her spiting made smell the face of the two brothers the cacapa. then they had no money more to by bread and the they would cut the goat in an other sance with the knife of the bread and cut the goat in two.

"then in the morning the goat was as before cut in two and she was vomiting they made come Carnot and he couerd her".

Such is the "explication of the goat". It is, of course, influenced by a Biblical myth: the judgment of Solomon, the two mothers claiming the same living child and the King's decision, in order to settle the dispute, to give each claimant a half of the child.

Let us first turn our attention to the goat. In a country house in the suburbs of Paris, where she was born, the little girl had dwelt until she was three years old, almost as long as her nurse had remained with her. There she had played in the grass on the sand near that nurse, who seemed to have been a very good wet nurse, feeding the child at the breast almost until she was a year and a half! The good warm milk from the nurse's breast she no doubt often drank in the shade of the summer garden. That country house remained a family property, and when the girl's father had moved to Paris, she was taken there each summer on some hot days to play in the garden of her baby years. There one could find fruit on the fruit trees, eggs from the hens in the hen-roost, but more impressive than all of these, in that garden the gardener and his wife possessed a marvellous animal. The snow-white fairy-like creature grazed on the garden lawns, fastened to a long rope, looking at the oncomers with her long golden slit eyes—and when the little girl approached her she was told: Mind the horns! For the white goat lowered her long head adorned with two curved horns and threatened to attack whoever came near. Only the gardener's wife could approach and milk her. From the long hanging teats she filled a big bowl with white foaming milk and offered it, still warm, to the little girl. The peculiar taste of the goat's milk! There was something fairy-like about it, it was so different from the monotonous, tasteless everyday cow's milk.

And it was found and drunk in the same garden where the nurse of former days had so generously fed her nursling! For the child's mind, two kinds of associations linked the nurse and the goat: both were givers of milk, both gave it in the same garden.

So it came that the *deadimannishfon* goat represented the woman who, in her early years, had nursed the child.

And now to Kami and Kama. The master of the horses of the father's stables, the presumed lover of the nurse, was in fact the half-brother of the child's father: an illegitimate uncle. Thus the little girl had had two successive oedipus complexes—the horseman and the nurse, and her real father with her dead mother. Kami and Kama, the two brothers of the story, no doubt express that fact. And they both appear as very sadistic men, in accordance with the classical infantile sadistic conception of coitus. They are not very nice to the goat. They grab at her, they both want a part of the goat, and cut her in two.

But what they do to her is in fact a reproduction of what the little girl saw the horseman do to the nurse. The brothers cut the goat in two with a knife that "had cutten bad smalling rockfort". The knife is not difficult to identify: the knife is phallic. The bad smell is related to the infantile theory of the cloaca where the child believed the penis to enter in sexual intercourse, which she had often witnessed. And it is because she is "cutten" with such a phallic knife that the goat the next morning is 'stikend again". Thus it happens to women after coitus. They appear again "complete".

Now about the "rockfort that grew *on* the goat". It ought probably to be translated: "that grew *in* the goat". The result of coitus can be pregnancy. The child's real mother here looms behind the nurse. That mother had been made pregnant through coitus. And she even died from it, in childbirth. She became a *deadimannish goat*. Though it is *fun* to say it, that fun is very serious. A kind of macabre humor.

The goat of the tale, anyhow, tries to escape such a doom. That is why she is made to smoke. Smoking here appears as a means to provoke abortion. For smoking when one is not accustomed to do so makes people vomit. Pregnant women also vomit. The little girl had just seen an aunt of hers pregnant and vomiting. And that vomiting had been interpreted by her as being some effort to "get rid" of the dangerous, death-bringing fetus. Moreover, the nurse, had she become pregnant, would no doubt have wished to "vomit" the fetus up as her husband was away and as a result she would have lost her post. Through these trends of thought winding through the unconscious, the goat could become *"the smoking deadimannishfon goat"*.

Anyhow, the sadistic brothers manage to cut the goat in two in a more efficient way: in cutting her in another sense. Here we think of the famous story of Münchhausen, in French translated under the name of Mr. de Crac. This Mr. de Crac is so rash that wanting to cut a slice of bread for his lunch in a forest with a big knife, at one stroke he cuts himself through the waist and cuts through the tree he is leaning against. The little girl had a picture book where he could be seen doing so, with the upper part of his body flying up in the air. Mr. de Crac was very thin, he was pictured with a waist so thin that the most elegant women might have envied it at that time of screwed-in waists. Of these women it was sometimes said: Her waist is so thin that she seems as if she were cut in two! So is the goat of the tale in her exquisite feminine masochistic way!

And this time the goat does not only *seem* cut in two. She is actually cut in two she remains so until the next morning. Does the real mother of the child, who died as a result of coitus, in childbirth, here reappear? The mother died, and her death made her widower rich—she had been a rich heiress and her husband inherited a large part of her fortune. This might be the reason why the goat's spitting makes the face of the cutters smell "the cacapa": excrements are classical symbols of gold and possessions. And it is because they have "no money more to buy bread" that the men cut the goat with "the knife of the bread". They want to get money, to get rich, to inherit from her.

Though the little girl revelled in these sadistic fantasies, she all the same had a good and kind heart. She wished to give her tale a happy ending. So she finally appeals to the supreme good earthly father, that is to the head, at that time, of the French State, to the President of the Republic, Sadi Carnot. He comes, as a deus ex machina, and cures the goat of her sexual vomiting and of her being cut in two; that is, Carnot saves the goat from death.

At the time of this analysis, the child's nurse, in her far distant French province, had long since died. But the old horseman, the master of the horses of the father and his half-brother, was still alive. He was then eighty-two years of age, a still vigorous, robust old man. Of peasant origin, with the simple devoted clan-like propensities of his race, he had remained devoted to the little girl he had played with in her youth. The patient went to see him, as she often had since he had been pensioned by her father. There, one evening, she asked him to tell her many particulars about her family—their family one might say—and about her early years. She also questioned him about her nurse. He spoke enthusiastically about the beautiful peasant woman. And then the patient dared to ask directly: "It it true, what was said in our house, that you were my nurse's lover?" The old man began: "What a slander! Would I have so abused your parent's confidence! *Your* nurse! I would never have done such a thing!" And the old man explained how the child's mother, before her fatal confinement, had, said he, entrusted the child to his protection . . . That was why he had often come up to the nursery at any time of the day—for he lived out of the house—and remained there contemplating the baby in her tiny cot.

The patient did not try to get more information from the old man for the time being. However, a few months later she invited him to come to see her again. Now, in her own house, she reproached him for not having been truthful. "You have been my nurse's lover though you denied it. I know it is true . . . I shall tell you how I know it. I have of late studied how to understand dreams. Well, in my dreams I found the dim memory of having *seen*, as a child, adults indulging in sexual acts . . and one of them was *you*. I also wrote little books when I was seven, eight, nine years old; they contain fantastic stories which can only thus be understood. I therefore *know* it. I do not accuse you—on the contrary, I ought to be grateful to you for it. Strange to say, it has been shown that the faculties of observation, of intelligence, are often derived in great part from such early sexual impressions.

So I am indebted to you however strange it may seem, for part of the intellectual faculties I may have . . . But I beg you to tell me the truth. I cannot think ill of you for it, and it would be of considerable scientific interest. Tell me the truth . . ."

And the old man, looking at the woman with some fear, said slowly: "I shall not say yes . . . but I shall not say no. That is all I can say." After the patient's continued insistence and after some last hesitation, the old man added, " *She* wanted me . . . she ran after me. Then I did my man's duty . . ."

The old man then gave a detailed account: of sexual intercourse in full daylight, until the child was about two years old; of different modes of sexual activities, including fellatio, as the *Mouth Pencil* suggested; and of the continuance of the sexual relationship with the nurse, after the second year of the child's life until she was dismissed from the house; but in this second period at night, in the dark, as was suggested by other stories in the little books, where ears and hearing played a prominent part.

The value of this case lies in the exceptional coincidence of the internal and the external evidence concerning an analytical reconstruction. Several factors had to work together in order to achieve this result: firstly, the survival of one of the actors of the primal scene; secondly the fact that, instead of being some awe-inspiring and self-restrained father, he was an illegitimate but devoted uncle, with simple, primitive and sincere inclinations, able to confess with not too great shame his former instinctual activities; lastly the scientific, almost compulsively enterprising spirit of investigation of the patient, in part derived precisely from these early observations which in its turn it helped to ascertain.

INDICATIONS FOR CHILD ANALYSIS

By ANNA FREUD (London)

Introduction

Since 1905, when a phobia in a five-year-old boy was first treated by psychoanalysis, the father acting as intermediary between child and analyst, child analysis as a therapeutic method has had a stormy and checkered career.[1] There is hardly a detail that has remained uncontested, that has not at some time become the starting-point for controversy.

In some respects child analysis revived the same objections that the psychoanalytic treatment of adults had to meet and overcome a full decade earlier.

1. *The sexual prejudice.*

At the end of the last century the conception of a sexual origin of adult neurosis ran counter to all the current prejudices. However, no one went so far as to deny altogether the existence of adult sexuality, although medical and lay opinion failed to concede it the importance it deserved. On the other hand, everyone violently objected to the possible existence of a sexual life in childhood. Psychoanalysis had laid itself open to the reproach of over-estimating the role of sexuality in the adult and to a similar charge of inventing an infantile sex life, contrary to the facts then known and accepted by physicians and educators. Thus the existence of an infantile sexuality had to be established and proved at the same time that its importance in the development of the neuroses of childhood had to be demonstrated.[2]

1. S. Freud, "Analysis of a Phobia in a Five-Year-Old Boy," *Collected Papers*, III.

2. S. Freud, *Three Contributions to the Theory of Sex, Nervous and Mental Disease Monograph*, 7, 1916.

2. *The fear of immorality as a consequence of psychoanalytic treatment.*

A second argument originally used against the analytic treatment of adult neurotics was based on a misconception of the psychoanalytic process itself. It was thought that the constant preoccupation with instinctual tendencies which is inherent in the analytic work, the release of these tendencies from repression, and their consequent emergencies in consciousness could have only the one effect of their expression in actions, i.e., the fulfilment of the instinctual (sexual and aggressive) wishes which had been kept under repression before the treatment. According to this argument, psychoanalytic treatment would lead directly to immorality and licentiousness. It needed much patient and lengthy demonstration to convince the public that this was not the case; that, on the contrary, unconscious tendencies were deprived of most of their power when an outlet into conscious thought was opened up for them: relegated to the unconscious, these instinctual urges had been out of reach; uncovered, and lifted to the conscious level they automatically came under the patient's control and could be dealt with according to his ideas and ideals.

The same objections that had been successfully refuted with regard to adult patients arose again in full force when child analysis made its first appearance. The argument was now advanced that the child could certainly not be trusted with the same discretion in dealing with his reawakened instinctual tendencies as the adult. Surely the child would want to make full use of the license offered him in the analytic situation and would give free rein to his instinctual urges inside and outside of the analytic hour. Or even if his intentions were otherwise, his attempts at restraint and adaptive behavior would be entirely overrun by the instinctual forces let loose through the agency of analytic treatment. Fears of this kind were expressed not only by doctors, teachers and parents, but were shared to some extent by certain analysts who thought it quite possible that child analysis might need some special form of educational guidance as its constant implement and counterpart. But, as experience proved, this was not necessary as often as it had been expected. It was demonstrated repeatedly that when a child's ego and superego were both severe enough to produce an infantile neurosis, they could also, with some help, be relied on to deal with the sexual and aggressive impulses that emerged from repression after the neurosis had been analyzed successfully. Fears of this nature are more justified when the object of child analysis is not a neurotic, but a dissocial, delinquent, or otherwise deficient character.

3. *Controversies about the technique of child analysis.*

It became obvious immediately that the classical analytic technique was not applicable to children, at least not before the age of puberty, or at best pre-puberty. Free association, the mainstay of analytic technique, had to be counted out as a method; young children are neither willing nor able to embark on it. This fact affects dream-interpretation, the second main approach to the unconscious. Children tell their dreams freely; but without the use of free association the interpretation of the manifest dream content is less fruitful and convincing. The child analyst frequently has to supply the links between the manifest dream content and the latent dream thoughts according to his own intimate knowledge of the child's inner situation at the time of dreaming. Furthermore, it is impossible to establish the same outward setting for the analytic hour. Children placed on the analytic couch for the purpose of relaxed concentration are usually completely silenced. Talk and action cannot be separated from each other in their case. Nor can the patient's family be wholly excluded from the analysis. Insight into the seriousness of the neurosis, the decision to begin and to continue treatment, persistence in the face of resistance or of passing aggravations of the illness are beyond the child, and have to be supplied by the parents. In child analysis the parents' good sense plays the part which the healthy part of the patient's conscious personality plays during adult analysis to safeguard and maintain the continuance of treatment. Appropriate substitutes for free association were accordingly the prime necessity in establishing techniques suitable to the varying needs of different phases of childhood. The first divergence of opinion between child analysts arose about this matter. Certain child analysts (Hug-Hellmuth in Vienna, Melanie Klein in Berlin and later in London) developed the so-called play technique of child analysis, a method that promised to give more or less direct access to the child's unconscious. According to this technique, the child's spontaneous play activity with small toys offered by the analyst for free use within the analytic hour, was substituted for free association. The individual actions of the child in connection with this material were considered to be equivalent to the individual thoughts or images in a chain of free association. In this manner the production of material for interpretation became largely independent of the child's willingness or ability to express himself in speech.

Other child analysts (on the European continent and in the United States) were reluctant to employ this play technique to the

same extent.   Although such a method of interpretation allowed certain flashes of direct insight into the child's unconscious, it seemed
to them open to objections of various kinds.   Like all interpretation
of symbols (for instance purely symbolic dream interpretations) it
had a tendency to become rigid, impersonal and stereotyped without
being open to corroboration from the child; it aimed at laying bare
the deeper layers of the child's unconscious without working through
the conscious and preconscious resistances and distortions.   Furthermore these analysts refused to accept such activities as actual equiva-
lents of free association.   The free associations of the adult patient
are produced in the set situation of analytic transference and, although
they are freed from the usual restrictions of logical and conscious
thought they are under the influence of the patient's one governing
aim to be cured by analysis.   The play activity of the child is not
governed by any similar intention.   This leads to the further open and
controversial question as to whether the relationship of the child
to the analyst is really wholly governed by a transference situation.
Even if one part of the child's neurosis is transformed into a transference neurosis as it happens in adult analysis, another part of the
child's neurotic behavior remains grouped around the parents who are
the original objects of his pathogenic past.   Considerations of this
nature led a large number of child analysts to evolve techniques of a
different kind.   They worked on the various derivatives of the child's
unconscious in dreams and daydreams, in imaginative play, in drawings, etc., including the emotional reactions of the child, both in and
outside of the analytic hour.   As in adult analysis, the task was to
undo the various repressions, distortions, displacements, condensa-
tions, etc., that had been brought about by neurotic defense-mechanisms
until, with the active help of the child, the unconscious content of
the material was laid bare.   Such cooperation with the child naturally
presupposes the extensive use of speech.[3]

The method of symbolic interpretation of play activity that
Melanie Klein devised for her technique was later taken over by psy-
chotherapists and widely used in England and America under the name
of "play therapy".   But in these instances it was deprived of its full
original meaning, since it was used without reference to an analytic
transference situation.

3. Detailed accounts of the two different types of child analysis are contained in
Melanie Klein's *Psycho-Analysis of the Child*, International Psycho-Analytic Library,
No. 22, 1932; and in Anna Freud's *Introduction to the Technique of Child Analysis*,
Nervous and Mental Disease Monograph, 1929.

4. *Controversies concerning the appropriate age for child analysis.*

Differences in the manner in which child analysis was practised inevitably led to differences in opinion concerning the age at which the therapeutic method was applicable. The decisive factor in this respect was the use of speech. Melanie Klein and her followers repeatedly expressed the opinion that with the help of play technique, children can be analyzed at almost any age, from earliest infancy onward. When the faculty of speech in the child is of major importance for the treatment, it is hardly possible to contemplate analysis before the age of two or three. The majority of cases treated with the Vienna-Prague-Berlin techniques (as distinguished from the Kleinian techniques) were considerably older than that; many of them were analyzed at the height of the oedipus complex (four or five years) or in the latency period.

5. *Controversies concerning the range of application of child analysis.*

Here again a wide difference of opinion exists between the school of Melanie Klein and the former Vienna school of child analysts, many of whom are at present working in America. Child analysts of the former school express the view that every child passes through phases of grave abnormality (psychotic states, depressions, etc.) in infancy, and that normal development in later stages can best be safeguarded by early child analysis, by analyzing the psychotic residues of the earliest stage whenever outward circumstances permit. The former Vienna school, on the other hand, is of the opinion that the application of child analysis may well be restricted to the most severe cases of the infantile neurosis which every child experiences at one time or other before entering the latency period. With all other children, the application of analytic knowledge to their educational handling may prove sufficient to guide them through the intricacies of their instinctual and emotional development.

The Evaluation of Infantile Neuroses

1. *Selection of cases.*

Those who do not share the opinion that analysis should be universally applied to all children are faced with the task of selecting their cases, that is, of assessing the seriousness of the various manifestations of infantile neurosis. In practice, child analysts of today have little opportunity to determine this matter by their own judgment. The question whether or not a child should be analyzed is usually decided for them, and not infrequently for inadequate reasons. Children who are severely ill are often withheld from treatment because their parents, with whom the decision lies, know too little about analysis, or are frightened by the little they do know; because the parents are reluctant to have the intimacies of their own lives exposed to the analyst; because they fear the sexual enlightenment of the child; because they, especially the mothers, are unwilling to see a stranger succeed with their child when they themselves have failed. Sometimes the reasons given are very superficial: analytic hours would clash with school hours; would take up the time otherwise given to sport, handicraft or some other occupation, from which the child usually has ceased to benefit because of his neurotic disturbance. The most decisive factor is frequently the matter of time and distance. To accompany a child to and from a daily analytic hour is a heavy burden on the mother; if long distances aggravate the issue, this factor is often prohibitive.

On the other hand, a number of children are sent into analysis, not because they suffer from an excessive form of infantile neurosis, but because their parents, either as analytic patients themselves, or as practising analysts, are more apt than others to detect and evaluate signs of neurotic behavior whenever they appear. They readily decide upon analytic treatment at an early stage to avoid for their child the graver forms of neurotic suffering which they know only too well from personal experience. Their positive decision for treatment, like the above mentioned negative decision against treatment, is based on a personal attitude rather than on an objective assessment of the child's disturbance.

The child cases actually in treatment in our day, either in child departments of psychoanalytic clinics or in private practice, are thus a more or less chance selection, not a representative selection of infantile neuroses that are most in need of therapeutic help. It is to be expected that these conditions will change when knowledge about the mental development of the young child becomes more widespread, that is, when parents and physicians understand at least as much about the importance of instinctual, emotional or intellectual setbacks in the child's development as they understand now about its bodily illnesses. The assessment of the disturbance and the decision as to whether treatment is indicated or not will then be left to the psychiatrist or psychoanalyst, as it is nowadays left to the pediatrician in all cases of organic disturbance.

(a) The factor of neurotic suffering.

The question whether or not an adult neurotic seeks treatment is in the last resort dependent on the amount of suffering his neurotic symptoms cause him. For this reason neurotics undergo treatment more willingly than, for instance, perverts. A perversion disrupts normal life as much as a neurosis. But the perversion brings satisfaction, whereas neurotic symptoms are painful.

The statement can be maintained in spite of the fact that every neurosis is also a source of pleasure for the individual who is afflicted by it. The pleasure that the patient derives from the distorted gratification of repressed wishes, that is, from his symptoms, is not experienced as pleasure by his conscious system. The conscious pleasure, on the other hand, that neurotics often enjoy owing to the consideration they receive from their environment, a sense of importance, etc., is of a secondary nature and not really inherent in the illness. Whenever this secondary gain from the illness becomes greater than the neurotic suffering itself, the patient will be unfit for treatment, or will in most cases quite openly refuse to be treated. The existence of neurotic suffering is an important prerequisite, if it is not indispensable, for the attitude of persistence and determination that a patient needs to carry him through the difficulties of an analytic cure.

In dealing with cases of infantile neurosis one realizes that neurotic suffering is not present in the child to the same extent; and that whatever the amount of suffering may be, it is equally divided between the child and the parents. In some instances it is only the reaction of the parents to the symptom that brings home to the child, secondarily, that he suffers from a symptom. Such is the case, for instance, in the frequent feeding disturbances of childhood. Children become bad eaters for reasons that originate in their early mother-relationship, in their reactions against their oral-sadistic and their anal-sadistic tendencies, etc. The normal intake of food is thus made difficult or impossible for neurotic reasons. The child, left to himself, would gladly put up with this symptom and eat less. Mothers, on the other hand, suffer acutely from anxiety caused by this behavior of the child and, in their turn, inflict suffering on the bad eater through reproaches, scoldings, forcible measures, etc. The same occurs in the neurotic bed-wetting of childhood. Children under a certain age tend to show indifference toward this symptom while the adult environment suffers badly on its account; the amount of pain it causes the child depends on the reaction of the environment. The night terrors of children (*pavor nocturnus*) usually cause consternation and anxiety to the parents while the afflicted child himself remains unmindful of them. Temper tantrums are disturbing to the family; for the child himself they are often a welcome outlet. Neurotic display of aggression and destructiveness, as they occur in the initial stages of an obsessional neurosis, are most disturbing symptoms to the family; the child rather indulges in them. His attitude in this respect resembles that of an adult pervert more closely than that of an adult neurotic.

Acute neurotic suffering is felt by the child in all states of anxiety before a consistent defense against it has become established. When anxiety is once warded off, either by phobic or obsessional mechanisms, the amount of the child's suffering depends again on the reactions of the environment. Many mothers fear the child's anxiety as much as the child does himself. Consequently they do not oppose the child's phobic or obsessional arrangements; they even help actively in various ways to reinforce them. They help the child avoid the danger situations in which anxiety arises; they adapt themselves to bed time ceremonials and to eating, dressing and washing obsessions, etc. Their object is to spare the child the suffering inherent in his anxiety, and simultaneously to avoid the violent outbreaks that ensue whenever an obsessional act or phobic precaution is opposed or prevented. There are thus many infantile phobias and obsessional neuroses that exist under the surface and that are not felt as acutely painful by the child although they cause endless trouble for the mother.

During the time of mass evacuation in England, 1940, many children became neurotic sufferers after separation from their parents. It would be erroneous to conclude that they had all acquired a neurosis due to their traumatic experiences. In many cases their neurosis had merely not been in evidence while they lived with their mothers; acute anxiety and suffering appeared when they had to live with people who were less willing or able to show consideration for their phobic and obsessional arrangements.

To sum up: the presence or absence of suffering cannot be considered a decisive factor when making up one's mind about the treatment of a child. There are many serious neurotic disorders that the child bears with equanimity; there are less serious ones that cause pain. Since the decision to seek advice for the child normally lies with the parents, an infantile neurosis is more likely to be brought for treatment when its symptoms are disturbing to the environment. The parents will be guided in their assessment of the seriousness of the situation by the impact of the child's neurosis on themselves.

They show more concern, for instance, about aggressive and destructive states than about inhibitions; obsessional acts are taken more lightly than anxiety attacks, though in reality they represent a more advanced stage of the same disorder; bedwetters are taken to clinics more regularly than any other group of cases; the beginning stages of passive femininity in young boys, though often decisive for their whole future abnormality, are almost invariably overlooked.

(b)   The factor of disturbance of normal capacities.

An adult neurosis is not only assessed subjectively according to suffering, but objectively according to the extent to which it damages the two main capacities of the individual: the capacity to lead a normal love and sex life and the capacity to work. Patients usually decide to come into treatment when one or both of these functions are severely threatened.

The question arises whether there are any functions in the child's life, the disturbance of which is an equally significant indicator for the seriousness of the infantile neurosis.

The child's love and sex life, as revealed by psychoanalytic studies, is not less extensive and certainly not less intensive than that of the adult. But, after the first severe repressions of early childhood have occurred, it is inhibited in its aims. Though centered according to objects (oedipus complex), it is diffuse in its manifestations (component instincts), not organized under the primacy of any single one of them. Furthermore, it lacks a climax in its expressions, the disturbance of which could be taken as indicative of disturbance of function. The intactness of the child's sexuality is therefore more difficult to gauge than that of the adult. To measure the child's capacity for object-love we can only measure his libidinal urges directed toward the outer world as against his narcissistic tendencies. Normally after the first year of life object-love should outweigh narcissism; satisfaction derived from objects should become increasingly greater than autoerotic gratification. An infantile neurosis can seriously interfere with these proportions. But the assessment of these factors in the diagnosis is too subtle and too complicated to be of immediate help as an indication for treatment.

It is equally difficult to find in the child's life a parallel for the disturbance of work capacity. It has been suggested by many authors that play is as important for the child as work is for the adult, and that consequently a test of the child's ability to play is indicative of the extent of his disturbance. This view seems to be borne out by the fact that neurotic children are invariably disturbed in their play activity. With certain types of neurosis imaginative play is excessive, at the expense of constructive play. In its initial stages this is sometimes construed as an asset by the parents, as the sign of a specially vivid imagination and of artistic gifts. But when such play becomes repetitive, monotonous, and interferes with all other kinds of activity, the neurotic element is unmistakable: it is a sign that the child is fixated at a certain point of his libidinal development.

Although the child's capacity for constructive play is the nearest substitute for the adult capacity to work, the two functions remain so far removed from each other that it is hardly justifiable to give them an equal place in the diagnosis. Since play is governed by the pleasure principle, and work by the reality principle, the disturbance of each of the two functions has a different clinical significance.

(c) The factor of disturbance of normal development.

It is thus unpractical for the evaluation of an infantile neurosis to use the same criteria that we apply in the case of an adult. Childhood is a process *sui generis,* a series of developmental stages in which each manifestation has its importance as a transition, not as a final result. Its tasks and accomplishments cannot therefore be compared with those of the more static stage of adulthood. There is only one factor in childhood of such central importance that its impairment through a neurosis calls for immediate action; namely, the child's ability to develop, not to remain fixated at some stage of development before the maturation process has been concluded. The suggestion is therefore to assess the seriousness of an infantile neurosis, not according to its damage to the activities or attitudes of the child in any special way or at any given moment, but according to the degree to which it prevents the child from developing further.

2. *Libidinal Development.*

(a) The sequence of libidinal development.

On the basis of our present knowledge it is possible, even in a cursory examination, to establish whether a child's libidinal development corresponds to his age level. We roughly know the age limits for the pregenital organizations of the libido, and for some of the subdivisions. Gross disturbance in the order of events, or a child's failure to progress from any of these transitory stages when he is neither organically nor mentally deficient, points to serious neurotic interference.

But wide individual variation and the scantiness of our knowledge prevent us from making anything beyond rough estimates on this basis. Normally, we have to take into account the extensive overlapping between the various organizations. The oral phase, for instance, persists for months after the anal-sadistic organization has come into being; anal-sadistic manifestations do not disappear with the beginning of the phallic phase. The latency period is usually in existence for one or two years before the tendencies of the first infantile period fade into the background. It would, for instance, be erroneous to conclude from a persistence of oral or anal forms of autoerotic gratification into the fourth or fifth year, that the child has failed to reach the phallic level. It never happens that the libido expresses itself wholly in the manifestations of the latest phase of development; some part of it invariably remains attached to earlier modes of expression. To ensure normality it is sufficient if the major proportion of the libido reaches the organization appropriate to the age of the child. The manifestations of this level then predominate over the earlier ones, though never as fully as the genital tendencies of adult sex life predominate over the pregenital tendencies.

There are more reliable data on which an opinion about the libidinal development of a child could, theoretically, be based: namely the fantasies that accompany the child's masturbatory activities. But practically this is of little help for the diagnosis. Such fantasies are always hidden, very frequently unconscious, and only laid bare in the course of an analysis, not in a consultation.

(b)   The intactness of libidinal development.

The libidinal normality of a child is judged also according to the fate of the individual component instincts. We would not expect any of the component instincts to be completely absent from the clinical picture (if the child is neither organically nor mentally deficient) except as a sign of severe neurotic disturbance.

But again, individual variation is sufficiently great for us to be cautious in our conclusions. The component instincts (including tendencies like exhibitionism and scoptophilia), or rather their manifestations, are not visible to the same degree in all children; nor does any individual child present us with equally clear pictures of all the different libidinal tendencies. Usually some of the component instincts are clearly in evidence, others remain faint and shadowy. With some children, cruelty, exhibitionism, or greed, may appear to have played no appreciable part in their lives; with others these urges may be unmistakable, while other component instincts are seen only on closer observation. Individual differences of this nature are based on constitutional factors, and are not due to neurotic interference; but they create points of special libidinal interests in the child's life, so-called fixation-points, which play an important rôle in later neurotic development.

(c)   Neurotic interference with libidinal development; the factor of spontaneous recovery.

Neurosis in an adult damages the intactness of the sex organization; an infantile neurosis also interferes directly with the forward movement of the libido.

In the beginning stage of a neurotic conflict the libido flows backward (regression), and attaches itself once more to earlier libidinal wishes (fixation point), in order to avoid anxiety that has arisen on a higher level of sex organization. The ego of the child thus finds itself confronted with primitive desires (oral, aggressive, anal), which it is not prepared to tolerate. It defends itself against the instinctual danger with the help of various mechanisms (repression, reaction-formation, displacements, etc.), but if such defense is unsuccessful, neurotic symptoms arise which represent the gratification of the wish, distorted in its form by the action of the repressive forces. While these symptoms persist, they are the central expression of the child's libidinal life.

From the developmental point of view it is immaterial whether such symptoms are a little more or a little less painful. What counts is that with the onset of the neurotic disturbance the libido has been arrested in its course. Instead of moving on toward more adult levels, it has been forced backward, and important gains have thereby been relinquished. Qualities and achievements that depend directly on the stage of libido development are lost. The child who regresses to the oral level, for instance, simultaneously reverts to the emotional attitudes connected with it: he becomes once more insatiable, exacting, impatient for wish fulfilment, "like a baby". Regression from the phallic to the anal-sadistic level destroys the hardly acquired attributes of generosity, manliness and protectiveness, and substitutes for them the domineering possessiveness that belongs to the earlier libidinal level. But progress is made at the same time in other spheres that are not influenced directly by the neurosis. The child grows bigger and more intelligent, and his development becomes inharmonious since this growing body and mind are tied to an instinctual and emotional life that cannot keep pace with it. The need for treatment seems urgent at this stage, not because the neurosis is in itself so severe, but because the presence of the neurosis hinders libido development.

On the other hand, this impression of a serious interruption is frequently misleading. After a shorter or a longer duration, symptoms may suddenly lose importance; the fixation may dissolve and the libido, freed from restrictions, may resume its normal progressive flow. The child has, as the popular saying goes, "outgrown" his neurosis, and therapeutic help has become unnecessary.

As analysts, who collect their evidence from adult cases, we do not readily believe in the spontaneous cure of a neurosis, and we view such appearances with distrust when they are brought to our notice. We know that neuroses can, at best, change their manifestations. Neurotic anxiety, for instance, can disappear, but only to reappear later, centered around a different object or topic. Changes in life circumstances can alleviate a neurotic condition in various ways. Neurotic suffering can be exchanged for ordinary suffering; for instance, the real loss of an object through death can take the place of the imagined loss of love from that object, and thus make a particular symptom unnecessary. A masochistic desire, which at one time manifests itself in neurotic symptoms, can at another time find satisfaction in organic illness. Inhibitions or obsessional restrictions that cripple a patient's activity may be given up when he is, for instance, in prison or in a concentration camp, that is, when he lives under crippling and inhibiting circumstances. A neurosis can further be relieved through separation from the love-object onto which it has transferred its central issues; but such relief will be temporary, and the neurosis will soon reestablish itself completely when a new transference has taken place. Happenings of this kind, though often described as spontaneous cures, are merely slight fluctuations within the neurotic arrangement itself.

On the basis of our theoretical knowledge, there is little reason to expect the neuroses of adults to clear up spontaneously. The neurotic symptom, as a compromise between two opposing forces, can only alter when decisive changes take place, either in the instinctual tendencies or in the ego and superego of the individual. Neither kind of change is likely to happen in the adult. The infantile wish, to which the patient has regressed, will remain potent. The ego will keep its repressive energy (unless a serious deteriorating process sets in). Furthermore, the whole process is anchored in the unconscious, and therefore not accessible to influence from conscious levels.

This is the point at which the conditions of an infantile neurosis are completely different. The child's libido organization is, as described before, in a fluid state, the libido moving on continuously toward new positions. A component instinct that is charged with libido in one phase may be devoid of interest at another. The child need not remain hopelessly tied to any fixation-point to which it has been led back through regression. If the fixation is not excessively strong, the libido has a good chance of freeing itself again, carried forward by the next wave of development. This possibility is greatest at times when the biological urges are of especial strength, as they are at the onset of the phallic phase (four to five years) and of puberty.

It is a common error to believe that as a result of the strengthening of the ego children become more neurotic in the latency period. On the contrary, the latency period marks a definite decrease in infantile neurosis. At that time the strength of the infantile sex wishes dies down, partly for biological reasons, partly owing to the frustration of the child's oedipal wishes. This lessens the need for defense against the instincts and alters the compromise-formations between ego and id which lie at the root of symptom formation. Many infantile neuroses therefore disappear at approximately that date, their spontaneous cure being due to these quantitative changes.

Puberty is rightly regarded as a time when numerous neurotic disturbances may be expected to appear. It is less well known that puberty also removes certain neurotic symptoms that are typical for the years preceding it. This refers especially to the neurotic behavior of boys who all through early childhood and latency fight against repressed wishes of a passive feminine kind. Their behavior is characterized by anxiety, due to their repressed castration wishes, and by a superficial and noisy aggressiveness which is a reaction against the underlying passivity. Puberty brings a biological increase in genital masculinity which, while it lasts, puts the anal, passive and feminine tendencies out of action. This is a spontaneous cure in the real sense of the word: the neurosis not merely changes its form, but the underlying unconscious forces themselves undergo alterations. It depends on future developments whether the former constellation of instincts will come to the fore again in adult life; in this case the neurotic defense against it will be reinstated.

There are other typical examples of infantile neuroses which almost invariably disappear before adolescence: bedwetting, and some of the common eating disturbances. They also are swept away by the libidinal changes before or in puberty. Certain disorders affecting sexual potency, and certain nervous disorders of the stomach may, much later, appear in their stead, if the adult genital sex organization is not strong enough to maintain itself.

To sum up: the decision as to whether a child needs therapeutic help or not can be based on the state of the libido development. An infantile neurosis can be treated as a transitory disorder as long as the libido organization of the child remains fluid and shows progressive tendencies. Infantile neuroses disappear whenever the normal forward movement of the libido is strong enough to undo neurotic regression and fixation. When the libido constellations become rigid, stabilized, and monotonous in their expressions the neurosis is in danger of remaining permanently. This means that treatment is indicated.

This view, that child analysis should be used only in cases where there is slight or no hope for a spontaneous recovery, is opposed to that of many analysts who hold that child analysis may be used prophylactically to remove the pathogenic fixation-points.

3. *Neurotic Interference with Ego Development.*

The threat which the occurrence of an infantile neurosis constitutes for the libido development is so apparent that it has not escaped notice. The same danger is less obvious in relation to the development of the ego. On the contrary, it is generally believed that neurotic development in children is associated with an especially good, frequently an especially early, blossoming of this side of the child's personality. It is left an open question whether it is the infantile neurosis that, in one of its results, overemphasizes the side of the ego forces, or whether it is an early ripening of the ego that predisposes the child to a severe infantile neurosis.

The following is an attempt to examine the question whether a childhood neurosis helps or harms the development of the ego; what the interactions are between the two processes; and whether the degree of harm done to the ego can serve as a further indication for the therapeutic use of child analysis.

(a) The quantitative factor in ego development.

A neurosis can affect the ego quantitatively, that is, in its strength.

The term "ego-strength" is not meant to denote an absolute quantity of ego forces which are, in themselves, not measurable. It refers to the relative efficiency of the ego with regard to the contents of the id (instinctual drives) and to the forces of the environment with which the ego has to deal. This ego strength varies repeatedly in the course of normal development. In the beginning of life the instinctual drives are of overwhelming strength and the first crystallizations of an ego are completely under their domination and at their service. The child's growing awareness of the outside world, the beginnings of his ability to retain and connect memory traces, to foresee events, to draw conclusions from them, etc., are used exclusively for the purpose of instinct gratification. The better the ego development of an infant, the better are his chances to gratify his desires and to use the outside world for the fulfilment of his wishes. This undisputed reign of the instincts does not outlast early infancy. As a result of his strong emotional ties to the parents, the child soon begins to consider their wishes, which are frequently in opposition to his own. To the degree in which he is able to identify with his parents, his ego develops hostile attitudes towards his instinctual demands and attempts to oppose and manage them. Simultaneously the ego begins to correlate conflicting emotions and tendencies instead of giving alternate expression to them. This means suppressing one or the other side of them (love or hate, active or passive desires, etc.), and creates new conflicts between ego and id. But although all these efforts are made by the ego to assert itself against the instincts, no real ego superiority is established in the first period of childhood. The pull of wish-fulfilment is still too strong, and the principle that governs the child's life remains to a large extent the pleasure principle. It is only the final frustration of the oedipal wishes, with the consequent fading out of the early libido organizations, that changes the situation decisively in favor of ego strength. While the sex drives remain latent (latency period), the ego assumes superiority, directs the actions of the child, establishes the reality principle, and effects the first real adaptation to the exigencies of the outside world. Ego and id have now reversed their positions. But the new order is by no means permanent. Ego superiority is overthrown again as soon as the first signs of adolescence appear. Because of the biological increase in pregenital tendencies during pre-puberty, and genital tendencies during puberty, the libidinal forces rise in strength. Throughout adolescence ego forces and id forces struggle with each other for the upper hand, a combat that is responsible for many of the conflicting and abnormal manifestations of that period. It is impossible to predict before the end of adolescence whether the individual will emerge from this struggle with a strong or a weak ego, but this uncertainty is normal and necessary. It is essential for the development of a rich and vivid personality that this part of character formation (the establishment of a definite proportion between id strength and ego strength) should not be terminated too early. The changing flow of libidinal development should, while it lasts, find scope for at least transitory expression without being too crippled by the dictates of a strong ego. On the other hand, every new gain in the ego achievements should contribute something toward altering the balance between ego and id and mark a further step in perfecting a sensible management of the instincts.[4] The personality of the child will develop as long as the relationship between ego and id remains fluid and changeable.

The incidence of an infantile neurosis acts like a calcification in the middle of a living organism. Every neurotic symptom represents an attempt to establish an artificial balance between an instinctual wish and the repressive forces of the ego, a balance that is rigid and, once established, not open to correction. If symptoms multiply and the neurosis organizes itself into a coherent structure, the whole relationship between ego and id becomes hopelessly paralyzed.

Another and more direct manner in which infantile neuroses reduce ego strength is due to the regression that occurs invariably at the beginning of symptom formation. Libidinal regression is always accompanied by a certain amount of ego regression; ego strength is to a degree dependent on the phase of libido development. The oral organization of the libido, for instance, always goes together with a special urgency of wishes and impatience for wish-fulfilment. That means, practically speaking, that a child who regresses from the genital to the oral level simultaneously regresses from ego strength to ego weakness. Or, to put it differently, regression from the genital to the oral level implies regression from the reality principle to the pleasure principle.

The neurotic child may thus, at first glance, appear to possess a strong ego. But this appearance is misleading. The child's ego is committed to definite and irreversible attitudes toward instinctual drives, in order to maintain the delicate balance necessary for symptom formation. But his ego is in reality weaker than that of a normal child since the id forces have gained a more or less lasting victory in the disguise of symptom formation.

(b)   The qualitative factor in ego development.

From the first months of life onward the ego develops from a mere receiving station for dimly perceived stimuli into an organized center where impressions are received, sorted out, recorded, interpreted, and where appropriate action is undertaken. A separate part of the ego fulfils the task of supervising thoughts and actions from

4. A little girl of four-and-a-half, when asked to behave and control herself nicely on a certain occasion in the absence of her nurse, answered sensibly: "I think I can manage."

a moral point of view (superego). The essential ego functions in this respect are: *testing of inner and outer reality; building up of memory; the synthetic function of the ego;* and *ego control of motility.* All through childhood a maturation process is at work which, in the service of an increasing knowledge of and adaptation to reality, aims at perfecting these functions, at rendering them more and more objective and independent of the emotions until they can become as accurate and reliable as a mechanical apparatus. In the last resort, an individual's efficiency in life (under less civilized conditions, his chance of survival) is determined by the perfection or imperfection of these ego functions.

But simultaneously with this maturation process another, even more powerful, tendency is at work in the child. These ego achievements are wholly acceptable to him as far as they serve instinct gratification and provide some mastery over the environment. But it soon becomes evident that this new way of functioning brings at least an equal, if not an overwhelmingly greater amount of pain, discomfort and anxiety. Each one of the new functions has its disagreeable consequences. The faithful testing and recording of outer reality reveals to the ego the existence of countless alarming possibilities; the outer world is shown to be full of frustrations, disappointments, threats. The testing of the child's own inner reality reveals the existence of forbidden and dangerous tendencies which offend the child's conception of himself and therefore cause anxiety. The sorting and interpretation of stimuli as they arrive leads to a sharp distinction between the child's own self and the objects outside; before this faculty is developed, the infant has been able to feel himself at one with the world around, to ascribe anything pleasurable to himself, and anything disturbing as "outside". The development of the function of memory is equally. disturbing, since it aims at retaining memory traces irrespective of their quality; the infant gives preference to pleasant memories and rejects painful ones. The synthetic function of the ego, which aims at unifying and centralizing all mental processes, is opposed to the free and easy manner in which the infant lives out its most divergent emotions and instinctual urges either simultaneously or alternately; as, for instance, loving his parents, and hating them; being a passive baby in need of comfort from its mother at one moment, only to confront her as an active lover and protector the next moment; destroying possessions, and then immediately afterwards desiring and treasuring them passionately. Lastly, a strict ego control of motility permanently deprives the instinctual forces in the id of their former free expression.

Strictly objective functioning of this nature heightens the feeling of tension and anxiety for the ego. On the one side, the libidinal forces in the id, represented by the component instincts of infantile sexuality, are felt to clamor for satisfaction. On the other side, the child is aware of the threat of punishment from the adults in the outside world, or of the loss of their love, should he indulge in forbidden sexual or aggressive wishes and actions. From the side of the superego, i.e., from within, the ego is flooded with feelings of guilt and self-criticism whenever it fails to live up to its own standards.

The weak and immature ego of the child fails to stand up to the impact of these dangers. It consequently attempts to undo its own achievements as fast as they are made. It tries *not* to see outside reality as it is (*Denial*); not to record and make conscious the representatives of the inner urges as they are sent up from the id (*Repression*); it overlays unwelcome urges with their opposites (*Reaction-Formation*); it substitutes for painful facts pleasurable fantasies (escape into *Fantasy-life*); it attributes to others the qualities it does not like to see in itself (*Projection*); and it appropriates from others what seems welcome (*Introjection*); etc.

Normally these methods are used to a moderate degree in every childhood to defend the ego against anxiety. A certain retrograde movement in the development of the ego achievements is, therefore, the rule. It does no more than to create a certain amount of subjective and faulty functioning, which is usually overcome with the beginning of the latency period when the position of the ego is strengthened and anxiety lessens.

But events shape themselves differently if acute neurotic conflicts intervene either in the preoedipal phases or during the oedipal phase. In the face of excessive anxiety the ego makes excessive and more lasting use of the defense mechanisms at its disposal. Therefore, the harm done to the ego functions becomes considerably greater and is of more permanent importance.

Examples of the excessive use of the method of *denial of outer reality* can be found when the child is confronted with the facts of the difference of the sexes, which give rise to penis envy and castration anxiety. Under the pressure of these painful emotions the ego waives *reality testing,* pretends to see what is not there (for instance, a penis on the mother), or ignores what is in plain view. (A little girl, on watching her newborn brother's penis, said, with satisfaction, to her sister: "He has a belly-button just like us," thus remarking on their similarity instead of admitting the obvious difference between them.) Denial makes still greater inroads on reality testing where the central subject of observation of parental intercourse is concerned. Under the influence of their oedipal jealousy children will refuse to realize that their parents have a sex life with each other, and will uphold this denial in spite of all other advances in knowledge of biological facts, of propagation among animals, and even of the facts of life when they concern strangers. Evidence of such denial can be found in countless fairy tales, myths, religious beliefs, etc. Under neurotic conditions it frequently outlives the latency period and adolescence and continues into adult life. But even normally, as long as children avoid admitting reality in this all important respect, they are not free to use their full intelligence for becoming acquainted with outer reality. (An adult neurotic, by profession a medical man, began his analytic treatment with the following words: "My parents never had anything to do with each other." Since he was a child in a long line of brothers and sisters, there was evidently no truth in his statement. But it contained the key to his neurotic and bizarre behavior which made his dealings with the real world somewhat unpredictable and unreliable.)

Examples of excessive use of the method of *repression* are by now common knowledge. Repression occurs invariably when a young child finds himself faced with the intolerable frustration of the component instincts of his early instinctual life. It is easier for the child to stand the clamoring for satisfaction that comes from the id when the representatives of the instincts are refused admittance into consciousness, i.e., are repressed. Since all instinctual manifestations are interrelated, such repression extends in ever-widening circles until ego and id become entirely estranged from each other. What the neurotic child knows about his own inner life is frequently negligible; at best it is scanty and faulty. *Awareness of inner reality* cannot be maintained under these conditions.

The most instructive instance of neurotic defense doing harm to an ego function is the complete obliteration of childhood memories due to repression. To uphold belief in the asexuality of the parents, or to blot out coitus observations, or scenes of seduction, etc., the memory traces of whole periods of life are removed from consciousness, thus damaging the objectivity of the function of memory, and disrupting and disconnecting the individual's relationship to his own past. Normally all children remove the memory traces of their earliest years in this manner, to spare themselves the memory of their primitively aggressive, and crudely sexual infantile reactions; but this infantile *amnesia* should not cover more than the first years of life. (A young neurotic girl was able to remember most of her past childhood, with the exception of two years during the latency period, the memory traces of which were completely absent. Her analysis revealed that during this period her widowed mother had been unfaithful to her dead father, a fact the child had tried to ignore.)

Excessive use of *projection* is usually made by neurotic children when dealing with their hostile feelings against father or mother. They either ascribe these tendencies to the parents themselves, to another child or to an animal, etc. When used in a normal degree this defense method is an important transitory help in the development of the personality. Used excessively it once more blurs the newly-made distinction between the child himself and the world outside. (A child of two-and-a-half years was subject to violent temper tantrums directed against her mother substitute; she would shout, throw things at her, etc. When she began to make attempts to overcome these tantrums, she suddenly got hold of the rocking-horse of the nursery, rushed it against the nurse, shouting: "Naughty Jane, Jiji bit you now." When the nurse said: "Oh no, the horse will not bite me, it is not cross with me, but you are," the child laughed and said: "No, me not cross, only Jiji.") Similarly children ascribe their bad feelings to the "big bad wolf", or some other outside agency, with the result that they themselves can feel all "good" and loving.

Another defense method for dealing with the negative side of the child's ambivalence against the parents is the *splitting of the personality*, with the resulting damage for the *synthetic function* of the ego. For certain periods many children go so far as to invent special names for their "good" and their "bad" selves, though normally they retain the knowledge that both the good and the bad child are themselves, with a vague feeling of responsibility remaining for both. In an outstanding case of this kind, a girl of six referred to her bad side consistently as "the devil" and had ceased to feel any conscious responsibility for the devil's thoughts or actions.

One of the most important advances in ego development during early childhood is the *control of actions* by the ego itself. This is withdrawn when too many actions become invested with symbolic sexual or aggressive significance. The ego then tries first to inhibit them and if unsuccessful, withdraws from certain forms of activity altogether, leaving the control of motility in these respects to the forces of the id. The child then presents a picture, partly of *inhibitions*, partly of unreliable, unpredictable functioning, that is not adapted to reality. (A little girl of three was hardly able to use her hands for any practical occupation. She would stretch them out in front of her, uplifted as if to ward off actions, her fingers spread wide apart. In this manner she kept herself from committing the aggressions against her little companions with which her mind was constantly occupied in fantasy.) Many boys are greatly disturbed in their urinary function by guilt feelings that arise when they have to touch the genital. They withdraw from action because for them it implies the wish to masturbate. A boy of eight was unable to use a knife at table since he had the fantasy of cutting his mother with it; but withdrawing from this action was of little help since his aggressive wishes dominated other acts also; for instance, holding a stick, etc.; accordingly, many activities suddenly took on the meaning of passionate attacks on his mother.

The common *escape into fantasy*, which is of the greatest help to every child, is used excessively under the pressure of neurotic conflicts, and can then become the basis for a complete withdrawal and estrangement from the real world and its demands.

This interference with the ego functions is of greater importance in childhood than under otherwise similar conditions in the adult neurosis. It occurs while the maturation of the ego is still in process. The function that is most directly attacked by infantile neurosis is kept back from further development, at least temporarily, while the other ego achievements continue to mature. Accordingly ego development becomes one-sided and inharmonious.

The particular defense mechanism employed and the consequent ego damage depends on the type of infantile neurosis. In the various forms of hysterical neurosis anxiety is warded off predominantly with the help of repression. This may account for the fact that children of the hysterical type frequently possess a faulty and unreliable memory with consequent difficulties in studying: damage to the function of memory has spread further than the emotionally dangerous memories with which the ego tried to interfere. Obsessional children usually have an excellent and undisturbed memory; but, owing to the excessive ego interference with the free expression of their anal-sadistic tendencies, they are estranged from their own emotions, and are considered cold and unresponsive, even when other than these primitive aggressive-sexual manifestations are concerned. Phobic children deal with their anxieties by withdrawal from their danger-points. They tend to withdraw from many forms of activity altogether and give up motility, far beyond the original range of neurotic danger. As a consequence they frequently become altogether retiring and clumsy in their actions, with passionate and unpredictable outbreaks whenever the motility is governed by the id forces instead of the ego.

With this point of view in mind, it may be possible to assess the seriousness of an infantile neurosis, and with it the need for treatment, in an indirect way, through the harm done to the ego functions by the extensive use of one or several of the neurotic defense mechanisms. There is no reason for alarm or interference when one or another of the ego achievements are reduced or retarded in their development or temporarily put out of action. This is a normal and inevitable occurrence. But such retardations may become lasting; or several, or all, of the important ego functions may be severely attacked at the same time. If a child shows a faulty knowledge of the outer world, far below the level of his intelligence; if he is seriously estranged from his own emotions, with blank spaces in the remembrance of his own past beyond the usual range of infantile amnesia, with a split in his personality, and with motility out of ego control; then there can be little doubt that the neurosis is severe and that it is high time to take therapeutic action.

Conclusion

In the foregoing pages an attempt has been made to find indications for the therapeutic use of child analysis not so much in the neurotic manifestations themselves as in the bearing of these manifestations on the maturation processes within the individual child. Emphasis is shifted thereby from the purely clinical aspects of a case to the developmental aspect.

When diagnosing cases from this point of view, the child analyst or child psychiatrist has to be as intimately familiar with the normal sequence of child development as he is with the neurotic or psychotic disturbances of it. He is actually faced with the task of judging the normality of the developmental process itself.

It is an open question how much help diagnosis of this kind can receive from academic psychology. The various mental tests so far devised assess circumscribed aspects of ego development; they are nearly indispensable in cases where a differential diagnosis has to be made between mental deficiency and defective awareness of reality through excessive denial. The Rorschach test goes furthest in inquiring into the state of libido development and its disturbances. Other tests try to disclose the fantasy life of the individual. It is to be expected that in time further testing methods will be devised to cover an increasingly wider range of factors on which a satisfactory diagnosis of infantile neuroses can be based.

At present our analytic knowledge about the developmental processes on the libido as well as on the ego side is still very incomplete. Besides, too little is known about the interactions between them, beyond the fact that a precocious ego is especially intolerant when coupled with the primitive pregenital component instincts. We are only slowly learning to distinguish the various characteristics that mark a neurotic disturbance as either transitory or as permanent, although this distinction is of extreme importance for our diagnoses. Not enough is known about the relation between the development of the purely intellectual factors and the other important functions of the ego, etc.

Until these gaps are filled by more clinical data from the psycho-analytic investigation of individual children, it will be necessary not to confine examinations to short cuts of any kind, helpful as they may be in furnishing additional data, but to adhere to the former, lengthy, laborious, and groping methods of individual approach.

CLINICAL NOTES ON CHILD ANALYSIS

By BERTA BORNSTEIN (New York) [1]

About twenty years ago the suggestion that the training of every analyst should include child analysis was seriously discussed. Since every analytic case leads into the conflicts of childhood, and since every neurosis in an adult is based on a childhood neurosis, this idea seemed not without justification. The analyst who had had first-hand experience with children would be on less strange ground in analyzing adults. His understanding of the adult's unconscious would be increased and it would be easier for him to comprehend the strange character of the transference reactions. Since the unconscious is less concealed and seems to be less repressed in children we expected to penetrate to material of the very first years, which in adult analysis could only be concluded and reconstructed. However, this expectation was disappointed. The suggestion to analyze children was taken up only by a few analysts, but even these dropped the experiment after one or two cases. It was difficult for them to find any access to the child. The child neither talked of his current experiences nor seemed in the least interested in his past. He even brought far fewer recollections than the adult patient. And worst of all, the adult analyst felt helpless against the child's refusal to bring free associations.

In brief, the dissimilarities between the analysis of an adult and the analysis of a child are more striking than the similarities. The differences are obviously rooted in the conscious attitude of the child. The id of the child and of the adult are alike, but the ego of each is unlike. This unlikeness makes it necessary to approach a child differently from an adult.[2]

This necessity for a different approach becomes apparent from the beginning of the analysis. The child patient is often brought into

---

1. From a course of lectures given at the Institute of Psychoanalysis, 1942-1943.

2. A. Freud, *Introduction to the Technique of Child Analysis* (Vienna, 1927), Nervous and Mental Disease Monograph, 48, 1929.

151

analysis against his will. Frequently it is not he, but his environment, that suffers from his symptoms; and even if he does he may reject our help. The analyst and his procedure are strange to him. As a little girl put it, "The minute I saw you I knew that I was trapped."

The child's distrust of the analyst has to be replaced by a positive relationship that will enable the child to sustain the trials of analysis. In this preparatory period, we try to approximate the young patient's situation as closely as possible to the conditions that have proved helpful in adult analysis. We try to change his external compliance into inner willingness, we try to convey to him the insight he lacks. The means we employ vary, of course, in each case, and many an analytic session may not resemble any therapeutic procedure. We follow the child's interests and participate in his activities and thus, with a minimum of direct questions, we are introduced into his world, and are enabled to observe his attitudes and reactions.

Occasionally our endeavors to give the child insight are of no avail. Ruth, who introduced herself with the words quoted above, had stopped bedwetting the very moment she heard her mother make the first appointment with me over the telephone. Since she did not suffer from her character difficulties she could not understand why she had to be treated. She had consciously decided not to cooperate and to deceive me in every way. As some of her symptoms appeared and disappeared independently of our interviews, I never failed to congratulate her on achieving these miraculous cures, assuring her that I hoped sometime to learn from her how they came about. Two years later the girl confessed that she had attributed the disappearance of her bedwetting to some magic power of mine. Secretly she hoped that by a similar trick I would make her give up her masturbation as well. On this basis of mutual esteem for each other's magic powers, Ruth fought her way into analysis.

The most startling difference between the analysis of adults and the analysis of children concerns the phenomenon of transference. As a rule the child does not develop a transference neurosis; and therefore we frequently are deprived of many of the rather loose transference reactions which in adult analysis lead back to childhood material that cannot be verbalized. It is important to point out that in psychoanalytic literature in general, and even in Freud's writings, the word *transference* is used with various meanings. Two of them may be more clearly differentiated. Transference, in the broader sense, may comprise all that goes on in the relation between patient and analyst; in a narrower sense it may mean certain emotional attitudes of the patient to his analyst that repeat patterns of his infantile relationship to his parents. Transference in both senses occurs in child analysis. The analyst may become the target of many of the child's sexual or aggressive impulses, and occasionally and within a limited scope he may play the part of one of the parents. And yet, as a rule, no transference neurosis in the proper sense of the term arises.[3] The symptoms are not centered around the analyst's person nor around happenings during the analytic session.

There is good reason why the child does not develop a transference neurosis in the strict sense. There is no need for him to repeat his reaction vicariously since he still possesses his original love-objects, his parents, in reality.[4]

We are also deprived of the other main access to unconscious material, since the child is unable and unwilling to produce free associations. The analysis of his play supplies a partial substitute for these free associations.

The following episodes from a case history will illustrate what this method has to offer, and at the same time show why we prefer not to interpret play directly.

The play of an eight-year-old boy indicated from the very beginning of his analysis his oedipal problems, his sexual excitement, and his subsequent fears. For a period of weeks he assumed the roles of captain, general, or director of a theatre, in his hour. Usually the general was killed in action, the captain drowned while saving a ship, the theatre director prevented from receiving the applause of the audience as the theatre burned down just at the moment when he appeared on the stage.

In these actions the boy revealed the conscious wish to be a grown-up man, and his unexpressed doubts concerning his capacity ever to reach that stage. We could only surmise, however, that the catastrophe that took place in his game stemmed from his unconscious hostility against his father. One day the boy asked me to take a part in his play and prefaced his request with an explanation: "Let's play that you are a friend of mine, my girl friend, I am on leave and I am twenty-one years old. Let's pretend you give me some whiskey and we smoke cigarettes. But while we are pretending, let's make a real fire." He immediately started to do so. He did not include the usual catastrophe in

3. See B. Rank, "Where Child Analysis Stands Today", *American Imago*, 3, 1942, p. 41 ff.

4. Melanie Klein and her followers assume that the absence of transference neurosis in child analysis is due to the nature of the introductory period. (See "Symposium on Child Analysis", *International Journal of Psycho-Analysis*, VIII, 1927.) However, it seems more accurate to say that while the introductory period may disturb our interpretations of the child's transference reactions, it does not account for the absence of a transference neurosis.

his play this time, but it showed up in an unforeseen way, namely, in a slip: while preparing the fire he broke an ash tray. He was terrified and inconsolable to a degree quite out of proportion to the incident, to my reaction, or to the reaction he might expect from his parents at such an occurrence. He pleaded with me not to let anyone know about this incident, thus betraying that the breaking of the ash tray had an unconscious meaning for him. It had aroused his fear of retaliation which became clearer when we learned later that his idea of sexual intercourse was linked up with fantasies of violence, to overwhelm a woman, to break into her and to injure something in her.

After the incident the boy ceased playing and was depressed. Suddenly he said, "I am afraid I'll never grow up. Some grown-ups are grown-up when they are born. Or at least they are strong as soon as they are born. Or at least they have the intelligence of grown-ups. And some people have to be told what to do until they die." He elaborated these thoughts, but finally ended the session with a rebellion against the idea of always remaining a little boy. He withdrew the statement about people who are born as adults, saying, "After all, that can't be. No one can be born grown up." Suddenly he burst out in anger, "And I do not believe in anything any more. I do not believe in Columbus, I do not believe in Washington, and I do not even believe in Abraham Lincoln."

During the following sessions he replaced the dramatic play of being a great man by verbal elaborations of his conflict about the existence of Washington and Lincoln. During this period he developed a strong interest in biographies. His believing or not believing in great men depended on the daily variations in his relationship with his father. If he was on good terms with his father, he was interested in the life histories of his heroes and insisted that even the deeds of mythological heroes were true. If he had any reason to be dissatisfied with his father, because the latter, for example had censured him for something, he doubted the existence of the great men. We understand therefore that his not-believing in great men means: I cannot and do not want to bear the comparison between them and me, between my father and myself. By denying their existence he removes them, spares himself the comparison, and expresses in this mild manner his death wish against his father, which at this time was remote from his conscious mind.

His ambivalent attitude toward his father did not come closer to consciousness for a long time. One day he again did not believe in Washington; we had just discussed the war situation and he said, "There is only one way Hitler could lose this war. If his own people turn against him." I misunderstood him, thinking that he was speaking about a revolution against Hitler, but he corrected me. "I don't mean the people who don't know him, the common German people. I mean, what would happen if Hitler's family turned against him because he is so bad—his brother or his sister or his uncle, or even his parents." And then the child pondered, "Can a person be so bad that even his parents turn against him? Do you think that Hitler's parents would? But what if they really hate him?" He shuddered with fear and said, "Imagine, his father would come and take a knife and shoot him in the back, maybe when he does not know it." Then, checking with reality again, he decided, "I do not believe a father could do that, not even to Hitler." In the conversation following we learned about a few incidents that proved to him his own ambivalent feelings toward his father. When I asked him, "Can you imagine that a son may sometimes think of doing something evil to his father?" he became pensive and answered, "Well, he may think of it but he will never do it."

All this child's libidinal wishes, doubts, and fears were indicated in his game. Their specific content, however, showed up in detailed form only later, in his reaction to the accident with the ash tray, in his discussions, and in the use of his historic interest. The disaster in his play may have expressed his death wish against his father as well as his fear of retaliation. The latter fear came unambiguously to the fore in his fantasy about Hitler, and further showed the manner in which he tried to ward off the death wish. He projected his own aggressive impulses onto his father: It was not he, the son, who was turning against his father, but the father who turned against the son. The question, "Could a father come with a knife and shoot his son in the back?" and the subsequent fear of being attacked from the back by men on a dark street, indicated his longing for passive homosexual submission to his father. This, too, may have been suggested in the child's play—expressed by the inevitable debacle—but it could be discerned only in retrospect. At the time of the play, it was even more remote from the boy's consciousness than was the aggression stemming from his normal oedipus complex.

While we did not interpret the boy's play actions we were able to give explanations of his ambivalent attitude toward his father in the discussion of general problems and of specific incidents at home and during the analytic hour. One day, for instance, when I insisted on his refraining from hitting me or building fires, he grabbed a cigarette and smoked it defiantly. Soon his mood turned into elation, as he concentrated on producing an ash stick as long as possible without letting the ash drop. At that time the child had already gained insight into the sexual pleasure he experienced in gradually increasing his tension by provoking dangerous situations. Thus we ventured an interpretation, pointing to his fear of erection and the damage he expected from it. The child's response led to remembering incidents that had caused this fear, namely, his active castration tendency toward his father. He suddenly remembered that his father occasionally used to smoke "long ash sticks" at his demand. "But once, you see," the boy said, "I just couldn't help it; by mistake, by pure accident, I kicked Daddy and the long ash stick fell down, all over his suit. And was he mad at me." In telling the story he felt amused, but also criticized the lack of humor his father had shown on that occasion. Immediately thereafter, however, he enumerated all the kind things his father had done for him, thus protecting himself from further eruptions of his aggression against his beloved father.

The fact that material observed in the child's play actions is bound to show up in other manifestations as well, is not the only reason that makes us unwilling to give immediate and continuous interpretations.[5] Among the main reasons are the following: The multiplicity of mean-

5. The technique of child analysis as developed by Melanie Klein (*The Psycho-Analysis of Children*, International Psycho-Analytic Library, No. 22, 1932) relies on this type of interpretation.

ings in a child's play is likely to lead to misinterpretations. Without a
thorough knowledge of the child's past and present life situation a
play cannot be fully understood. It is comparable to a dream containing familiar symbols to which we lack the dreamer's associations. In
both cases we prefer to postpone the interpretation. But even if, under
favorable circumstances, the play permits detailed insight into the
child's conflicts and the ways in which he tries to master them, we
should still hesitate to interpret the symbolic play actions because of the
significance of play in general. As we know, play is the first important
step in the process of sublimation. Continuous interpretation of its
symbolic meaning is likely to upset this process before it is well established.[6] For the same reason it seems preferable not to interpret children's drawings, stories, or other forms of sublimation directly, but
instead to use them as a valuable source of information about the child.
At a later stage we may employ the knowledge gained from plays,
stories, and drawings, just as we use the knowledge gained from the
observation of his symptom-formation and his resistance.

We know from experience that the method of continuous interpretation of play action and its symbolic content may lead to an undesirable over-sexualization. I had occasion to observe a child who had
gone through such an analysis. In spite of her excellent intelligence
the girl conspicuously lacked the capacity to sublimate. She had completely sexualized her ways of play and thinking; her theoretical interests were restricted to the reproductive processes. It is true that the
patient had been a sexually over-stimulated child before she came into
her first analysis at the age of five. But the technique of symbol translation had augmented her compulsive preoccupation with sexual material, as we learned during the second analysis, begun at the age of
eleven. She introduced herself by handing me a note which read: "I
want a piece of milk chocolate—I mean, I want to have a piece of your
white breast." She was startled when she got a bar of cholocate and
when no reference was made to her abuse of analytic interpretation.
With this child I had to depreciate symbolic interpretation and the use
she made of it. The flight into symbolism and the insistence on sexual
topics was gradually understood as a facile way of eluding narcissistic
disappointments in everyday occurrences. Thus the child would talk
openly about her masturbation and about the attendant fantasies which
contained hardly distorted variations of the oedipal theme, but it was
only after considerable working through of her resistance that she

6. See review by Sandor Rado of Anna Freud, *Einführung in die Technik der Kinder-
analyse*, in *Internationale Zeitschrift für Psychoanalyse*, XIV, 1928, 4, p. 545.

became aware that the flight into obscenity relieved her of the burden of apparently unimportant experiences. For instance, her teacher once praised another girl's paper and read it to the class. It was on that day that she came to her session with her breasts prominent and asked me "Don't you think my breasts are attractive?" and then embarked on long daydreams in which men followed her on the streets.

It should be clear from this material why in her case our procedure was one of devaluating symbolic interpretation and minimizing her insistence on sexual topics.

Most cases, however, require a procedure that, at least on the surface, seems the opposite of the above. Only a long course of analysis leads to those conflicts in which sexuality is involved.

In the moods of a ten-year-old girl a certain periodicity became conspicuous. All her activities fell into a rhythmic swing between great efforts and sudden discouragement. While with all children such instances of behavior are occasionally prevalent, with Ruth they were ubiquitous. The new notebook was a model of neatness until the first blot discredited the resolve to keep it clean. A bedwetter, every new sheet was to her a challenge to a complete change; a nailbiter, she set herself a term at the end of which she would stop biting nails—for instance, as soon as her thumbnail had grown long. There was a period during which she tried to take the analytic rule seriously. When she broke the rule once she let down completely. The repetitious sequence of resolve and defeat led gradually to the idea that so general a pattern had developed from a particular root. At this time it became appropriate to discuss the problem of masturbation directly. At first, the child bluntly denied even knowing anything about masturbation. But when she asserted that her mind was completely blank she started pulling her lips with great intensity. We learned eventually that this was a new favorite game that she played with her friend. They both produced skillful poems about morons, which Ruth recited to me. Pulling lips and inventing stories about morons became for weeks the subject of analysis. Eventually the interpreting question, "Aren't you poor kids—haven't you any other fun from your bodies than pulling your lips?" brought about the confession of mutual masturbation with her friend, as well as of a form of masturbation that she practised alone and that consisted in pulling her labia. It had taken months before Ruth was convinced that she could trust me with this confession. But by the time it came she had gained insight into the character of her struggle against her impulses.

Naturally, it might have been possible to interpret the conflict earlier and to carry interpretation further. This was avoided so as not to overwhelm the child by a verbal onslaught. She might have understood what we meant but she certainly would have withdrawn the budding confidence, which we had to win with such difficulty; and we might have forced her into ever more petrified defenses. Understanding this danger, we proceeded by following one of the basic rules of

psychoanalytic technique in its adaptation to child analysis: we interpreted the defenses before we interpreted the nature of the impulse.

The struggle of the ego against the instinctual drives reaches its
peak in the latency period. The child does not want to be reminded of
his impulses and therefore conceives analysis as a danger. It is in this
period that we encounter resistance at its strongest. In contrast to
earlier conceptions, however, it is no longer regarded as a disturbing
factor. On the contrary, with two essential factors missing—free association and the transference neurosis—the utilization of the defenses
which the ego erects against the impulses has become one of our most
important tools in child analysis.

While we do not here deal with the theory of defense mechanisms in general, it seems appropriate to stress one aspect: the defenses
are not only directed against dangers coming from the environment or
against instinctual demands, but also against the affects associated with
both. If we succeed in understanding a patient's particular defense
against his impulses we are able to deduce how he will treat his affects.
Vice versa, we may deduce from his attitude toward his affects how he
will treat his instincts.[7] This consistency is especially important in
child analysis. The child may lie about his daily experiences; but by
observing his affects and their transformation we make ourselves independent of his voluntary cooperation. If emotional reactions are distorted, as, for instance, when the child shows a friendly smile instead
of disappointment, or if he says, "Who cares!" or "Skip it", when we
expect him to be unhappy, we know that the normal course of affects
and impulses has been upset. By minute observation we may gradually
learn which situations in particular cause the child to hide or to transform his affects, and—in favorable cases—with whom the child identifies in his defense.

Ruth, whom we have mentioned above, had learned to conceal her insatiable
demands which were related to her wish for a change of sex. Any present she
received was likely to reinforce this wish; and yet, she demonstrated exaggerated
enthusiasm for every little gift or favor. Her reaction was obviously insincere.
In inquiring into what had caused her to reverse the affect of disappointment
into its opposite we learned that her grandmother used to announce presents
with a high-pitched, insincere exclamation, "Look, Ruth, what Granny brought
for you!"—producing a lamb chop, for instance; clearly not what the child
expected. As the grandmother used to arouse her highest expectations, the

7. Anna Freud follows up this parallelism between a patient's defense against his
instincts and against his affects, his symptom-formation, and his resistance, in *The Ego
and the Mechanisms of Defense* (Vienna, 1936) London, 1937.

child experienced continual disappointment. But identification with the grand-mother's hypocritical attitude offered her a welcome solution for an earlier dilemma. As a little girl she had been prone to manifest her discontentment with presents, had been scolded as ungrateful, and threatened with never again getting anything. The imitation of grandmother's insincerity permitted her to reverse disappointment into over-joyfulness.

At the time of Ruth's analysis this behavior was so automatized that she was unaware of any hypocrisy. Only after we realized the origin of her attitude was she able to examine similar reactions. One of Ruth's symptoms was severe constipation and subsequent incontinence. The contrast between her external compliance with her mother's demands and the rebellious attitude retained in this symptom aroused our interest. Ruth's mother frequently interfered with her daughter's freedom. For example, she made doctor appointments without first consulting the girl. Ruth never objected and never showed signs of resentment at home. But on such days she came to her session gloomy, whiney, and pre-occupied with time. She looked at her watch every five minutes, and in feverish excitement she cancelled or changed appointments for months ahead. In explor-ing this behavior we discovered, to the child's surprise, that beneath her apparent obedience she hid hatred and fury against her mother. The rebellion, however, had been reversed into its opposite.

This reversal in her affects served us as a means of access to her fantasies which revealed that the same mechanism of reversal was applied toward her impulses. Medical examinations had always been a cause of fear to Ruth, so much so that she tried to keep injuries secret until they developed into serious infections. The expectation of medical examinations provoked masochistic fantasies. During analysis when these fantasies pressed to the fore, the usually well-mannered child ordered the servants around and spoke in a coarse and often offensive tone to her schoolmates. She was thrown into fits of rage if she lost a game. On such days her whole appearance had an air of rigidity. Occasionally this rigidity collapsed and the girl admitted that she wanted nothing more than to be a Raggedy Ann doll. She became relaxed and soft, and pleaded with me to do with her whatever I wanted: "I cannot move one muscle without your help." In her fantasies she imagined herself as a maid mistreated by her mistress, or a child pursued by witches. She thus had turned her aggressions against her mother toward herself. Sadism was reversed into masochism. What is more, every single detail was distorted by the same mechanism of reversal. Thus, in her fantasy a witch robbed her of her clothes: in reality it was she who coveted her mother's wardrobe, which she even con-sciously envied. It is interesting to observe how in her effort to ward off her unbearable masochistic fantasy the warded-off element of sadism reemerged.

With a child so frightened of analysis that she refused for many months any cooperation, it was of the greatest value to recognize one of her defense mechanisms. This opened the way into analysis and permitted us to follow the fight between ego, instinct, and affects, in actual operation. And only after the analysis of the unconscious dis-tortions of affects and impulses was she prepared to reveal her conscious lies.

In most cases, fortunately, it is somewhat simpler to recognize and to translate this mechanism. Two enuretic boys reacted to every defeat with a complete reversal of behavior. Castration fear was replaced by an exaggerated show of masculinity. Peter, at six, was unable to report in analysis that he had wet the bed; instead he would act as a policeman, drunkard, or a bull. The other boy, eight years old, would on similar occasions smoke cigarettes or produce fits of temper. In both cases aggressive outbursts were the alternative to extreme submissiveness, sadism was substituted for masochism, and vice versa.

Anna Freud has directed our attention to another mechanism of defense, namely the *identification with the aggressor*. This mechanism must be distinguished from what we usually mean by identification, the process that serves the child in subjugating his instincts. In order to maintain a positive relationship to the ambivalently loved parents the child identifies with their demands and prohibitions, a process in which part of the child's aggression is bound. But the identification with the aggressor serves a different purpose, namely to ward off a danger coming from outside. The child tries to conquer his fear of external objects by appropriating the very characteristics of the aggressor, which have aroused his anxiety. In assuming these qualities the child is changed from the one who is threatened to the one who threatens.

A five-year-old boy was frightened of wild animals; he consequently rushed into my house roaring like a tiger. For a period he called himself a poison-maker, talked about nothing else but poisoning people and prepared supposedly poisoned drinks for me. His greatest fear at this time was that of being poisoned by the bad tasting medicine his father gave him. A stereotyped yawning of his mother frightened him; he believed that she would eat him up. He imitated this gesture for weeks until the understanding he gained in analysis reduced his fear.

Sometimes the child may assume a *prophylactic* aggressive attitude; he takes over an aggression that he anticipates. This variation, although well known to us from everyday experience, is harder to trace to its causes, but its interpretation is of considerable therapeutic value.

A thirteen-year-old patient abused me for "getting too much money" for her analysis. She became increasingly agitated, finally calling me a crook and a cheat. She said she would not mind my receiving the fee for sessions in which she worked, but I should be made to refund half of the money for hours in which she cooperated only half of the time. This strange reaction was caused by an incident that had happened the previous day. She had invited a few children to a roller-skating party for which her mother had offered to pay in order to keep the children from going to the movies. The children nevertheless had suddenly decided to see a picture and the mother refused the money. Thereupon the child had bought the tickets from the change of a five-dollar bill which she was supposed to return to her father. She tried hard to forget the episode, but feeling guilty and anxious lest her behavior be condemned as embezzlement, she turned against me a criticism that she expected from her family.

Another child, Nancy, applied this mechanism consistently to every dangerous situation. After Pearl Harbor she was frightened that Japanese and Germans would invade the United States. She came proudly to her session and boasted of just having smashed the headlight of a car in front of her house. My interpreting question, "Why, are you afraid anyone would do that to your car?" caused her to reveal little by little the motives of her tension: the dangers that threatened her family if the Nazis came to this country.

Once she took off her shoes and stockings and began to pick her toes. She took the dirt to her nose and mouth and looked at me challengingly. Before I had said a word her facial expression changed from childlike indulgence to refined loftiness. When at that moment I happened to wipe my forehead with a handkerchief she remarked disapprovingly, "Aren't you ashamed to wipe your forehead with a handkerchief?" The discrepancy between her demands of others and her own behavior with regard to etiquette was striking. Although she knew exactly that certain things were not done she was not willing nor able to comply with the requirements of "manners". Fearing my disapproval, however, she anticipated my criticism, identified with the expected aggression, and reprimanded me for a trifling matter that lay in the same sphere as her own behavior.

In general, she devoted all her ingenuity to discovering faults in others, sometimes projecting her own deeds or intentions on them, but sometimes detecting weaknesses in others with photographic accuracy. In the trolley car, she counted the "deadheads" and denounced them. She entered a room in which guests were assembled and immediately would point to the one woman who had a run in her stockings. She knew that her mother fought a compulsion to scratch her head. Nancy, in a joking threat, would exclaim, "Bad habits! Mommy," until her mother burst into tears. From smallest indications she concluded what crimes other people had committed. Since the crime to her was masturbation, and since her masturbation revealed itself in such minor defects of behavior, she was constantly looking for them in others. Her turning into a detective served to ward off her almost paranoid fear of being watched and caught at her masturbation. Her intolerance of displeasure coming from outside equalled her inability to bear her feelings of guilt.

Before Nancy had resorted to the described mechanism, identification with the aggressor and projection of her own misdeeds on others, she had tried to evade feelings of guilt by crude denials of facts and actions even though she knew she had been observed. One of her symptoms at that stage was compulsive exhibitionism and stealing. She lacked a conscious feeling of guilt for both. If caught, she sometimes said, "Forget about it. Every child does it," or

"It's quite all right." Sometimes, however, she bluntly denied the facts. Consciously she was proud of being a girl. In her analysis she talked in a parrot-like manner about the advantages of being a female; she would express her disgust with boys and their ugly sex organs, but suddenly she would say, "Anyway, I, too, have a penis. Why shouldn't I? I can be just like the boys. I even am."

The *mechanism of denial* which in the phallic phase is used to ward off insight into the sex difference was preserved in full strength up to the tenth year in Nancy's case. Her denial of unpleasant realities was supported by the attitude of her home environment. Although several dramatic events occurred during Nancy's earlier childhood, her family carried on the pretense that everything ran smoothly and was in good order. What the girl denied most vehemently was the divorce of her parents and the sickness of her mother. When the latter had to be hospitalized, Nancy was never told why she disappeared. Years later, insignificant happenings, such as a weekend trip or her mother's headache, caused the girl to fear that her mother might suffer a "nervous breakdown", might become seriously ill or die. These fears led us to material showing that the girl knew of the hospitalization mentioned above and its causes. Faced in analysis with this fact she denied it and maintained the pretense that her mother only had a sore throat. In spite of this evasion her preoccupation with her mother's illness was expressed in a compulsive interest in the problem of menstruation. The adults of her environment had treated this problem with the same secretiveness with which they had treated the mother's illness. Nancy developed the idea that these two factors were related to each other, which aggravated her fear of menstruation. She denied this fear, however, and told everyone that menstruation must be the most beautiful experience in life. By incessant talking about it she tried to keep off the more dangerous subjects of adulthood and mental disease.

Usually the mechanism of denial is employed as an escape from pain intruding from the outside world. Children who use it extensively may become more and more alienated from reality, lose what power they have to correct external conditions, to overcome obstacles, and to bear any harder blows of fate. Unable to tolerate the disagreeable, they are more exposed to the consequences of even minor accidents. Thus they are driven continually to extend the mechanism of denial until they apply it to difficulties within themselves as well as to external conditions.

In the case of a seven-year-old boy all essential character traits were largely determined by this mechanism of denial.[8] It permeated his entire life pattern. We traced it from early childhood, where it was still to be considered as a normal phenomenon, to the latency

8. This case is also reported by the author in "Ein Beispiel für die Leugnung durch die Phantasie" ("An Example of Denial in Fantasy"), *Zeitschrift für psychoanalytische Pädagogik*, 1936, 4/5.

period, where it took an exaggerated form, and constituted the core of the boy's neurotic symptom.

The child was brought for treatment because of a tic and numerous fears. Though his fears were so considerable that he sometimes trembled in panic and held fast to his mother, he would assert that he was not afraid. At school, he avoided taking sides, indulged in ideas of "pacifism" and strenuously objected to contests of any kind. His peace-loving nature was ridiculed and subjected to severe trials by his school-mates. In discussing this situation the child pretended not to care about the jibes and blows of the other boys, but his efforts to belittle them were belied by rising tears. His denial was an attempt to protect himself from anxiety and suffering. Only in dreams and in occasional attacks of night terror did his anxiety break through undisguised. In his waking life he had succeeded in denying it to himself and others. He even maintained the illusion of a carefree friendship with people who seemed dangerous. He had such a relationship for several years with his father, with whom he was on a footing of affectionate comradeship. Father and son played a game of make-believe, which was essentially a mutual daydream. It played an important role in their daily life, and was continued in letters during the father's long absences from home. The game flourished especially when the boy was between four and six years old. Its theme was that a giant or wicked magician wanted to steal a little boy's toy. The giant was very crafty and cunning, but by observing his tricks closely the boy grew even more cunning than he. He always managed to get his toy back—and in such a way as not to offend the giant. In fact, they remained good friends. This capacity for keeping the giant's friendship was reported by the patient as "the cleverest thing of all".

The daydream came to an end before the child's sixth birthday. It was replaced by fantasies of a fearful monster who threatened the boy when he lay alone in his bed at night. He kept this fantasy and the fear it inspired secret, not even admitting it to his father. The fear of the monster was the end-product of an unsuccessful struggle against masturbation. Shortly before the outbreak of the fear the teacher had surprised the child in a sexual play, which consisted of a punching gesture toward the genitals of a little girl: he was reprimanded and threatened with being sent home. His fears spread, and though up to this time he had been free and sincere he now became shy and secretive. He developed a fear of death, and a tic which bore the imprint of his particular mechanism of denial. It consisted in his first closing his eyelids and then casting his eyes back until only the whites showed. With these movements he was saying symbolically, "I see no danger. Therefore no danger is present." The danger referred to his awareness of the sex difference.[9]

When the boy visited the zoo shortly after the incident in which he was reproved by his teacher, he showed great fear of wild animals. Within a few hours, however, he appeared to have mastered it. In his analytic session on that day he demonstrated his method of regaining control. He played with toy animals, talking to the lion and the tiger, of whom he had been so frightened in the morning, in a friendly, loving tone. I called his attention to the fact

9. The tic was of course over-determined. I do not here discuss its other meanings.

that he was not talking to the animals as if they were wild dangerous beasts that might leap upon him at any moment; he behaved rather as if they were very little children or birds whom he was trying to coax. Thereupon he explained very quietly that he was no longer afraid of them. "The animals are my friends, and we are on such good terms that they won't do anything to me." He did admit that they might be dangerous, but only to strangers—not to him, their good friend; they would in fact protect him against all enemies. His fear of the real animals at the zoo completely disappeared. He even became an enthusiastic visitor there. The fear had been overcome in the same way as his fear of the giant, by making friends with the dangerous object.

To summarize: the child had succeeded in denying his aggression against father and schoolmates. Enemies became friends and he could be carefree. His fear of the animals was managed similarly. He did not succeed, however, in mastering his castration fear by this mechanism. After the play with the little girl, and the reprimand, he reacted with an increase of his neurotic symptoms.

It was at the height of his neurosis that he gave the wild animals the job of protecting him against the monster. He surrounded his bed with toy animals and with imaginary ones. But the animals did not keep their promise of protection; when the monster clamored most loudly for his rights, they failed the child. For several weeks he practised his trusty denial; he kept insisting that the monster was nothing but a pet dog that would harm no one and that everyone should love. "The monster is my friend," he said, just as he had said that the giant and the wild animals were his friends. However, he could not keep up his pretense. At this stage of the analysis, when we acted the theme of the "pet dog", he took the role of the dog which its mistress should pet and speak nicely to, until the dog would suddenly sit up on his hind legs and jump against his mistress like a terrible monster with seven tails and seven heads. Then the boy screamed, "I'm a monster! I'm a monster!" A monster with seven tails and seven heads, so big that the whole earth trembled when he moved to strike, is dangerous indeed. What did the monster represent? And why could it not be placated by the pretense of friendship that had appeased the other objects of fear? Giants and animals represented objects in the outside world. The monster, however, represented the child's own frightening impulse, and symbolized his erect penis. Friendship made the monster only more demanding. What the child was afraid of when he was alone in his bed was the increase of his general sexual excitement, and the increase of his sexual demand for his mother.

We gradually learned all the strange things the little patient had to do in order to protect himself against the monster, and how his attempts were doomed to failure. He made me play the role of a sleeping child who was repeatedly disturbed by the monster. It was no use for the child to hide his head under the covers, just as it was no use for the pet dog to lie quietly in the corner. It only made the monster grow more powerful. When at night the boy called his parents for protection, they merely comforted him and said that he had an over-active imagination. Though he felt the existence of the monster distinctly, his parents did not even notice it—they treated the little boy as he made me treat the dog in the game. Their disbelief hurt him most of all. But being a "pacifist", he did not blame them for their lack of help. He even excused them, saying, "They really can't know it exists, because it is a coward. It hides from grown-ups and grows small again." It was still worse if he called the maid for help against the monster. She was quite willing to take part in playful tussling and scuffling during the day (thus contributing to his sexual excitement), but at night, when he needed her help, she only scolded and threatened him for waking her. Consequently he was forced to renounce the help of human beings. He tried to master his sexual excitement and fear by other means. He did sums when the monster approached; he recited the multiplication table, or a poem, but the monster drowned him out. Quick as he was, the monster was always quicker, and set a pace with which he could not keep up. In the language of the real struggle this meant, "My sexual excitement is so great that all my efforts to combat it are in vain. It is too big for me (my penis is erect) and I am frightened." Thus he had turned to his animal-idols, surrounded his bed with them, and tried to fall asleep. These animals, as we have seen, had once been objects of fear; they represented the parents who with their kindness and friendliness only increased his sexual desire, and his subsequent fear. It therefore was understandable why even the good, protecting animals should suddenly turn to evil ones and make common cause with the monster.

In this changing of the helpful animals into wicked beasts we see the failure of the child's attempt to call good what was wicked. He had tried to deny the existence of an enemy in order to undo his own aggressive sexual tendencies.

The same mechanism of denial was used to withstand various undesirable affects. One day the boy visited friends whose wealth made a great impression on him. He spoke with admiration of their power and was not aware of any personal envy or jealousy. Suddenly, however, he developed an intellectual interest in a better distribution of money. As he put it, "The best thing would be if money didn't exist at all . . . why should there be some people who are rich and others who are poor? Why should people have to be unhappy because they have nothing? Everyone in the world should have the same, then everyone could live in peace and friendship." (Just as the giant and child had become friends and had shared knowledge and cunning.) The next day such considerations were no longer necessary. He had by then identified with his wealthy friends to such a degree that he talked about their wealth with as much pleasure as if it were his own. As his father's knowledge had made him powerful, so the riches of his friends added to his own ego-feelings, his self esteem.

It was interesting to see his identification break down. It happened when he believed his friends' power to be shattered after a policeman stopped their car because they had violated the speed limit. When the additional news came that lightning had done some insignificant damage to a barn on their estate, the borrowed self-assurance vanished. If his friends had to suffer anxiety as he did himself, there was no longer any reason to identify with them. Simultaneously, the self-confidence which he had acquired in his identification and which had made him appear balanced for a few days, disappeared. His symptoms of anxiety returned once more, and he was again the little boy who always strove to remove the sting of unpleasant affects by denying them.

Summarizing what has been described, we may say that unpleasant reality was elaborated into a system of denial: There are no enemies, i.e., *I do not have to be afraid.* There are no bad people, only good ones, i.e., *I do not feel any conflicts.* There is no difference between rich and poor, i.e., *I do not have to be envious.* The technique of this extensive denial was as follows: Make friends with the dreaded enemy by becoming as artful and clever as he, and then you may participate in his power; make friends with the envied rich people and enjoy with them the advantages of their wealth; make friends with your own instincts, your monster. If that fails, call in the aid of protecting animals, the good superego—share and participate in the accepted morals of this world.

However, these methods of elaboration did not suffice to control high degrees of excitement, such as masturbation and sexual aggression towards the mother.

At the height of the oedipus complex, the child cannot evade his strong impulses as he has evaded the dangers of a tolerant outside world. The child's skill in elaboration by denial collapses, and he becomes neurotic. In analysis, he has to learn to reconcile the demands of the id with those of the ego. He cannot accomplish this by the mechanism of denial but only by a genuine reconciliation between the two opposing forces.

ANALYSIS OF PSYCHOGENIC ANOREXIA AND VOMITING IN A FOUR-YEAR OLD-CHILD[1]

By EMMY SYLVESTER, M.D. (Chicago)[2]

According to Abraham the decisive factors in the psychogenesis of melancholic depression are the following: The constitutional make-up, libido fixation on the oral level with sibling rivalry as an important factor, and disappointment in the mother which takes place before the dissolution of the oedipus complex. A basic disturbance in the libidinal object relation is a predisposing factor. Hostility against the mother whose loss as an object precipitates the illness remains the central conflict. The coprophagic impulses represent self-punishment and also the cannibalistic impulse to devour the destroyed object. They arise from the fixation on the oral sadistic level which necessitates strong defenses against the excessively strong impulses of sucking, biting, and chewing.

This case presents observations which, while showing striking resemblances to the psycho-somatic entity of anorexia nervosa reveals the structure of the melancholic depression as postulated by Abraham, *in statu nascendi*. The causal connection between the somatic manifestation of disturbed intake and the central psychological problem of threatened object loss is demonstrated in the onset, course, and cure of the neurosis of a four-year-old child. The disturbance of physiological function in one phase of this patient's illness assumed such dramatic proportions as to lead to prolonged and intensive exclusively medical treatment. The somatic manifestation, however, will be seen to be only a single aspect of a comprehensive emotional disturbance that closely corresponds to the reconstruction of childhood experiences as suggested by the analysis of depression in the adult.

1. Read before the Chicago Psychoanalytic Society, November, 1941, and before the American Psychoanalytic Association, May, 1942.
2. From the Department of Neuropsychiatry, Michael Reese Hospital.

When first seen in the Children's Hospital in August of 1940 the patient, a little girl four years old, was a pale, extremely emaciated child with a weight of only twenty-three pounds. The turgor of her skin was poor, her face had regular attractive features, but the expression was old beyond her years. She smiled rarely, her lips were tightly pressed together most of the time. Finger-sucking was excessive and rhythmical rocking of the body was frequently observed. She was shy, listless, and withdrawn and she hardly spoke. Her speech was babyish. From time to time, apathetic behavior changed into hyperactivity that appeared incongruous with her nearly marantic condition.

On the basis of her physical examination, the pediatricians considered the following causes for her pernicious vomiting: cyclic vomiting, congenital abnormalities of stomach and duodenum, dysentery, tuberculosis, enteritis, coeliac disease or hairball. Secondary symptoms were: anemia, avitaminosis and deficiency diarrhea. The diagnosis of high intestinal obstruction was most seriously entertained and apparently confirmed by a series of x-rays of the G. I. tract which showed spasm of the duodenum with dilatation distal to the spasm and associated stasis and regurgitation. Stomach and small intestines appeared normal. The plan of treatment was to build her up through blood transfusions and parenteral feeding in order to perform an exploratory laparotomy. Shortly after admission to the hospital the diarrhea stopped and vomiting occurred at irregular intervals only. A second series of x-rays showed no stasis or regurgitation. There was, however, irregular filling and irregular dilatation which, it was felt, were still compatible with duodenal pathology. Gavages and aspirations were prescribed through which the child went with "surprising calmness". When all the laboratory findings, including B.M.R. and blood cholesterol, were negative and the third series of x-rays failed to show any pathology while vomiting still occurred and the child continued in her debilitated condition and with her "peculiar" behavior, she was referred to the psychiatric service as a case of "possible schizophrenia in a child with undiagnosed organic pathology".

Investigation of the onset and development of her illness revealed the following: in January, 1940, six months prior to her admission to the hospital, the parents noted a personality change in the little girl; she talked less, became cranky and disobedient, was withdrawn, refused to take responsibility for her personal care. She also started to suck her fingers excessively, a habit that had been marked during her babyhood. Her appetite became irregular. She developed food fads, preferred liquids to any other diet, and while sometimes refusing nourishment, at other times she would eat voraciously. This was alarming to the mother since previously she had considered the patient to be the most mature and best trained of her four children, even more matured than the two older ones, a brother of seven, and a sister of five. Nevertheless, the mother could not allow herself to be too concerned about the patient because she was again pregnant; in January, the second month of this pregnancy, she started to vomit severely and was diagnosed as suffering from toxemia of pregnancy. Subsequently, the child was scolded severely when she developed the habit of eating dirt: from the earth in the yard and from flower pots first, then ashes from the stove, and pieces of paper. Vomiting started soon after this and was at first considered to be food poisoning. In May, 1940, when the patient already had lost some weight she was seen in the Pediatric Clinic where phenobarbital was prescribed. She was not seen again until July when the gravity of her condition led to immediate hospitalization.

These data were obtained from the mother who, at the age of twenty-five, was having her fifth pregnancy within six years. As has been indicated, the patient is the third child, has a brother three years older, a sister two years older, and two younger siblings, a brother only thirteen months younger than the patient and a baby sister whose gestation precipitated the patient's illness and who was born while the patient was under treatment. At the time of the original presentation of this material the mother was pregnant with the sixth child. Our patient, who is now well, has been uninfluenced by this despite the fact that the mother has again suffered from vomiting and toxic symptoms.

It appears that the patient, of all the children, had the shortest period of unshared baby care. The parents were very young when they were married. The mother is a shy, quiet woman who had known many deprivations in her own childhood. She felt that the patient resembled her more than any other of her children. The mother had a depressive episode with vomiting and anorexia in puberty. The patient's father has been very dependent on his older sisters and now is dependent on his wife. He is described by the mother as "gay and easy-going, more of a child than a man". He worked irregularly and on and off he was on relief. When the patient was nine months old and the mother in the fifth month of her fourth pregnancy, the husband forged relief checks and for this he was in prison until the patient was nearly three years old.

All the siblings present neurotic disorders. The older brother, age six at the time of the study, is described as serious and old for his age, too thin, quiet and withdrawn and "too easy to manage". The next child, the oldest sister, is demanding, clinging, bossy, very sure of herself and the father's favorite. The younger boy is whining, babyish, needs much attention, and bites the mother. All three "weaned themselves" and are feeding problems. The older boy bites his nails and the other children suck their fingers. All the children developed fast and are attractive and of good intelligence. They all showed extreme reactions to the birth of the last child and all but the patient have continued with their disturbed behavior.

The patient was delivered normally, at full term, following a pregnancy which, like all others, was unwanted and attended by severe vomiting. Until the age of four months she developed well on breast feeding. As the mother then became pregnant again, she had to be weaned. Excessive thumb-sucking set in immediately and the most drastic measures against it were of no avail. Her development, as compared with the other siblings, was accelerated. She started to talk at seven months and was completely toilet trained at nine months.

When she was thirteen months old she had a slight attack of measles which coincided with the mother's return from the hospital after the birth of her younger brother. Our patient's prolonged convalescence could not be ascribed to any physical sequelae of this illness. She lost considerable weight over a prolonged period, gave up walking, resumed soiling and wetting and became a feeding problem. She had temper tantrums whenever the mother nursed the baby and was difficult to manage.

The mother, who had a hard time, being left alone with four small children, handled these episodes with more strictness than she herself found advisable. She was therefore very gratified, when at the age of two, the little girl became over-solicitous for the younger brother, insisted on sharing her food with him and became very grown up, reliable, and self-sufficient. Her development continued along these very "pleasing" lines until the father's return. She showed remarkable intellectual achievement, took complete care of herself and was very eager to help in the house.

When the father returned she at first refused to go near him while the older children took full possession of him. The older girl soon became the father's favorite. The father was moody and despondent, stayed in bed late, and took up most of his wife's time. The latter, despite the great demands he made on her, was very eager to humor him.

The patient had slept with the mother until the father returned. She reacted so violently to sleeping in a cot by herself that the mother had to take her back into her bed. Subsequently the child developed a very annoying habit: while in bed and whenever otherwise unoccupied she would wrap the longest hair on the left side of her head around her fingers, and suck them. This habit became so intensive that she soon developed a bald spot. She also showed a marked tendency to separate her parents in her wish to sit or sleep between them and in other attempts to divert the mother's attention from the father. The personality change described above occurred gradually from now on.

The treatment of the child extended over a period of seven months including two interruptions of two and five weeks respectively. There have been no direct contacts with the child since treatment was terminated in February of 1941 but the monthly follow-up visits by a social worker have shown that so far the therapeutic results have been sustained and the child's development progresses normally.[3]

While under treatment she lived on the general ward of the Sarah Morris Children's Hospital. Contacts with her family were limited to weekly visits of the parents. Her contact with the sibling substitutes among the patients, and with the parent surrogates among the hospital personnel determined to a considerable extent the content of the analytic material. Treatment under such abnormal conditions involved a number of technical problems that I shall not discuss here. But it is necessary briefly to describe the set-up and the persons who constituted the child's environment while she was under treatment.

The ward had room for five children who, with the exception of our patient and of a three-year-old boy, stayed for a short time only and mostly were confined to their beds. Philip alone, a rather well-adjusted, active and intelligent boy who suffered from megalocolon, remained the patient's constant companion through the larger part of the treatment. The patient and Philip had use of a sun-porch, a bathroom and a playroom, where they also took their meals. There they

3. The most recent home visit made in December of 1944 confirms this. According to our last report the patient continues in excellent physical and emotional health. She attends school regularly, gets good grades, is outgoing and sociable. Her relationships with parents and siblings are good. Since her discharge from the hospital three younger children—one girl and two boys—have been born without causing any untoward reaction in our patient.

were joined by other children who were well enough to be about. The nursing staff consisted chiefly of student nurses who changed services frequently. The patient, as well as all the other children, had regular physical examinations by the interne and the medical staff on rounds.

During the first session the solemn little girl appeared surprisingly independent and self-sufficient. She devoted herself exclusively to play with plasticine which she molded and smeared on the furniture while producing grunting and belching sounds. She did not respond when spoken to. Her awareness of the analyst's presence manifested itself only in her grabbing plasticine out of the analyst's hand and in a fiercely defiant look when she attempted to eat the plasticine. No resistance was offered to this but candy was placed on the table when she repeated it. She ate the candy rapidly and greedily, asked for more and more, and after stuffing herself demanded to be carried around and rocked in the analyst's arms. The aggressive smearing was handled by acceptance and the offer of candy seemed to substitute gratification for self-punishment.

Being carried around and allowed to stuff herself with candy in addition to actual satisfaction meant reassurance, and enabled her to bring her first confession in a very impressive performance with a set of dolls. The father doll fed clay balls to the whole family, and the mother doll and the doll representing the patient herself vomited. She repeated this play throughout the whole session, at the end of which she made her first verbal communication, a request to be called by her older sister's name rather than by her own.

What she expressed was this: Her own and her mother s symptoms are alike and are connected with the father. She evidently identified with the pregnant mother and disclosed her oral impregnation fantasy. Confession, however, is followed by denial. When she asks to be called by her sister's name she expresses the wish to be the father's favorite and to be free from symptoms.

This request, demands for candy, and direct pleas for the analyst's attention in the way of feeding and cuddling were the chief content of the subsequent sessions over a period of a week during which she was entirely free from vomiting. But when her mother, on visiting day, informed her of the birth of the new sister and brought her a big baby doll as a gift she had a severe attack of vomiting. The new doll was brought to the treatment room and left there apparently unnoticed for many days. Two of the analyst's dolls were broken in the same session and she introduced a new game which consisted in distributing food equally among a number of small dolls. Her stuffing with candy took on quite extreme forms and a new element entered into her relationship to the analyst: She searched the analyst's pockets and the desk drawers, investigated the analyst's mouth, kissed and bit her and increased her demands to be fondled and carried around. She again threatened to swallow plasticine and when prevented from doing so stuffed it into little boxes, requesting that the analyst remove it and make "babies" out of it. These she crushed immediately and distributed as food to the other dolls. Hiding under the analyst's hospital coat became another frequent game. Following the next visit of her mother she had an attack of wetting and soiling.

We see that the enjoyable security of getting undivided satisfaction from the analyst is interrupted when she learns about the birth of the new sibling and she reacts with manifestations similar to her disturbance after the birth of the next sibling.

The meaning of her investigation of the analyst's mouth appeared explicitly when she asked that a "real big" doll be made, referred to it as "mother" and with marked excitement started to look for "the baby inside" She began her investigation by enlarging the doll's mouth, then suggested looking into the doll's stomach and finally requested that a tiny doll be hidden there. Urgent questioning showed her need to be reassured that no new arrival was going to destroy the present fully satisfactory relationship.

She now proceeded to develop, in her play, theories about impregnation: The mother doll ate large quantities of plasticine and when the analyst, in response to a question, denied that this was going to make a baby, she had the father doll and the mother doll kiss each other and again asked the same question. The next step in her play was to put father and mother to bed together with the father lying on top of the mother. The father then stepped on the mother, making her cry out. The mother doll now broke into pieces and had to be fixed by the analyst, after which the patient delivered the baby through the mother's abdomen and put it on the mother's breast.

We note several elements pertaining to her sex theories: The first is a fantasy of impregnation through eating. The oral concept is maintained in the second phase of her play, the gratification being given by the father. In the third and final, repeatedly staged phase of the play her sado-masochistic ideas about the primal scene become evident. However, the significant point is that the rage against the pregnant mother evokes these fantasies and these are benevolently modified only when the analyst forgivingly repairs the mother doll. As long as the child is assured of the possession of the kindly analyst she can allow a doll baby to be born and to nurse.

During the first period of the treatment her intense wish for gratification by way of the undivided possession of a mother figure was clearly expressed. The way in which her requests were met by the analyst allowed her temporarily to renounce her symptom.

On the basis of this security, through gratification, she became able to disclose some of her aggressions in the second period of the treatment. Progress is noted when she succeeds in crystallizing her destructive wishes by the creation of an impersonating figure. This shows that she no longer is fully overwhelmed by her impulses but, with the help of a supporting relationship, has acquired some distance from them and has thus made her first attempts at controlling her impulses. These attempts are, however, not yet sustained attempts and she still has to resort to regressive solutions.

During this period the material dealt with the problem of the sex difference. Her attitude was quite clear: whereas previously she had modeled sexless babies and mothers she now wanted girls and boys. They were correctly identified initially, but with obvious excitement the female doll was invariably adorned with numerous penis figures attached to head and upper chest. These creatures were stubbornly and defiantly referred to as "girls". Her whole attitude at this time assumed a clearly masculine tone. Regularly, following the modeling of the so-called "girls", she played aggressively with gun and flashlight which were used to attack the analyst. Vomiting occurred again during this period.

Her masculine identification apparently served the purpose of safeguarding from the danger of being displaced by a boy in her relationship with the analyst.

She next created the figure "Whoof". Whoof was a little lead dog of whom she was very fond at first. She insisted that the analyst address him in endearing terms. To start with, Whoof was very gay; he jumped around and barked; but subsequently he became quite nasty, chasing little toy-pigs and dolls. He started to devour them and became quite voracious. Impersonating him, the patient talked in a deep voice, accompanying this performance with much grunting and belching. Whoof bit and killed the whole family of dolls. He refused pieces of plasticine that the analyst offered him on the patient's direction. Only big lumps of plasticine that the child herself forced on him placated him temporarily, "until tomorrow when he will start again". The next day Whoof and the entire family were put into a box which the patient closed and rattled furiously. "They fight," she said. Upon opening it with many precautions she decided that "he killed them all" and "now I will do it too". She then proceeded to castrate a plasticine boy: "Now he's a girl," she said. Then she fed the castrate and said, "Now he's a boy again." The boy was then devoured by Whoof who got sick "because he had too much".

The significance of Whoof apparently is this: he shows her oral-aggressive wishes which are directed against the siblings, the little pigs and dolls, that he chases. It appears further that her concept of aggression is connected with her conception of the primal scene as indicated when she has the family fight in the dark box. Like herself, Whoof does not go without punishment: he becomes sick and vomits. Self-punishment for and denial of her destructive tendencies is expressed in the symptom of vomiting. Whoof becomes calm and docile after he has relieved himself.

Whoof and the little girl doll remained on the scene of action for some time. The child ate a lot without vomiting; Whoof, however, bit and had to vomit afterwards. Once the little girl even ate her spoon and thus became a boy. Then she got sick and when father and mother came to visit her she sat between them and ate. Her brother Gilbert, she played, also came and gave her the candy she asked him for. He was represented by a little boy doll with a golf club. While the patient insisted that he was really big and gave her everything she broke his golf club and fed it to the girl doll. Finally she selected all the broken or injured toy soldiers, put them in a box with the girl doll and said, "She gets all the candy from all the Gilberts."

This confession of her envious aggressive incorporative attitudes towards the males of the family shows her wish to be like the brother and father in order to be as close to the mother as they were and to have their advantages.

Now came a period of regressive play: she lay on the couch, kicked like a baby and talked baby-talk. She demanded that candy be fed to her. She apparently wishes to avoid the hostility connected with her rivalry and achieves this by regressing to a level at which gratification was not yet endangered by hostile competitiveness. Eating under such conditions does not call for punishment as the hostile meaning is eliminated. She is free from her symptom while this stage lasts.

The following period is characterized by new phenomena of ego-growth when her depressive reactions to the first separation from the analyst are worked through. It will be noticed that the maturing process becomes accelerated under the influence of actual and later of self-inflicted frustration. She has already learned during the process of treatment that satisfaction actually can be expected from the analyst as an outside object. This loosened the need for incorporation, and the tendencies that until now had been autoplastically expressed by the smooth muscles of the visceral tract emerge as alloplastic expressions of love and resentment within the interpersonal relationship of the transference.

The interruption of the treatment for two weeks brought on a severe reoccurrence of her vomiting. During the analyst's absence she resorted to excessive finger sucking, and seemed withdrawn and unapproachable on the ward. However, there was surprising progress in her speech development when treatment was taken up again. She started with an urgent request for candy and after this had been met returned to her play with plasticine: She asked that a boy be modeled, then requested that the analyst destroy him but quickly crushed the figure to pieces herself. She next modeled a number of "snakes", put them upright on the table and presented them to the analyst: "That's for you." She asked for more candy after ·presenting her gift and proceeded to press the "snakes" into the mother doll. The snake "bit" the mother, and finally was fed to the girl doll who then was used as a destructive tool with which to crush the other plasticine dolls. Then she proceeded to model a "mother" commenting that she had "both titties and stickies", putting the penis figure in place of the breasts. She claimed to be hungry because Philip, the little boy in the ward, had all the cereal, eggs, and ice cream in his stomach already. She crushed another plasticine doll and then kissed the analyst demonstratively, asking that we both feed the little girl doll. On the following day she made aggressive demands on the analyst. After eating her fill of candy, she snatched fountain-pen and comb from the analyst, she pulled the analyst's hair, and insisted that it was Whoof and not she who did all these bad things. She fantasied that her mother was going to bring her as presents "a big plate with cookies and a big high hat". Finally she refused to stay in the treatment room. For several days she reacted to each approach of the analyst by withdrawal and acute outbreaks of anxiety. But no vomiting occurred, her eating was normal, and she was in good contact on the ward. Then her behavior again changed. The violent screaming, which for several days had been her only reaction to the analyst's presence on the ward, stopped one day and with tears she stated: "I want to sew like you." Thus a new relationship was established. She carefully tried to imitate each of the analyst's movements. She was, however, still unable to accept any favors from the analyst; and when the purse on which the analyst was working was offered to her she pretended to throw it away because, as she said, "All the other children want it, it is an ugly purse." But she continued the pleasant situation of sewing together.

After the outbursts of ambivalence with which she reacted to the analyst's departure, she tries to create a new and more secure relationship through identification; her refusal to accept anything from the analyst at this time means that she not only denies her former possessive wishes but also wishes to exclude the conflictful sibling rivalry which had necessitated her vomiting.

Finally, she attempted to place herself in a position of guiltless receiving by shifting her interest from candy to bracelets, necklaces, and similar things which could further her identification with the analyst. Sibling rivalry took new forms: Philip was included in her play but quite subtly she arranged that his be only minor roles. Sharing food with him and other children became a protective mechanism, as was also her sharing of aggressions against the analyst by organizing groups to attack the analyst.

The material just presented needs to be understood in terms of the separation from the analyst. The patient had reacted to it with depressive behavior, increase in symptom, and finger-sucking. The interruption of the treatment is a recapitulation of the emotional situation at the onset of her neurosis, namely the separation from the mother by the arrival of brother and father. As then, hostility is activated. The anger against the analyst which results from the separation poisons the very source of her satisfaction; because the patient's ego is still too undeveloped to reconcile apparently incompatible libidinal and hostile tendencies. She therefore makes the best of it with temporizing measures: the presents she offers to me on my return are intended, on the one hand, to placate me, and thus preserve a good relationship, and on the other hand, to win me by showing that she has as much to offer as did father and brother. This is more primitively demonstrated when she requests that the analyst destroy her rival in the form of the brother-doll, in order to make possible her own close union with the mother-analyst. She indicates the latter when she presses the snakes into the mother-doll. When she models a doll with breast and penis she really models herself and indicates that the reason for her illness lies in her hostile incorporation of the brother and father as a means of securing for herself the relationship of which they have deprived her. These measures fail and therefore she has to turn away from the analyst in the period of hostile resistance described before. This last self-inflicted separation does not have the malignant characteristics of her original depressive withdrawal, because she is no longer fully overwhelmed by her hostile fantasies. It is for this reason that she does not have to resort to vomiting. Increasing ego-control becomes manifest in her attempt to solve her conflict with the analyst by identification. Superego factors become obvious in her attempts to be good and socially acceptable. Reaction-formation appears when for a time she has to pass on everything that is given to her. But when, later, she again asks for candy, adding "for Philip", the little boy who is the object of her most intense sibling rivalry, she shows a true conscience reaction. Aggression against the analyst and sibling rivalry now emerge again but they are handled on a distinctly different level. When she gets angry at the analyst she now no longer attacks her; her aggression takes socially acceptable forms as when, after tearing up paper or cardboard, she insists that we clean it up together.

Experimentation with these newly-acquired functions characterized the following treatment period. A number of passing tentative solutions appeared but the next step became established as within the transference she learned to differentiate between permitted and forbidden acts. For a time she developed an eating ritual. She requested that the analyst count "one, two, three, now" before she allowed herself to eat. When given wrapped candy she put it into her mouth without unwrapping it, commenting, "Eating paper is bad, take the paper out of my mouth." Removal and throwing away of the tinfoil became a repeated game that was followed by relieved laughter. Spilling water or dropping paper on the floor led to prolonged games of cleaning up in which the analyst had to participate actively. After eating candy she had to have her mouth wiped and she wanted to know whether crushing candy with her teeth was bad. She was over-concerned that the other children on the ward should get an even share of the candy she received and put a piece of candy in a box for each of them before she allowed herself to eat. She frequently challenged the analyst by pretending to be bad and she would take and pretend to keep articles in the treatment room and then would restore them with much laughter. This relieved laughter which had never been noticed before indicated that her experiment had definite value for her in establishing new security. In the transference the analyst became a person of new and different importance: at first she had been a person of whom unconditioned satisfaction could be and was expected. The difficulties that this had brought about have been shown. Now the analyst had to prove herself to be a protector against such impulses as the patient recognized to be forbidden. And by entering into compulsive play the analyst opened up a new era of permitted gratification: eating the candy whose tinfoil has been removed by the analyst is gratification in an approved pleasure, and assuredness of freedom from sanctions.

It appeared then that her somewhat extreme reaction-formations were only temporary measures and once learned and successfully applied could be given up again after they served the purpose of establishing her capacity for self-control. She was now able to admit her two most disturbing tendencies, namely, her receptive wishes towards the analyst and the sibling rivalry that arose from them and stimulated her hostility. The first was done when she showed the analyst her toy chest which contained the purse that had been given to her. She admitted, chuckling, "I pretended to throw it away— I kept it." The second was shown when in the analyst's presence she denied Philip a toy, explaining in a mature tone, "Philip, this is not for you, I may keep it." Evidently she is striving to find conditions under which keeping is permissible, another step in her attempts to separate good and bad.

She also gave up her eating ritual and became free enough to experiment with her aggressions against the analyst by frequently stressing that her shooting was only a game and surely would not hurt the analyst, though it was meant to frighten her.

Statements like these show that the previous attempts to differentiate between good and bad are the preliminary steps in her progress in reality testing, namely, the ability to distinguish between fantasy and fact.

In addition to her communications by play, verbalization become more extensive and direct. She now described an attack of vomiting with real insight when she reported that it occurred when Philip was presented with a birthday cake. She had taken the biggest piece and eaten only a few bites when she had to throw up: "Because it was too much and I was angry." She told about another attack which occurred after spanking Philip when he wanted to come to the treatment room instead of her.

The span of her creative activity widened considerably. She began to sew, to draw, to cut out and to paint. At the same time the analytic material as shown in her play now had direct reference to her conflict and its mastery: Whoof was cautioned against peeping into a house that was full of little dolls because it would make him "too mad", but later he was allowed to look together with the analyst. She said, "We look together and he does not bite any more." Still Whoof was accused of making candy "black and bad". She fought him with the analyst's help until he became harmless and ridiculous and she made fun of him.

In this play she shows clearly how her hostility stems from her sibling rivalry and how she can now face it because she feels secure in her close contact with the analyst whom she does not have to share. It was the same hostility against the sibling and the father that by projection made the mother bad and the candy unpalatable. When she is able to make fun of the representation of her hostility, she shows that she has acquired distance from it and that a new step in ego-control has been achieved.

She now, for the first time, began to show interest in men. She chatted with orderlies and internes and to the analyst bragged about the attention they gave her. With the decreasing intensity of her pregenital conflict, she had become able to enter into other relationships. This development, however, was checked by her reaction to a severe illness of Philip, her little brother-substitute. But it was in this phase of the treatment that reality testing became definitely established. Now the hostile implications of her relationship to mother and sibling were recapitulated and worked through.

Resistance was her immediate reaction to Philip's illness. She became very aggressive towards the analyst, called her "Bad girl— you make me keep things and now Philip is sick." For the first time she talked a lot about her mother who did not allow her to keep things for herself and did not make her bad. While she turned away from the analyst she showed great attachment to one of the nurses known for her neurotic strictness. However, she did not, as in the previous phase of resistance, reject all gifts from the analyst. She even requested them but looked upon them as coming from her own mother. Most of these presents she did not keep for herself but passed on to Philip. She said, "I have to give everything to Gilbert (her brother). Philip is sick. He got up without his pajamas. I saw his sticky." This confession was followed by an outburst of tears but with much relaxation. She called the analyst back and still, with tears in her eyes, suggested a game in which she insisted that the analyst had to laugh at the frightening faces she made. Following this confession the vomiting, which had been recurring during Philip's illness, stopped.

During this episode, she obviously has felt that her intense destructive impulses against this little brother-substitute have become real. She shows a conscious reaction when she blames herself for his illness and she tries to handle this guilt by projection of her hostility to the analyst. This new mechanism still leaves her free to receive without vomiting, and indicates considerable progress from the former mechanism of incorporation which had served to increase her conflict rather than to alleviate it. She attempts reality testing when she states that she saw Philip's penis, recognizing as it were, the fantasy character of her destructive wishes. But she has felt the necessity for reinstating the strict mother-image when she turns to the punitive nurse and she talks so much about her own mother because she feels that the analyst's permission to keep things has brought her into the dangerous situation of Philip's illness. She projects her own aggressive impulses to the analyst and in doing so displays a new mechanism in the mastery of anxiety. Again reality testing is attempted when the analyst is requested to respond to the patient's frightening grimaces with laughter. She wants to test out the analyst as a benign mother-image and she has to prove to herself that her aggressions cannot really destroy the objects of her environment. She obtains this proof not only from the analyst but also through the fact of Philip's survival.

Integration of the reality testing capacities became apparent in the next period: she took the role of the father, the analyst became the mother, and her doll became her own surrogate. The doll was bad; bit, spat, and vomited on the mother. The patient, as father, examined her with a stomach tube and decided that the doll was not bad but sick and had to be fixed in the hospital.

After Philip was discharged from the hospital she quickly found a new brother-substitute in Charles whom she robbed of his toys but with whom she faithfully shared her food. Hostility, it appears, was under ego-control but the basic meaning of this hostility against the sibling, namely, its reference to the mother's love, was recapitulated in the transference as follows:

She asked anxiously and repeatedly whether Philip and Charles were seen in treatment too, and continued her compulsive questioning in spite of all reassurance. She put much stress on having her hair fixed in a queer way with three little pig-tails sticking out. For long periods of time she lay on the couch, a gun in one hand and a flashlight in the other, and insisted on being fed and petted by the analyst. The baby role was finally ascribed to a doll and, while the patient occupied herself with good grown-up activities like drawing and sewing, she gave detailed orders as to the endless loving care of the doll. She said, "If she stays with you and you like her, she won't throw up."

It seems that Philip's discharge threatened her with similar separation from the analyst. Her own loss of the analyst must seem more likely to her if even the brother, the preferred rival in her home, can be sent away. The material expresses the question: How is it possible that I, who am a girl, can be loved in view of the fact that boys who I know are preferred are sent away? In the last quoted comment "If the doll stays with you and you like her she won't throw up" she clearly shows the connection between her symptom and her reaction to the loss of love.

She apparently found this reassurance and utilized it immediately, as her play showed: Whoof was put into the dark box with the entire family of dolls but he did not do any of them any harm. The two piggies no longer chased and bit each other but laughed and danced together. Security in the transference and more complete ego-control made unnecessary the need to destroy the siblings and allowed a full positive attachment to the mother-analyst.

The problem of the other instinctual tendencies which were looked upon by the little girl as bad and therefore capable of disturbing her relationship with the mother was worked through in the last phase of the treatment. At this time there had been the second interruption of the treatment because the whole ward had had to be discharged in order to prevent an epidemic of mumps. The patient had returned to her home for five weeks during which there had been only two attacks of vomiting, immediately upon her return. The mother reported that the patient showed interest in the new baby and, in contrast to the neurotic behavior of the other children in the family, appeared happy and content, so much so that the parents only reluctantly agreed to her return to the hospital for further treatment and insisted on taking her home at the end of three weeks of this second stay in the hospital. As learned later, the mother just then had found out about her new pregnancy and the fear that this would produce a further bad reaction in the patient, had finally induced her to allow the child to return.

The final period in the hospital then began with an angry resistance which in the end appeared to be a defense against the anxiety of the subsequent material. As her anxiety subsided, hiding and peeping games became very frequent: She cautioned the analyst against looking and covered herself with a blanket. She said, "I show you (what I am doing). You don't mind," and proceeded to suck one hand while she masturbated with the other one. She became quite exhibitionistic in her masturbation which occurred during the treatment only and was never observed on the ward. She also made repeated pleas for the analyst's admiration of her body. She talked freely about her mother, compared the furniture in the treatment room to the mother's new chairs, table, and davenport. Jumping all over the furniture, she informed me that her mother would not allow this behavior and that she had become angry when the patient had vomited on the new davenport. Once, while masturbating, she told me that at home she had gotten a licking. Then she said to me, "But you would not mind." She invented a game called "Who took the sticky?" in which she hid a pencil between two sheets of paper and recovered it triumphantly with the emphatic statement that she did not take it as it belonged to the doctor, to Philip, to Charles, and to Gilbert. She again played at tube-feeding the doll. The doll had it done as punishment for trying to swallow the tube. Then she sprinkled the floor with the same bottle and tube which she had used for the tube-feeding, and stated, "like a boy doing number one". After this had been discussed she decided to let the doll get well without washing her stomach, to sprinkle the floor "like a girl" without using the tube and to use the bottle as a symbol of the womb. She put tiny buttons into the bottle which, she then said, had been put there by Dr. B., who had become her favorite. She said "They grow there until they are big and come out." She developed quite a crush on Dr. B., bragged about his attentions to her, and insisted that he rather than the nurse should bring her to the treatment room. She called him "my doctor and not yours" and decided to save her candy for him. When the analyst gave her special candy for this purpose she clearly differentiated her relationship to the two objects of her attachment in referring to him as "my darling doctor" and to the analyst as "the good ice-cream lady".

Apparently the return to the home environment has served to stimulate sexual curiosity and sexual activity rather than to provoke again the hostile destructive envy of brother and father which had originally led to her illness and had necessitated the somatic symptom-formation. This constitutes real progress and makes it clear that the somatic symptom had been connected with pre-genital problems which are now worked through. The vomiting is now given up definitely. The analyst's attitude towards the newly discovered sources of pleasure in masturbation and peeping is tested out. But since the patient already is sure of the analyst's former acceptance she is able to anticipate new permissiveness. She says to me: "You don't mind" before she proceeds to the testing. She contrasts the analyst's understanding attitude with the mother's punitive strictness and shows that now she is well able to separate and differentiate according to the indications of reality.

Well integrated utilization of this permissiveness accounts for the next step she makes when she becomes attached to the interne. She is finally able to test out the possible consequences of her other presumptively bad impulses, such as genital and voyeuristic tendencies, after the anxiety connected with her hostile oral tendencies has been dispelled; and she shows realistic differentiation in her object relations to father and mother figures.

A series of quiet sessions followed during which she made great progress in various skills like sewing, drawing and building. "Doing things together" was the chief content of this period during which her symptoms had disappeared completely. She gave the impression of a normal, outgoing and happy child. She showed much interest in a set of paper dolls. "For fun" she dressed girls in boys' clothes but decided that they looked funny, called them silly and devoted much interest in the dolls' as well as in her own dresses.

It is no longer necessary for her to be envious of boys, she can accept her status as a little girl, and it becomes possible for her to make a non-hostile identification with the mother.

Thus she decided that the paper dolls were all her children until she should have a baby of her own, a real baby girl, who would be taken care of by the analyst. She became very much attached to a little kitten and when it scratched her, decided that it was "hungry and not bad". This is another proof of her benign identification with her mother.

When she was finally told that her parents wished her to go home she was somewhat angry but then asked for a farewell party in which all the dolls participated. She left with the statement, "Eating is O. K."

Summary

Recapitulation of the patient's emotional development shows severe traumatization during the course of her primitive dependence. The first trauma arose from the sudden weaning at the age of four months when her mother became pregnant. This resulted in simple physiological tension. The low degree of differentiation in the psychic apparatus of a four-month-old child still allowed solution by a short cut, as it were. Thus a substitute gratification, namely, thumb-sucking, was sufficient to achieve release of tension and mastery of the trauma. Though not yet representing a neurotic symptom this solution already may account for a certain amount of oral fixation and may have its bearing on the future choice of symptom. The next trauma occurred at the age of thirteen months when the next sibling was born. Again it took the form of a frustration of her anaclitic needs. A solution as simple as the former resort to thumb-sucking was no longer sufficient. Functions had already been acquired which could be lost. She gave up walking, habit-control, and whatever independence she already had achieved. She also may have prolonged her convalescence from measles in a tendentious way to procure the satisfaction she was deprived of. However, her regression failed to achieve its purpose and the precocious maturation she subsequently showed may be regarded as an attempt to master the environment actively where she had failed to do so passively.

This phenomenon of sudden jerky progress in maturation following the experience of frustration, was again observed during the analysis. On this basis it would seem that a more general deduction might be made about the connection between frustration of instinctual desires and the rate of ego maturation: given an individual who is constitutionally capable, disillusionment of the possibility of passive mastery forces an attempt at active mastery. One might refer to this process as maturation out of despair.

But in order to understand the acute upset that manifestly followed the father's return to the family, the patient's relationship to mother and siblings needs to be reviewed: From the very beginning this little girl had seen her mother as a person from whom gratification could not be expected unconditionally. The facts of her infantile history corroborate this. Her disappointment in the mother started with the early weaning. It flared up again when, after the birth of her brother, the mother did not fully satisfy the patient's regressive wishes. The breast which she had denied to the little girl was given to the next sibling, who happened to be a boy. She attempted to obtain for herself the gratifying advantages of her rival's position first by the wish to destroy him, and second, through the wish to become like him. This took the form of her destructive oral incorporative tendencies towards the brother, which were demonstrated in the course of the analysis. Incorporation thus became conflictful and therefore even the normal pre-ambivalent incorporative attitudes toward the mother which serve the biological purpose of nutrition became tainted with hostility. That is why she had so much difficulty, in the transference, in accepting the relatively unconditional gratification which her relationship to the analyst offered.

The father entered the picture as a new, more powerful rival for the satisfaction from the mother. The patient attempted to deal with him in the same way that she had dealt with the brother. But her conception of the sadistic role of the father in the primal scene led her to feel that to incorporate him and obtain his advantages in the relationship to the mother, could only lead to the destruction of the mother as the source of these advantages.

Thus we see that there is erected a double barrier to this little girl's relationship to her mother. In the first instance, through the influence of the brother's existence which had to be destroyed through her incorporative fantasies, eating became "bad". In the second instance, the return of the father, whose gratifying relationship to the mother she wished to have, made any relationship to the mother impossible because of its implicit destructiveness as derived from the primal scene.

The vomiting then appears as a defense against both aspects of the destructive incorporative tendencies and in a secondary way serves to restore regressively the dependent relationship to the mother.

Her neurosis thus showed the characteristics of a depression. The conflict arose on the oral level from her inability to integrate incompatible libidinal and destructive tendencies, both of which were expressed through incorporation. The need for oral satisfaction from the mother resulted in the wish to incorporate her as a love object; rivalry with the siblings and the father led to cannibalistic-destructive attitudes towards them. The aggressions were turned towards herself in her starvation and in her other self-destructive manifestations, such as the hair-pulling.

The decisive process in the treatment was the strengthening of her ego to an extent that enabled her to separate the loved and hated objects and to deal with them differentially on a realistic basis rather than on the former basis of a delusional fused incorporation. This was achieved in successive steps during the treatment. One might say that it led from the originally autoplastic manifestations of her organ-neurosis to the alloplastic behavior that she showed in the transference-neurosis.   On the secure basis of the transference, reality testing helped her towards ego growth and we saw the development of the emotional tendencies towards ego-acceptable forms. The dissolution of the pre-genital conflict finally enabled her to start on the way towards genuine maturity.

FORMATION OF THE ANTISOCIAL CHARACTER

By KATE FRIEDLANDER, M.D., L.R.C.P., D.P.M. (London)

The purpose of this article is to clarify the factors that may lead an individual in emotional stress to react with antisocial rather than with neurotic behavior. It is now generally accepted that none of the unconscious conflicts underlying criminal acts are limited to the delinquent. We know, for instance, that in many cases of kleptomania in women, the unconscious conflict that motivates the antisocial act is penis envy: the unconscious purpose is to take from the mother that which she has never given to the child of her own free will. We know also that this same unconscious conflict leads only rarely to stealing and more often results in neurotic conflicts, sexual disturbances and various character distortions. Unconscious feelings of guilt arising out of the oedipal conflict have been shown by Freud[1] to result in criminal behavior. Alexander[2] describes a dramatic case in which the criminal acts are clearly shown to be motivated mainly by this mechanism. Every analyst is familiar with a vast number of ways in which this particular conflict is expressed. Familiar to all is the formation of a masochistic character, in which suffering is achieved without actual punishment by law. It is of interest to study the rich case material Healy[3] presents when emphasizing the importance of mental conflict in the causation of antisocial behavior.

Psychoanalysts have thus far stressed the similarities between neurotic and delinquent reactions rather than investigated the difference. Foulkes, in a recent publication,[4] is one among many who do so. The reason for this seems twofold. First, the similarity between the

1. S. Freud, "Some Character Types Met with in Psychoanalytic Work", *Collected Papers*, III; and "Criminality from a Sense of Guilt", ibid., IV, p. 342 ff.

2. F. Alexander and H. Staub, *The Criminal, the Judge and the Public*, London, 1931.

3. W. Healy, *Mental Conflict and Misconduct*, London, 1918.

4) S. H. Foulkes, "Psychoanalysis and Crime", *English Studies in Criminal Science*, Cambridge, 1944.

neurotic's unconscious impulses and the overt actions of criminals, and second, the similarity in structure of certain delinquent and neurotic symptoms allowed psychoanalysis to make a contribution of great importance to criminological research. The conception of the "born criminal" was discredited and the psychological foundation of antisocial behavior was established. Second, the majority of cases investigated by the psychoanalytic method showed neurotic symptoms in addition to the criminal behavior. The fact that they existed in combination may indeed have been the very reason why these cases were singled out for investigation.

Although the difference in behavior between delinquents and neurotics has of course not been wholly overlooked, it has never sufficiently been subjected to special investigation. In the literature on the subject the question has long been asked why one person becomes neurotic and another delinquent and whether the answer lies wholly in psychological areas. Alexander[5] is inclined to stress differences in the material environment of neurotics and delinquents. He states that "if earlier emotional dissatisfaction in the family situation is combined with social discontent, antisocial behavior rather than neurotic symptom formation is likely to result". He bases this conclusion on the fact that the unconscious conflicts in criminals whom he analyzed were in no way different from those of neurotic persons. Aichhorn,[6] without directly discussing the difference between the neurotic and the delinquent, describes certain purely psychological characteristics common to the majority of delinquents. He believes that environmental factors lead to delinquency only when a "state of latent delinquency", i.e. psychological preparedness for antisocial reactions, already exists. In a recent sociological research into the origins of delinquent behavior, other investigators conclude[7] that environmental factors give rise to antisocial reactions only if a "susceptibility" to delinquent behavior has previously existed. Clearly all these authors are referring to the condition that Aichhorn has called the "state of latent delinquency".

I had occasion to analyze a boy between seven and nine years of age who before and during the analysis had showed character traits uniformly found among delinquents. For delinquents, satisfaction of instinctual desires is invariably more important than satisfactions gained from an object relationship; their impulses demand

5. F. Alexander and W. Healy, *Roots of Crime*, New York, 1935.
6. A. Aichhorn, *Wayward Youth*, London, 1936.
7. Saunders, Mannheim and Rhedes, *Young Offenders*, Cambridge, 1942.

immediate gratification; postponement is impossible, and their regard for right and wrong is wholly subordinated to instinctual satisfactions. Hence their unreliability, the ease with which they lie, and the apparent defect in their moral code. These character traits common to all delinquents and present whether or not their behavior is complicated by neurotic conflicts are worth studying more thoroughly, because they are the greatest obstacle to psychoanalytic or any other kind of treatment of the offender. In my opinion, they distinguish the delinquent from the neurotic.

Billy's mother sought advice because of difficulties the boy had presented for about a year-and-a-half. She described him as having been a pleasant, amiable child up to the time he was five years old. After that his behavior slowly changed. He became dirty, cruel to animals and younger children, disobedient and negativistic at home. Recently he had begun to play truant from school. He did not get on with other children, teased the younger boys and provoked older ones to such an extent that they finally drove him home crying like a baby. He stayed out late at night when sent on an errand, and time and again came home or not as he pleased. No measure the mother could apply, from moral lectures to spankings, had the slightest effect upon him. At home he very often behaved like a much younger child: refused to wash himself or bathe and was afraid to sleep in a room alone. Though he showed great ingenuity in outwitting his mother, his school attainments were very poor. At the age of seven, when he was brought for treatment, he had not yet learned to read and write.

The following is Billy's story as it came to light during the two years of his analytic treatment.

He was the only child of middle-aged parents of the lower middle classes. The marriage had never been happy. The mother came from a higher social level than the father and prior to her marriage had been in love with another man for many years. Only when the hope of marrying the man of her choice had definitely vanished did she consent to marry the father, a man of the working class. Even then she did so against the wishes of her family. The child was born after two years of marriage and for another six years the parents lived together, quarrelling frequently. When the boy was about four-and-a-half years old an incident occurred that disturbed the parental relationship profoundly. The mother went out one day for a walk with the boy and met the father in the company of a woman with whom he had previously lived. In a fury of jealousy the mother, without even greeting her husband, turned away, taking the boy with her. Thereafter she refused to speak to the father or to hear his explanations, which were simple enough: he had met this woman after not having seen her for years, and could not pass her by without a word. Though at times the mother was willing to believe this story, when it was transmitted to her by her own mother, she insisted nevertheless that the father had broken his word given before their marriage, never to see this woman again. From then on, she treated her husband with utter contempt, rarely condescending even to speak to him. In response he broke off their sexual relations. Though they maintained a joint household there were weeks when the boy did not see his father at all. At this time air-raids were so frequent that mother and boy slept many nights in a shelter; family life, when there was any, was further complicated by the presence of many of the mother's relatives who had been driven by war conditions to seek a haven in her home. After the blitz had subsided somewhat the boy shared a room with his mother and grandmother, while the father was consigned to a room of his own. For a short time during the child's analytic treatment marital relations between the parents were resumed, but after a further quarrel caused by the fact that the father had contracted debts, the relationship again deteriorated and shortly before the end of treatment the father left the house. In the meantime the mother became intimate with a man more nearly of her own social class who lived nearby. Whether there was a sexual relationship was not ascertained, but the mother and at times Billy also, spent more time in this man's house than in their own.

This was the family atmosphere in which Billy grew up. Countless scenes, quarrels and discussions with the various members of the family took place in Billy's presence. The mother could not believe that small children understand the conversations and conflicts of grown-ups and therefore took no measures to insure privacy which was difficult anyway because of the close quarters in which they were all living. After the parents' first separation the boy became the storm center for their quarrels and he, on his part, played one parent off against the other, taking bribes from both. When Billy first came for treatment, he openly hated his father, regarding him merely as a source of money. Every small service rendered had to be paid for in cash.

There was nothing very outstanding in Billy's early development. The birth was normal, he walked and talked at the usual time. He was bladder and bowel trained very early and the mother was especially proud of this achievement. However, he started wetting the bed again when he was four years of age and continued to until about six months before the beginning of analysis. For a short period during treatment, when he was removed from his mother for a week for the first time in his life, he wet again, but stopped after about a fortnight. In spite of the fact that he was clean so early, when he was eight his mother was still obliged to accompany him to the toilet and to wipe him clean. When he started to masturbate, however, he met with a different reaction: his grandmother told him that his penis would be cut off unless he stopped. At the same time all questions about sex were left unanswered and discouraged as "dirty". The mother was completely opposed to my telling him anything, because she considered him much too little to understand and because it would spoil his innocence. Urged by my explanations, she gave her consent, but the next day sent a letter by the boy withdrawing it and at the same time told him not to listen to any explanations I might give him. Only much later did her real reason for this attitude become clear. For some months before Billy came for treatment, he had been exhibiting himself in the presence of both his mother and his very strict grandmother and had also been using "dirty" language. He talked about his penis getting hard, about wishing to put it into the mother's mouth, and he constantly tried to draw attention to his genitals. This happened usually when the mother bathed him and though consciously she was very worried about this behavior, she continued to create situations in which he could display himself. He also came into her bed in the morning, lay on top of her and talked about his genitals. The mother was afraid that any sexual enlightenment might increase his exhibitionistic tendencies and that he might use his knowledge to shock her mother and other people who came to the house. Here she was right. For a short time after he had learned certain sexual facts in the analysis he used this knowledge exactly as she anticipated. He stopped this, however, and also stopped exhibiting himself when the mother's attention was taken up with her new man friend and when she no longer bathed him nor let him come into her bed.

The mother's personality and her relationship to Billy of course played a paramount role in the boy's emotional development. Clearly, she herself was emotionally disturbed. She was an intelligent woman, very tall and broad, and as dominating physically as she was mentally. She could not accept advice because she could never accept any views other than her own. Opinionated and quarrelsome, she led an isolated existence, having made enemies of everyone around her. Even the school teacher who had seen her only once was convinced that the boy's difficulties were entirely due to his mother's attitude. Certainly the outstanding feature in the mother's relationship to the boy was ambivalence. She had never been separated from him even for a single day until he came for treatment. During the blitz the thought of sending him out of London had never entered her mind. Yet she was constantly concerned with his physical condition, insisting, contrary to the facts, that he was exceedingly delicate. Though she catered to his greediness (he had an enormous appetite) and constantly yielded to his wish not to be left alone she had no idea of the boy's other needs. He had no suitable toys, there was insufficient play space in the excessively clean and tidy house, and she was adept at suppressing all masculine activities. She would have preferred to have had a girl child, a fact frequently reiterated in the boy's presence. Once when I visited the boy during an illness, she drew my attention to his photograph at the age of two and asked me in his presence whether he did not look like a nice little girl. The playmate of Billy's childhood was a girl cousin, six months older, who was constantly extolled as a shining example of all the virtues. Before coming to treatment Billy had been girlishly dressed, his blazers and overcoats buttoned at the wrong side; and he was not permitted to go out to play with other boys in the street nor to join the Cub Scouts because he might mix with rough children. His mother wanted him to keep quiet at home and to help her with her house work.

Despite nagging, despite constant picking on him for being "dirty" or "silly", despite smacking him when he did not obey, Billy's mother was entirely unable to remain firm once she had forbidden something. In the end he got what he wanted. Billy himself was quite conscious of the way he handled his mother in order to win out. After long explanations I succeeded once in persuading her to try not to forbid the boy what in the end she would allow him. But she could not stick to the plan. Somehow she was convinced that there was something "wrong with the boy's brain", an idea probably unconsciously connected with the fact that he was not a girl. Her hostility to him became especially clear whenever there was any sign of progress in the treatment. When for a time he came home punctually, she at once trumped up another complaint and it was only by chance that I learned that the tardiness had disappeared. When I told her that he had been able to read a whole page in a book he had never seen before, she teased and challenged him to prove it. When he misspelled one word she was triumphant and Billy did not go on. Thus she proved to herself that he really could not read and that he was stupid. She was, as we know, much concerned about the boy's health, yet at least three times during the treatment he came with a high temperature which she had overlooked. On other occasions she kept him at home with a cold or other minor complaints. Though she did her best to suppress any signs of boyish behavior in the child, she was equally annoyed by his whining and cowardice. Billy, of course, lied whenever it suited him, just as she did. She complained of his untruthfulness though she constantly incited him to lie to me or to his teacher. She complained when he stayed away from school, though she kept him home whenever it suited her convenience, in order to buy him a hat, for example. This inconsistency was impervious to change and there was of course no hope of modifying her sado-masochistic behavior to which he responded readily in accordance with the pattern of his own development.

Billy, was very tall for his age, good-looking in a slightly effeminate way, shy, but friendly when I saw him for the first time. He was quite willing to come to see me and soon sensed that I wanted him to tell me all sorts of things. Equally quickly he had made up his mind not to do so. He was very pleasant as long as he was allowed to do exactly as he wanted, and especially as long as I did exactly what he wanted me to do, such as, for instance, playing a game and allowing him to cheat. The moment I wanted him to talk he became rude, aggressive, and generally uncooperative. This attitude was apparent from the beginning of the treatment and became more marked as time went on. He tried to establish the same sado-masochistic relationship with me that he had with his mother. He was entirely uninterested in school life and learning or in what was going on in the outside world unless it specifically served his desires, and bored with information about animals, plants or human beings. He had no hobbies. However, his choice of activities during the analytic sessions soon showed the interest with which he was preoccupied. Whatever materials were offered, bricks, plasticine, drawing books, were used to dramatize a conflict. There were always two parties, represented either by him and me, or by toys, and these two parties fought it out until one or the other adversary, or both were killed. His play with airplanes was of the same kind; he imagined them crashing into one another,—and there his interest stopped. This instinctual interest lacked the signs of sublimation common to most boys, the wish to distinguish various types of aircraft or to understand their construction.

Analysis showed that this fantasy represented Billy's conception of intercourse. The sex relation between the parents was interpreted by him as a sadistic act, and it was evident that he felt considerable anxiety about its consequences. According to his fantasy the man is hurt by the act. When this was discussed he drew pictures of Hitler minus an arm or leg; frequently thereafter he came to the session showing some recently acquired bruise. But he also supposed that the woman gets hurt. This idea was reinforced by observations of menstruation, and fixed in his mind by a cover memory: he remembered his father having once, after a quarrel with his mother, crushed her foot by slamming the door near which she was standing. This the mother verified. It was an accident, but she was positive that no quarrel had preceded or followed it.

This fantasy engrossed Billy entirely, and as the analysis of it proceeded it was possible to draw conclusions as to his instinctual development: A partial regression to the anal-sadistic phase was expressed not only in the sadistic interpretation of intercourse and in his sado-masochistic object-relationships, but also in his open cruelty to animals and smaller children. The regression was as usual due to a strong castration fear, aroused not only by actual prohibitions, but also by the mother's attitude toward all boyish activities and, especially, toward the father. The break between the parents occurred at the height of the child's oedipal conflict and demonstrated to him the danger of identifying with the father. The anxiety was increased by the fact that after the separation he shared the mother's bedroom—which stimulated his oedipal desires anew.

Further analysis showed that the boy's hostility towards the father was a defense against his passive wishes. On occasions this passive-feminine attitude was quite open: he would run after air force men in the street, walking beside them admiringly and talking in a friendly way. Occasionally there were older boys to whom he would behave in a similarly passive-feminine way, in contrast to his usual provocative manner. He would wander around parks talking with boys whose requests he would blindly fulfil. It was important that these boys be strangers and that he never talk to the same boy twice.

Such a regression to the anal-sadistic phase with a passive feminine attitude towards the father is by no means an unusual outcome of the oedipal conflict. It explains the boy's aggressiveness which was partly a defense against his passive wishes, and partly a means of direct instinctual gratification. It does not, however, explain his antisocial tendencies.

It has been mentioned that ever since he was six-and-a-half years old Billy had stayed out late at night, played truant from school and been generally unmanageable at home. On various occasions in the company of other boys, he damaged property and looted bombed houses. When we discussed this behavior he shrugged his shoulders: no policeman had seen him and therefore it did not matter. As is typical of antisocial children, he resisted every attempt at reeducation. Neither friendliness nor punishment had any effect on him. He continued to lie unscrupulously to get what he wanted. During one period in the treatment he transferred this behavior to the analysis: he came unpunctually, often toward the very end of his hour, always ready with a lie to explain his lateness. He ran around the room doing things he knew I must stop, such as burning paper on the electric stove and tearing down curtains. Often he arrived with a knife, a razor blade, a stick of wood, etc., that he had taken from some rubbish heap. To him all these objects represented the penis; this was his way of reassuring himself that his genitals were intact.

It is of course true that certain features of his antisocial behavior might be explained by the course of his instinctual development. His aggressiveness and obstinacy were, as has been noted, partly a defense against his passive wishes, and partly the result of sado-masochistic object relationships. However, conflicts arising out of the same kind of instinctual development are usually expressed differently.

I had occasion to study another boy of the same age and with the same instinctual development as Billy, and also engrossed in sado-masochistic fantasies and in the need to ward off passive-feminine wishes.

Peter also had a strong urge to possess objects representing the penis. But the way he set about to fulfill his wish was quite different. Every day in a most friendly manner he asked whether I would give him a knife or a little animal from the toy cupboard. At home he sought presents from visitors, asking whether perhaps they had a toy pistol or a similar object to give him. When these visitors were careless enough to promise anything he surreptitiously learned their telephone numbers, rang them up and asked whether he might come and fetch the toy. As in Billy's case, the object had to come from another person, but the way in which it was acquired was within socially accepted limits.

To make another comparison: Billy was well aware of the fact that when he was late I had to wait for him. One of the unconscious purposes of this behavior was to make me angry. The fact that I did not get angry aroused no guilt; on the contrary it drove him to take more and more liberties. Peter, the other little boy, was also occasionally late and for exactly the same reasons as Billy. Consciously he would be attracted by something he saw in the street; unconsciously he wanted to provoke me to punish him. But his attitude when he came was entirely different: he was sorry that he had kept me waiting and would explain to me what had caused the delay. There could be no doubt that though his unconscious desire was to create a quarrel consciously he very much feared to disturb our relationship.

The same difference could be observed in the attitude of these two boys during analytic sessions. Both were intent on expressing their sado-masochistic fantasies in play or action. Billy, in fact, refused to do anything else or even to try to understand what he was doing. Either he was permitted to do as he pleased without interference by the analyst's interpretations or he would do nothing at all. Peter, having understood what the analysis was for, was prepared to forego some of his pleasures because he wanted to please me. This motive, to please the other person, was entirely absent in Billy. It would not, however, be correct to say that Billy's aggressions were more intense than Peter's; if anything, the reverse was true. It may seem that Billy's transference was negative and Peter's positive. But outside the consulting room also, the reactions of both boys clearly reflected the same trends in their various object relationships.

Certain similarities and differences in the relationship of these two boys to their mothers are noteworthy. For both boys this relationship was the most important factor in their lives and separation from the mother, even for a short period, seemed quite unendurable. Billy's attitude to his mother has already been described. He wanted her to satisfy his desires and if she did not he was openly hostile. It was impossible for him to do anything to please her or to forego a pleasure even at the risk of losing her affection. If a desire arose in him, immediate gratification seemed of prime importance. Peter also felt hostility toward his mother if she did not conform to his wishes, and he resented not having her to himself all the time. But his aggressive feelings toward her were always disguised. Once he broke a favorite vase and for days felt extremely guilty though he was neither punished nor nor reprimanded.

The significant difference in the overt attitude of these two boys is not to be sought in the pattern of their instinctual development, but rather in their ego and superego formation.

Peter's conscience was in the process of becoming independent, that is to say, internalized. His neurotic symptoms were the result of an inner conflict, of the struggle between his desires, many of which were sadistic, and the prohibitions imposed upon him by his own severe conscience. The result was that he was a rather timid, shy boy, usually unaggressive, but with outbursts of temper and obsessional symptoms. He did not steal, not because he might be found out but because of his own sense of guilt. Although he wanted to provoke me, this provocation could only go on under the cover of acceptable social behavior.

There were no signs that Billy was ever restrained by conscience from the gratification of his desires. It is true that some of his instinctual wishes, such as his genital impulses toward the mother and his passive-feminine wishes towards the father, were repressed and that regression to the anal-sadistic level had taken place. But the regression permitted him still to have some direct sexual gratification by way of his exhibitionistic activities, and to experience punishment as not entirely unpleasant: doing right or wrong was merely part of his sado-masochistic relationship with his mother. Thus the amount of his antisocial activity was not governed by his own guilt feelings but purely by the chance of being found out.

Aichhorn,[8] describing this lack of independence on the part of the superego from the actual people in the environment as a characteristic disturbance in the character structure of his "aggressive group", has demonstrated how under the special treatment devised for this group, the first signs of internalization of the superego could be observed when the boys began to feel guilty about their behavior toward the adults in the institution.

This lack of independence of superego formation has more far-reaching results than the mere perpetration of antisocial acts. Normally, during the latency period new identifications are made with

8. Aichhorn, op. cit.

teachers and other persons in authority, which enrich the content of the superego and make it more and more independent of the actual parent figures. In a case like Billy's, where identification with the parents has not led to the internalization of their demands, the relationship to persons in authority does not lead to identification with them. Such a child simply transfers his sado-masochistic object relationship to all who are for him parent-substitutes. This gives him some instinctual gratification but does not lead to an enrichment of his personality.

The lack of independence of superego formation also explains Billy's reaction to educational efforts. During the latency period the usual methods of education proceed on the assumption that the child really wishes to conform—in contrast to the early years, when, as the educator rightly assumes, the child's instinctual urges are opposed to the demands of the environment. In the latency period it is the educator's task to strengthen the child's superego formation and to help it to become successful in its fight against the instincts; the child is usually eager to get this help which will prevent him from feeling guilty. Not so with Billy. For him being good simply meant giving in. He wanted what he wanted and felt no compunction when he got it. In his case, punishment did not lead to a strengthening of the superego but was felt either as instinctual gratification or as a frustration permitting the expression of further hostility against the person administering it.

It may be that defective superego formation is based on a disturbed ego development in which case it might be profitable to try to find the specific quality of the ego disturbance in Billy by comparing the ego activities of the two boys.

Billy and Peter both had an I.Q. of about 100. In both cases achievement was poor. Peter went to school and sat there daydreaming. Billy very often did not go at all and if he did was out to fight someone or to disturb the teacher. Interest in school subjects was absent in both boys because they were too much occupied in satisfying or warding off instinctual urges. Consequently little energy was free for sublimation. But there were differences as well. Peter consciously wanted to learn, and could read and write by the time he was seven. Though concentration on school subjects was unpleasant for him, he felt that he ought to try. However, his reading was handicapped because his attention was constantly distracted by the shape of certain letters which suggested objects used in his fantasies.

Billy, who felt the same displeasure when confronted with a difficulty, tried his utmost to avoid any repetition of such a disagreeable experience. He was extremely pleased when he succeeded in reading a word and was praised for it—a successful beginning of sublimating his exhibitionistic tendencies. But he was unduly displeased when confronted with a word he did not recognize: he shut the book and gave up. Whereas most children are able to bear the tensions of learning provided that satisfaction follows achievement, Billy could not bear any tension whatever, nor did the prospect of future gratification attract him. He behaved in this respect like a very much younger child, his ego still governed wholly by the pleasure principle.[9] One day, toward the end of his analysis, Billy said, "I should not have been late yesterday, then I would have been allowed to go out today. Now I cannot go out today and that is worse than if I had been on time yesterday." This was the first time that the boy was able to judge his actions not only from the standpoint of immediate pleasure, but also from the standpoint of future results. Such considerations are usually present in children very much younger than Billy and certainly by the age of nine the behavior of normal children has already come under the control of the reality principle.

At first glance it might appear that Billy was better adapted to reality than Peter. Billy could ride alone in the bus for long journeys, which Peter was afraid to do. Billy displayed shrewdness of judgment in sizing up the various people in his world and thus could use them to gratify his desires. He was able to get money out of any member of the household and then went off to shops to buy what he wanted. Peter would not have been able to do this. Billy's behavior in school was aggressive and "fresh" but he acted as if he knew exactly what he was after. Peter, on the contrary, was considered stupid at school where he did quite inexplicable things without considering the impression they made on others. Nevertheless his ego conformed better to the reality principle than did Billy's. Peter's actions were a compromise between wishes that he recognized as antisocial (they were very often aggressive wishes) and his superego. In spite of the fact that his unconscious conflicts had made him unable to cope with his real problems, his ego nevertheless functioned in harmony with the reality principle.

Both boys were very difficult to handle: Peter, because he suffered from fear whenever his mother went out and because he was absorbed in daydreams and difficulties with other boys; Billy, because he lacked any incentive to conform to the wishes of the world if they ran counter to his instinctual drives. He could not tolerate postponement but had to satisfy all his wishes, whether or not they were antisocial. Of course Billy had his own unconscious conflicts but it is significant that owing to the difference in ego and superego formation, these conflicts were expressed not in neurotic symptoms, but in antisocial behavior.

Defective superego formation seems to result from the failure of the ego to develop toward the reality principle. During Billy's analysis it was possible gradually to see the process reversed. Slowly he was enabled to wait for satisfaction,—a process that began when he made the remark mentioned about the results of his own acts. In time he began to identify himself with a father figure, his mother's new friend. Though he had known this man for over a year, it was

9. Aichhorn describes this behavior as one of the chief characteristics of the delinquent personality. op. cit.

only after the described change had taken place that he voiced the wish to become an engineer like this man, got on a friendly footing with him and could therefore be influenced. Thereafter he became eager to learn to read because it was only on this condition that this man would be able to train him later on.

Identification with the parent of the same sex presupposes the capacity to renounce instinctual gratification under the pressure of fear. But in order to take this step the ego must be able to withstand tension, and thus conform to the reality principle. In Billy's case an identification had taken place with the mother instead of with the father; and furthermore, this identification had never been desexualized. His castration fear did not lead him to give up or even entirely to repress his wishes for the mother. They reappeared after regression had taken place and in his exhibitionistic tendencies. Defect in superego formation is, in my opinion, due to the incapacity to give up instinctual gratification even under the pressure of castration fear: so that the internalization of a desexualized parent imago never takes place.

It therefore becomes increasingly apparent that it is a peculiarity of character structure that determines whether unconscious conflicts plus pressure from the environment will result in neurotic symptom formation or in antisocial behavior. A character structure like Billy's, with the ego still under the dominance of the pleasure principle and with an undeveloped superego, seems in every way typical of the antisocial character. It is similar to what Reich has described as "impulsive character".[10] Its outstanding features have already been emphasized by Aichhorn.[11]

Antisocial character formation does not exclude the development of neurotic conflicts. The ego may have developed towards the reality principle in respect to some instinctual urges and not at all in respect to others, and a partial development of the superego, usually of a still archaic superego, may have taken place. This allows the development of neurotic illness on the one hand and antisocial reactions on the other. The varying proportion of neurotic admixtures explains the manifold psychological pictures met with in delinquents. There is for example the "common offender", who may not show any neurotic illness at all and who demonstrates his antisocial reactions from the latency period onward, often without

10. W. Reich, *Der triebhafte Charakter* (*The Impulsive Character*), Vienna, 1925.
11. op. cit.

any interruption and not necessarily when provoked. Aichhorn's "aggressive youths" belong to this group. They show antisocial character formation in its purest form. In a second group of offenders, the antisocial character formation becomes manifest only under the stress of either environmental or emotional disturbances of some magnitude. Their delinquent acts are in no way different from those of the common offender, but the immediate cause of their behavior can often be found in an unconscious conflict. The majority of delinquents who become antisocial only for a short period in puberty and often become stable again afterwards, belongs to this latter group. In a third group, a neurotic conflict leads to a delinquent instead of a neurotic symptom, as in kleptomania; however, this occurs infrequently. In a fourth group, delinquent instead of neurotic acting out governs the behavior throughout life. These are the cases which Alexander describes as "neurotic characters" and a number of the criminals whom he analyzed show this particular disturbance.

It is not possible within the framework of this paper to investigate the possible fate and the many modifications that may still occur in antisocial character formation during the latency period and puberty. Intelligence, special abilities and the power of sublimation as well as environmental factors may still decisively influence the eventual form of character as it emerges after puberty. Further research into this problem should lead to a scientific basis for the treatment of anti-social children and young offenders, work already successfully begun by Aichhorn and Healy.

One may well ask what educational factors contribute most to antisocial character formation. If we are right in regarding the failure of the ego to develop towards the reality principle as the key to the disturbance, it becomes clear that an early enviironment that fails to exert consistent pressure on the expression of those instinctual urges, which, because they are of an antisocial nature must eventually be modified, tends to predispose an individual towards this character disturbance. In Billy's case ego development was influenced by the mother's inability to be consistent in the ways in which she gratified or frustrated the child's instinctual urges during the first years of life. I have mentioned her attitude towards early bladder and bowel training and, by way of contrast, toward Billy's phallic impulses. Under such conditions, there is no need for a child's learning to wait for gratification. This, as we have seen, is the necessary requisite for satisfactory development from the pleasure principle to the reality principle. Such total inconsistency in the

mother's attitude towards the small child's impulses is equivalent
to a constant alternation between an over-intense mother-child-rela-
tionship with too much gratification on the one hand and, on the other,
too abrupt a separation of the child from the mother when too severe
frustrations are imposed.   There are also many cases where because
of severe economic or other privations the mother cannot care for
her child satisfactorily.   Here the same disturbances of character
may result as in those cases where the difficulty is caused by personality
disturbances in the mother.

A very similar effect on the ego-development of the small child
can result from the display of unrestrained emotions among the adults
in his world such as open quarrels between the parents with overt
expression of violence, open sexual scenes and so on.   Such experi
ences will enhance the antisocial impulses of the small child and have
the same effect as a seduction.   At the same time, children growing
up in such an environment are as a rule strictly prohibited from acting
out their aggressive and sexual tendencies within the family.

As far as we know from childhood histories of delinquents this
parental inconsistency towards the instinctual urges of the child,
primarily as it emanates from the mother and secondarily from other
adults in the early environment, is rarely absent.   But in order to
be certain that this is really a specific factor in antisocial development
we must prove that these factors are absent in the early environment
of the individual destined to become neurotic.   This would need study
by a large number of analysts.   My own experience inclines me to
believe that although these factors may be present to some extent in
the early environment of neurotics they do not appear in their histories
as invariably as in the histories of delinquents.   Statistical investigations into the causation of delinquent behavior do not help to clarify
this point because investigations into a large number of cases cannot
be undertaken with the care necessary to establish the existence of
factors of that kind.   But it is perhaps interesting to note that
Burt,[12] Healy,[13] and Bagot[14] found the highest correlation of any single
factor with the incidence of delinquency in what they call "defective
discipline", and, more especially, in inconsistent discipline, too lenient
behavior alternating with too severe frustrations.   These investigations were undertaken with older children and young persons, but the
assumption could be made that the parents' behavior in this respect

12. C. Burt, *The Young Delinquent*, London, 1924.
13. H. Healy, *The Individual Offender*, London, 1915.
14. Bagot, *Juvenile Delinquency*, London, 1941.

does not change very much with time. It is of course also possible that in some cases the disturbance may be caused not so much by the mother's attitude as by the fact that all or some of the instinctual urges of the child appear in such strength that too much gratification on the one hand and too severe frustrations on the other are unavoidable under ordinary circumstances.

To sum up: By a comparison of certain psychological reactions in two boys of the same age, with the same instinctual background and approximately the same intelligence, I have tried to show that development toward antisocial character formation is caused by a specific character structure. This character structure does not exclude the development of neurotic conflicts but it may explain why in some individuals neurotic conflicts do not lead to neurotic but to delinquent symptoms. The mother's attitude towards a child's early instinctual manifestations caused either by her own personality or by environmental factors and especially when augmented by the display of violent emotional outbursts among the adults of the early family setting may be a specific etiological factor leading to this disturbance.

THE FANTASY OF HAVING A TWIN

By DOROTHY T. BURLINGHAM (London)

A common daydream which in spite of its frequency has received very little attention to-date is the fantasy of possessing a twin. It is a conscious fantasy, built up in the latency period as the result of disappointment by the parents in the oedipus situation, in the child's search for a partner who will give him all the attention, love and companionship he desires and who will provide an escape from loneliness and solitude.

The same emotional conditions are the basis for the so-called *family romance.* In that well-known daydream the child in the latency period develops fantasies of having a better, kinder and worthier family than his own, which has so bitterly disappointed and disillusioned him. The parents have been unable to gratify the child's instinctual wishes; in disappointment his love turns into hate; he now despises his family and, in revenge, turns from it. He has death-wishes against the former love-objects, and as a result feels alone and forsaken in the world. This is a situation the child cannot endure; he seeks a way out of his loneliness and finds solace in a daydream. He creates a new family in imagination and builds up a wonderful life around these new imaginary parents who fulfill the wishes (though not the crudely sexual ones) that were denied by the real parents. If these daydreams are analyzed, the resemblance of the new imaginary parents to the real ones can be recognized although they are very much disguised. Details contained in the fantasies can be traced back to experiences of an earlier period of the daydreamer's life, when the child was still happy, before emotional conflicts had disturbed him, when he felt completely secure in the possession of his parents, dependent on his mother, proud of his father, and when there was no need in his life for other consolation.

Another group of daydreams, the *animal fantasies* of the latency period,[1] originate in the same manner in response to the oedipal conflicts. The child takes an imaginary animal as his intimate and beloved companion; subsequently he is never separated from his animal friend, and in this way he overcomes loneliness. This daydream is constructed in much the same way as the family romance, with this difference: the child does not here choose a new family, does not repeat a similar experience under improved conditions, but chooses a new companion who can understand him in his loneliness, unhappiness, and need to be comforted. This animal offers the child what he is searching for: faithful love and unswerving devotion. There is nothing that this dumb animal cannot understand; speech is quite unnecessary, for understanding comes without words. These animal fantasies are thus an attempt to substitute for the discarded and unloving family an uncritical but understanding, dumb, and always loving creature.

In the story of *Little Lord Fauntleroy* by Francis Hodgson Burnett,[2] the typical child-animal relationship is described. The author creates a situation where the child is separated from his mother and is therefore extremely lonely. In this situation the child meets a dog and the two make friends. In the scenes between them the dog's awareness of the boy's feelings of homesickness and of pity for others, are stressed. This understanding seals the friendship between them, and thus the child acquires a companion to lessen his loneliness.

In the autobiographical story *Waelder und Menschen* (*Woods and Men*) by Ernst Wiechert,[3] the author describes his friendship with a crane when he was a boy of seven years. He says of this friendship that man and animal could not have been more affectionate to each other in he garden of Eden. "We awoke when the sun rose, and greeted each other like two lovers . . . When I had to go away, it stood at the gate and complained of its loneliness. When I returned, it seemed as if it wished to embrace me . . ." The author describes himself as a child, lying in the grass after his midday meal: "It came and stood at my feet; it let itself down onto its knees, stretched its long neck once more, as if it were on the moor, to see whether an enemy was about. Then it lay down, so that its body lay between my arm and my heart, and it hid its head on my breast. From its throat came a continuous dreamy murmur of complete blissful happiness. I stroked its blue feathers as I would stroke the cheeks of a child . . . It seemed as if I were never nearer to God as in the moments when I stroked the feathers of the crane as it lay on my heart, as if we had the same mother."

1. For a dicussion of animal fantasies and animal stories see Anna Freud, *The Ego and the Mechanisms of Defense*, 1937, Chapter VI; and Kate Friedlander, "Children's Books and Their Function in Latency and Prepuberty", *American Imago*, 3, 1942.
2. Scribners, 1896.

3. Albert Langen, München, 1936. Passage below translated by this author.

Child and crane are thus described as if they were lovers; or a mother with her child; or two brothers.

Before the crane is ever mentioned in the story, the author describes the death of his youngest brother. He tells how his mother called him and another brother to the bed of the dying boy. She tells them to kneel down and pray. His brother kneels obediently, but he himself draws his hand away from his mother's and remains standing. He says of this experience, "It is dreadful to know that I remained like an outsider while my mother and brother prayed to God."

This passage throws light on the meaning of the crane fantasy. The death wish against the younger brother, which prevented him from praying as his mother wanted him to, made the boy feel guilty and an outcast; he thought that he had forfeited his mother's love. The gift of a baby crane soon afterward gave him the opportunity to build up a mother-child relationship with the bird. He identified himself with his mother, and he mothered the crane as he had longed to be mothered; and in identification with the crane he was now able to correct his former behavior. The crane even goes down on its knees; it can love and be blissfully happy; it can even love its brother. The longing for the loving mother whom the child had lost because of his own evil wishes is the basis of this animal fantasy.

A little girl in the latency period had a very disturbed relationship to her mother. She had continual daydreams of a better relationship, but in the presence of her mother she could only hate her and provoke her to severity. This ambivalence caused the child great sorrow. When especially angry at her mother, she would withdraw to a fantasy of possessing a dog who would love her devotedly, who would not question or criticize her, who would have understanding for her wicked actions, hostile thoughts, and even dangerously aggressive intentions. In other words, the dog would be aware of her conscious wish to love, and in spite of its additional knowledge of her inability to fight against her unconscious aggression, would love her.

It is evident that the imaginary dog replaces the mother whom she cannot love and who, she feels, cannot love her. She cannot live without love, and the dog now gives her what she longs for, at least in fantasy.

The *fantasy of having a twin* contains the main characteristics of these two groups of daydreams, the family romance and the animal fantasies. They are, as mentioned above, a reaction to the disappointment in love that is experienced during the oedipal phase. The child, unable to accept the inevitable disappointment and the resulting withdrawal of his love from the love-objects, escapes into a fantasy world. The twin is conjured up, not in an attempt to improve on a former experience, as in the family romance, but to take the place of the lost love-object and so to alleviate suffering, as in the animal fantasies.[4] The image that the child creates is, this time, not an animal but a child similar to the daydreamer himself, a twin. This twin is meant to fulfil many of the daydreamer's longings, above all to keep him from solitude and loneliness. The child with a fantasy twin has a constant companion, just as the child who owns an imaginary animal never lacks companionship. As in the case of the animal fantasies, the two share everything, good and bad experiences, and complete understanding of each other; either speech is not necessary, or they have a secret language; the understanding between them goes beyond the realm of consciousness.

The new element in the twin fantasies is the fact that the lost love-object is replaced by a being who is like the daydreamer himself. This aspect of similarity, or identity, plays a large part in the various twin books, adventure stories, and novels. For instance, in the *Twin Books*, by L. F. Perkins,[5] written for children in the latency period, stress is laid on the identity of the twins, especially in the first of the series. They are described as being so alike that "it is impossible to tell them apart, their own mother cannot . . .", and that "they almost get mixed up about it themselves". The author further emphasizes their alikeness by letting them wear similar clothing and by giving them similar-sounding names (Monnie and Mannie). However, this identity is not a continuous element in the stories, but is brought in, as it were, incidentally, from time to time.

In a novel called *Christopher and Columbus,*[6] seventeen-year-old girl twins, the main characters in the story, are first described as being very much alike, and often mistaken for each other, but are later characterized as being very different. One is efficient and healthy, and holds herself responsible for the other, who is beautiful, delicate and helpless. This story begins with the loss of the twins' mother through death. The twins live out a mother-child relationship, as do the child and crane in Wiechert's story (where the loved mother is felt to be "lost" because of the child's bad behavior). The happy companionship of the sisters remains undisturbed until one of them falls in love. One twin is in complete despair at the thought of losing the other. The emotional situation of loss of a love-object is thus created again. The author, as if under a repetition-compulsion, brings the twins together again in due course. The motivating force behind the story is the search for the inseparable companion, based on a feeling of loss and loneliness.

---

4. It should be kept in mind that these fantasies of having a twin are not the same as the actual relationships of twins to each other. The description of twin fantasies given here is only part of a more extensive study of twins, which will appear later.

5. Houghton-Mifflin, 1911-1935.

6. 1929, by Countess Mary A. B. Arnim-Russell, the author of *Elizabeth and Her German Garden*, Macmillan, 1931.

A further element in many daydreams of having a twin is that of the imaginary twin being a complement to the daydreamer. The latter endows his twin with all the qualities and talents that he misses in himself and desires for himself. The twin thus represents his superego. In the above-mentioned book *Christopher and Columbus* this point is brought out repeatedly. Christopher and Columbus are given dissimilar characters; in their relations with a third person they talk and behave as complements to each other. They are as two halves of one person, or as two sides of his nature; one twin representing the expressed, and the other, the unexpressed thoughts.

In a similar manner the twin figures can represent the two sides of an emotional conflict. This occurs in the story of Esteban, in *The Bridge of San Luis Rey,* by Thornton Wilder.[7]

The twin brothers, Manuel and Esteban, are characterized by the author in a way that is typical of all twin fantasies: absolute identity in appearance, a secret language, telepathy between them a common occurrence. It is an additional feature in this pair of twins that they are ashamed of being identical, which points to a forbidden (sexual) relationship between them. The first disturbance of their companionship occurs when one of them, Manuel, falls in love. The conflict between homosexual and heterosexual tendencies becomes evident. The other twin, Esteban, who feels forsaken and alone, tries in his turn to leave the brother; but Manuel, when he becomes aware of his twin's intention and of his misery, gives up the woman he loves. There is apparently no question in Manuel's mind which of the two relationships is more precious to him. The homosexual wins over the heterosexual side. But later, ill. and delirious, he curses Esteban for separating him from his love. His conscious and his unconscious tendencies struggle with each other. The unconscious heterosexual feelings break through in Manuel's delirium, while Esteban remains throughout under the domination of his homosexual wishes. The problem the author expresses by means of the twin brothers is the fight between the conscious and the unconscious, the homosexual and the heterosexual wishes, each twin representing one side of the conflict. The struggle in Esteban continues after Manual dies. Esteban cannot face life alone. He takes over his twin's name, trying in vain to unite the two personalities in one. Loneliness drives him to suicide. When this is interfered with, fate, as the power of the unconscious, provides a solution: Esteban is one of the victims of the Bridge of San Luis Rey.

A further important element in the twin fantasies is that of narcissism.[8] A child who feels himself thwarted and forsaken is

7. New York, 1927.

8. To be discussed more fully in a forthcoming paper. See also Otto Rank, "Der Doppelgänger" ("The Double"), *Psychoanalytische Beiträge zur Mythenforschung,* Vienna, 1919; and Hanns Sachs, "The Community of Daydreams", in *The Creative Unconscious,* Boston, 1942.

thrown back upon himself. He cannot imagine finding anyone more satisfactory than he is. He therefore creates a twin, an image of himself that he can love. This solution also acts as a cover for self-love and as a means of avoiding criticism and guilt. In the disguise of the twin the daydreamer loves himself; narcissism is hidden, and self-love appears under the mask of object-love.

There is still another use to which the twin fantasies may be put, that is, to express great strength and invincibility. This element is found in the adventure stories, in which the usual "hero" is replaced by a pair of twins. Two are able to do what one could not have accomplished alone, owing to their combined strength and power. There is some similarity between these fantasies and the fantasy of doubling or multiplying certain parts of the body, which occurs among children, especially in boys when they are passing through a phase of castration anxiety. In their fear of losing their penis or an arm or a leg, etc., they endow themselves with a surplus of these valuable attributes. The daydream of the twin hero expresses the idea: I am small and weak in the face of dangers, but if I were twice as big, twice as strong, twice as clever, there is nothing that I would not be able to do.

To sum up: all three fantasies, the family romance, the fantasy of having an animal companion, and the fantasy of possessing a twin, are found to originate in the frustration of wishes of the oedipal phase. Disappointment by the parents and withdrawal of love from them are the leading elements which seek expression and which the child tries to over-compensate and to undo. The relationship to the imaginary twin represents a partnership that is not threatened with separation. Although the element of loss crops up continually in the twin stories, reunion with the partner is invariably effected (in the case of Esteban it is reunion in death).

The twin fantasy has its further uses for expressing discord and unity within the personality itself, as shown in the examples of twins representing ambivalent tendencies and opposite instinctual wishes of various kinds.

THE UNCOMPROMISING DEMAND
OF A THREE-YEAR-OLD FOR
HER OWN MOTHER

By ELEANOR PAVENSTEDT, M.D. and IRENE ANDERSEN, M.S. (Boston) [1]

Betty came to the Children's Center at the age of three-and-a-half, referred by a children's agency because she had been declared unmanageable in a series of foster homes. The complaints were destructiveness, aggressive behavior toward other children and adults, poor toilet habits,,temper tantrums and running away. Only one foster mother had made some kind of contact with the child during the two years that she had 'been moving about. It seemed as though she had clung to her feelings for her own "Peggy-Mummy" from the time when, at eighteen months, she was first separated from her mother, and that she had resented everyone who tried to take her mother's place.

The mother had herself been an orphan from the age of eight. Infantile paralysis then caused her to spend the next eight years in a home for crippled children. From there she went to a wage home where she remained another eight years. She had an illegitimate son while there, whom she immediately gave up to her brother for adoption. Betty had the same father as this first child. The mother was sure he would marry her. He was intellectually and culturally superior to her and her family. It was a terrible blow when he married someone else during her second pregnancy. Several weeks before the delivery, the mother entered a maternity home where both before and after Betty's birth she worked in the kitchen. She had been well during pregnancy; labor lasted only six to seven hours; the delivery was uneventful. The mother had wanted a girl so much she was "sure it would be one". In the family where she had worked she had had almost sole care of another little Betty, the baby of her employer

1. From the Children's Center, Judge Baker Guidance Center, Roxbury, Mass.

(because of the post-partum illness of the mother) ; and she had come
to long for a little Betty of her own.

After the baby was born, she was nursed for five to six weeks.
During the first few days she did not suck readily; when she began
to nurse better, she fell asleep quickly and her toes were snapped to
awaken her several times during feeding.   When the mother got up
and around, she had no more milk.   There were supplementary bottle-
feedings almost from the start and the transition was easy.   Betty was
a happy baby, rarely cried, always loved to eat.   She always liked being
cuddled and the mother loved to cuddle her.   The mother gave Betty
what care she could before and after working hours and at noon, and
in between times the child was cared for by the nurses.

When Betty was six or seven months, her mother started putting
her on the potty.   Training progressed smoothly until nine months
when Betty had a case of roseola infantum.   She was kept apart from
her mother who visited her but was not allowed to pick her up or
feed her.   The mother was struck by Betty's apathy; the child lay quite
unresponsive; her only activity was to put a rubber kitten "under her
stomach" and bounce up and down on it.   After this illness she yelled
and screamed when placed on the potty.   There was a marked tendency
toward constipation.   Tied down to the potty chair, she usually managed to get off.   Suppositories were used but she retained them for
hours.   On the other hand, she began to take delight in smearing herself and her crib.   Her mother thought she did this because she loved
the extra tub, and spanked her for it a few times but Betty did not
seem to mind much.   When she began to walk she became the center
of attention of all the many employees.   She began having temper
tantrums when crossed.   She bit on several occasions, her mother as
well as others.

At eighteen months, Betty was placed in a foster home by a children's agency, since her mother continued to work at the maternity
home and it was felt that the child needed a normal home environment.   The mother persistently refused to give her up for adoption.
Betty was at first very unhappy, and standing up in her crib would
cry herself to sleep; but by the end of a week she appeared to be fond
of both foster-parents.   However, when the agency nurse visited in
the home, the foster-mother complained of Betty's thumb-sucking (for
which the child had been made to wear aluminum mitts at night), and
her totally inadequate toilet-training.   Whenever Betty was displeased
she threw herself on the floor and banged her head to the point of
bruising it.   She bit, scratched, pulled children's hair, and failed to

respond to any corrective measures. When her own mother visited, Betty behaved similarly toward her. After one month, the foster-mother felt unable to cope with these problems and repeatedly asked that Betty be replaced.

Two months later, Betty was moved to Mrs. B., the only one of her many foster-mothers whom she ever mentioned to us and to whom she had a definite attachment. Mrs. B. reported that she had to teach Betty how to have a bowel movement. It seemed that it had never occurred to Betty—now twenty-one months old—to go to the toilet for that purpose. Mrs. B. took her there right after breakfast, showed her how to bear down and sat with her until the bowel movement was accomplished. She was able to control the child's constipation by careful supervision, providing fruit juices constantly, laxatives and enemas quite often. Whenever the mother appeared, the child's temper tantrums and obstinacy reappeared. After six months of concentrated effort, the foster-mother succeeded in establishing toilet habits during waking hours only. Mrs. B. commented on the child's enormous appetite. Betty was placed elsewhere to give Mrs. B. a vacation but this placement was abandoned because the child's behavior was too difficult to bear; she was returned to Mrs. B. Then, when Betty took to roaming away, Mrs. B. (who preferred babies anyway) refused to keep her. In both of these homes, the foster-mothers attempted to cure Betty of biting, by biting back. Mrs. B. succeeded.

At two years, seven months (thirteen months after separation from her mother) she went to her third foster home, where she never adjusted at all. The early report that they all loved her because she was so affectionate indicates that she there had already established a pattern that we subsequently had frequent opportunity to observe: that of entering a new home with apparent radiant self-possession and friendliness. In this home where Betty remained ten months, her behavior became increasingly difficult. She turned on the oil stove, radiators and lights indiscriminately. She slapped, pinched and bit the children who would not give in to her. She tore her bed clothes and pulled the stuffing out of her pillow. Despite warnings and spankings, she wandered away; was headstrong and determined. Although she did not play with toys, she took them away from other children and often destroyed them. When petted she became rough, noisy and excited.

Betty's own mother visited her only a few times in this home, then stopped coming because "it was too far". When the child was brought to town for a clinical check-up at three years, two months, and there met her mother for the first time in almost half a year she reacted in a way that seems clearly to disprove the assumption that little children forget their mothers: she was quite demonstrative, and became much more active; she was very unhappy when her mother left and sobbed most of the way home and again at evening. Afterward she teased her foster-brother about his mother's not seeing him.

The mother's conduct had meantime become less and less acceptable to the authorities of the maternity home. She was drinking heavily and staying out late. Soon after the meeting with Betty, she was discharged; subsequently she also failed to keep a position with a friend of her former employer, even though she was offered the opportunity of having Betty live with her there. She began to get behind in payments for the child's maintenance, and failed to keep appointments with the agency. In the course of the spring and summer when Betty was referred to the Children's Center, there were only two letters from her saying she planned to be married to a sailor and would then take Betty home. These plans seemed so vague and improbable, and her interest in her child appeared to have dwindled so greatly, that no one felt she could be relied upon to play a constructive part in Betty's future.

The foster-mother was now demanding that Betty be removed from her home. The agency was at a loss to find another foster home and requested our advice concerning further care. In June, 1943, the child came to us for study and residential care. Until she could be admitted (and later when the Center was closed for a month) the most successful foster-mother, Mrs. B., was prevailed upon to keep her temporarily. Mrs. B. soon reported difficult behavior and temper-tantrums; in addition, Betty had diarrhea[2] to such an extent that Mrs. B. was obliged to put her into diapers again.

Betty was brought to Nursery School by various workers and as it was summer, children and adults were all in the yard together much of the day, so that contact with them was natural. She was charming to look at: a sturdy, energetic and vigorous little girl. All were struck by her impetuous and open-arm approach, and by the affectionate embraces she bestowed upon each new arrival. The following description illustrates her characteristic behavior:

A new volunteer whom Betty did not know arrived at the B. home to call for her; Betty immediately grabbed her hand and clung to it all the way to the

2. This was not true diarrhea but dribbling of small liquid stools during bowel retention, as will be later described.

Children's Center repeating "Mummy, Mummy" in a shrill excited way. On the street car she asked whether various men were her daddy and was delighted when an older man pinched her cheek and said that he would like to be. For the remainder of the ride, Betty chattered with him about all her mummies. Arriving at the Center she stared at the grocer and said "Daddy". Throughout she clung to the worker, kissing her frequently. Finally she went off to play, obviously aware of on-looking adults, playing up to them for admiration and affection. Her play was invariably the same: she was the mother, cooking busily for the father who would return home from work soon; when she could draw other children into her play she would assign to them the role of father and children, but when they tired and failed to fall in with her orders, she continued right on without them. She was careful not to soil her clothes, and gathered her household goods (tin cans, spoon, etc.) around her when she felt they were threatened. She seldom fought with other children unless seriously provoked and was protective and gentle with little children. There was a pushing quality about her every move as well as in her approach to people, that was remarked upon by all who observed her. Except for the play described above, her attention span was short. She made little use of toys and equipment.

Her problems appeared mainly in connection with her nap in Nursery School. She could not lie down or even sit on her cot, but roamed about noisily and actively interfered with the other children. When she was curtailed—by being taken into a separate room, for instance,—she usually had a severe tantrum: she trembled, chewed her fingers, cried convulsively, jumped from one foot to the other and shrank from whatever adult tried to calm her, refusing to be touched. Once, when she was roaming around, she sat down on the stairs and sobbed heartbrokenly. No one was able to divert her. As time went on there were sometimes entire days when she seemed gloomy and sulking and had nothing to say but "no". On such days she seemed at a loss what to do with herself. Trouble with elimination was noted almost from the start; on some days she had no movement at all; often while she was having one she would whimper helplessly, "It hurts." She ate very well and had no food dislikes.

She was much interested and very cooperative during all special examinations. Our pediatrician noted that she was well-built and self-confident. The only abnormal findings were hypertrophied tonsils. An electroencephalogram showed normal findings. On the Stanford-Binet, when she was four she had a mental age of 4.10 (I.Q. 121). Although she had a good vocabulary, her words were poorly formed: "I wanna do dis", "I ain't done yet", "Hey, hold dis".

When Betty came to live at the Children's Center at the end of July, her outstanding problem was going to bed at night. She took a great many things to bed with her but even then was not content to stay there. She would pace up and down her room, usually clutching a doll or a book. When she was removed to a room by herself she cowered in the corner of her crib like a little frightened animal, refusing to be touched. In the daytime she found it very hard to allow the adult in charge to give attention to the other children and often shoved them aside. Only when she herself assumed the role of an adult and helped care for them did she seem untroubled. She often did little practical things about the house, imitating adults. We observed throughout that there was remarkably little carry-over from "home" difficulties to school.

Very early on the fifth day in residence Betty called out "I want to go home. I go downstairs. I want to be sick." This call ushered in a period of extreme distress over her fecal elimination according to a pattern that was always noted when she moved to a new home, and often when she was threatened with a change.

At first her movements are small, hard and frequent, she shouts and cries on the toilet. Gradually she becomes very dependent, sucks her thumb, complains of abdominal pain, appears excited; she looks pale and strained with dark circles under her eyes. She goes to the toilet about every twenty minutes, complaining bitterly of pain, has the urge to defecate but obviously withholds her stool. During short periods off the toilet, she passes small amounts of very soft feces, smearing her panties and herself. Occasionally she laughs and coos and shows real pleasure at this. Before long local irritation appears, the pain increases, she screams on the toilet, holding her entire body rigid as a board, trembles and perspires. She pleads to be wiped by the adult of her choice. In a clean-up bath she laughs and shows obvious enjoyment. Her temperature remains normal until about the end of a week when she almost invariably develops an acute upper respiratory infection. Furthermore, although "I need to go" goes like a theme-song through her days, she sleeps soundly at night. The first two times the withholding was handled by enemas which produced enormous, very hard stools. At the height of these periods the rectal and genital region is very inflamed. The irritation is of short duration.

As we came to recognize the implications of this behavior we cut the episodes short by meeting her anxiety with understanding, as will be described below, and by early and frequent administration of mild laxatives.

A., our social worker, was at this time living in the Children's Center and because we were short-staffed, helped care for the children on occasional evenings and weekends. It so happened that the first time she took charge after Betty's arrival, Betty was already in the midst of one of her withholding periods. A. realized that Betty was suffering and regardless of the pleasure and attention the child was trying to gain by her behavior, A. felt that she needed complete acceptance and gave it to her. She cared for her as one would for a very small sick child, loving and babying her as Betty obviously wanted to be. After being wiped Betty held A.'s hand tenderly and hugged her. When the worker in charge of her returned to take over, Betty wanted to "stay with Miss A.", called for her each time she went to the bathroom, ran down the hall to assure herself that she was still in her room, insisted on having Miss A. give her her bath and put her to bed. On this occasion she played in bed for the first time and settled down quietly to sleep.

On the following day she enacted another characteristic scene. She ran after A. three times; and each time after a short visit was told that she was to remain with the group because A. had other work to do. The third time her thumb went into her mouth and she attached herself closely to the teachers in charge for the rest of the day. In the evening when A. came in to say goodnight, she seemed not to notice her. The next morning she packed her toy suitcase, went downstairs, and out of the house with the earnest intention of going away in the street car.

Since her bowel trouble was becoming very severe, she had to be separated from the other children and came under A.'s sole care for almost a week, during which A. did many of the things that Betty wanted. In return Betty was quite reasonable, although there were many brief periods of aggressiveness and over-activity. Almost immediately there appeared a trend that remained throughout this relationship; Betty talked again and again of being big like A. (who now became alternately "Mummy" and "Mrs. A."), of having big shoes like hers, of being beautiful like her, having hair, eyes, etc., like her; then *she* would be A. and would be the mother. At the same time she repeatedly tried to assure herself of A.'s continued care and talked of living with her indefinitely. She repeatedly played a game of leaving and returning. During her more difficult excited periods she was alternately affectionate and aggressive with A. This emotional swing was more pronounced when Betty rejoined the resident group and was prepared for the fact that A. was going away on vacation. She could not tolerate having another child close to A. and pushed him away. If A. persisted in doing something for the other child, Betty suddenly went off most affectionately with someone else to show she did not care. Now and again her shoes would turn up in A.'s bathroom, and her soiled clothes in A.'s hamper. When A. was about to leave Betty went into a terrific tantrum which no one could control. A. explained once more that she would return and that meanwhile Betty would stay in residence for awhile longer, and then go back to Mrs. B. She put some candies into her drawer for Betty telling her to come and get one every day. (Betty never confided this secret to anyone; at A.'s return the candies were gone.) After A. left Betty continued to ask for her, apparently never accepting her departure. During the remaining two weeks in residence she ate less well, sucked her thumb a great deal and generally gave evidence of restlessness and anxiety. The bowel retention recurred spasmodically but did not lead to as serious a disturbance as before until she returned for the brief stay to Mrs. B. who was obliged to put her in diapers.

Unfortunately the Children's Center had to close its residential quarters at this time for various practical reasons. For Betty this precipitated the very thing we wanted to protect her from, namely, another series of foster homes. At the same time, it provided us with a number of situations where we were able to make close observations of Betty with foster-mothers who were equipped with special training and understanding and who made an enormous effort to help Betty to adjust.

Mrs. B. had taken Betty in June and again in September, more or less against her will, to accommodate the agency. She now refused absolutely to have her remain. Since the agency could provide no foster home, Mrs. R. who had had charge of her in residence agreed to take Betty into her home until the return to town of a young mother, formerly a social worker, who was to be her "more permanent" foster mother. The child's maternal uncle offered to take her, but we were afraid of accepting the offer at this time because of Betty's emotional condition, lest we expose her to the trauma of being rejected by her own people. It was, however, our goal to prepare her to live with this uncle.

Just before moving to Mrs. R. Betty was visited by her mother for the first time since they had met at the clinic more than six months before. Unfortunately she told Betty that she was going to her uncle's where there would be a little boy whom she would call brother. Betty talked about this continually to Mrs. B. (where she still was) and was full of anticipation. The mother at this time was out of sympathy with our work, maintaining that Betty had no problems. She was planning to marry a sailor stationed in the West and then to have Betty with her. This still appeared to be a wish-fulfilling fantasy.

Since Betty had been unable to establish any enduring relationships and since it was felt that her contact with most adults was of a disturbingly brittle and superficial quality, we decided that a therapeutic situation unhampered by the demands of daily existence might help her to establish an attachment with some depth of emotion. At this time some of the people who had observed her felt that, in spite of apparently good constitutional endowment, her tendency to scatter her affection made her prognosis dubious. We recognized that just this quality would render difficult the establishment of a transference but hoped that in the course of the therapeutic process her anxieties could be resolved and her aggression worked through. As we shall see, the therapist's role became very secondary as regards the direct work with Betty, as she had already established a stronger attachment to A. than we realized at this time.

During her first hour with P. who had known her slightly in the early summer, Betty was engrossed with the idea that she had an uncle. She asked if the therapist had a father and a mother. She drew the picture below naming the various parts. When told she was about to move she denied it.

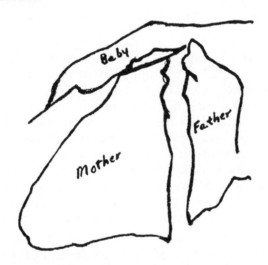

Betty took complete possession of the room into which she moved at Mrs. R.'s, as though she would stay there always. She was a "good little girl" for five days. As soon as A. returned, however, Betty ran and hugged her, saying she did not want to live with Mrs. R. "When can I live with you?" It was thought wisest for A. to withdraw as best she could to give foster mother and therapist a better chance to establish a relationship. The Nursery School teacher decided to assume a neutral role, since the difficulties in school were of a minor nature and since there were so many people involved already. On the sixth day when Betty was about to leave Nursery School, she had a severe temper tantrum, clung to A., talked incoherently and uncontrollably. From then on she ate and slept poorly, was very restless and resistant. On the twelfth day trips to the toilet became more frequent and she was headed for one of her typical sieges. In another few days she was a desperate little girl. A. was asked to resume her contact, since Betty had refused to come to the therapist's office following her first visit and was increasingly negative with Mrs. R. When A. went to her, she was on the toilet exhausted. A. told her she would go home with her and Betty put her head on A.'s chest and sobbed and sobbed. There followed a few days of slight fever with cold and sore throat. The pediatrician who had known Betty since birth diagnosed the condition as constipation with upper respiratory infection. As a result the child had a long week of bed care. A. visited her almost daily, was cuddled and stroked and kissed, and insistently called "Mummy". P., the therapist, was pleasantly received when she visited but remained quite unimportant. Betty calmed down and was again easy to manage. Amid a good deal of baby talk she told Mrs. R. she wanted to live with A.

A. prepared her instead for her entrance into Mrs. M.'s home where she was supposed to stay until we felt that she could go to her uncle's. When they visited Mrs. M. together, Betty had her eyes glued on A., and kept repeating that she would be only four blocks away from her. She came to her therapeutic sessions, but was restless and called the therapist Mrs. Brown (a name she had also given Mrs. R. the preceding summer), and announced triumphantly that A. was going to play with her today. When P. attempted to discuss her moving, Betty thrust a book into her hand to read aloud and sucked hard at a wooden toy in a very anxious way. Her excitement rose daily; she talked baby talk; in seeming confusion she tried to put her doll's dress on herself.

She was moved to Mrs. M., who by the end of a week was so worn out that she demanded Betty's immediate removal. After four relatively tranquil days the child had purposefully begun to scream to awaken Mrs. M.'s baby and had been totally unmanageable. When A. arrived at Mrs. M.'s insistence, Betty said, "Now I'm going to live with you."

We were at our wit's end to know what to do with her. Finally A. offered to have Betty live with her. This arrangement could only last for six weeks because her room would be needed but it seemed better than to send her to the uncle's at this point. Furthermore we all felt that it was an experiment well worth the effort in terms of research as well as treatment.

Betty settled down emphatically, announcing that she was going to live with A. forever. She resumed themes from the preceding summer: she would be big like A. Everything would be "ours". Betty told P. she was living with A. because she loved A. best. At night she wanted A. to sleep with her and sobbed deeply before she could let her go. At the same time she was extremely demanding, insisted on participating in all A. was doing, had temper tantrums and periods of negativism when she was denied anything. At other times Betty could not do enough for her new Mummy; she ate her supper for *her,* went to bed for *her,* and had a big bowel movement for *her*—she called A. into the bathroom and in proud excitement, hugging and kissing her, showed it to her as a present. Attempts to treat the feces casually were ignored, and Betty refused to have it flushed away for sometime. Whenever possible A. yielded to her demands so that there would be as little frustration as possible during this initial period.

Once again efforts to give Betty security were interrupted because her pediatrician felt that a scheduled tonsilectomy should be carried out before a week in her new home had elapsed. As soon as she was told about it, she complained of abdominal pain and started her trips to the toilet. The night before the operation she slept poorly, whimpering and crying out, "Mummy, Mummy" all night long. On her way to the hospital the next morning she asked whether her Peggy-Mummy would come to see her there. When A. came for her on the following day she pretended not to care and ignored her. Convalescence was most difficult because she so resented having A. leave her to go to work every day. She withdrew under the covers, cowered in the corner of her bed, ate almost nothing and had her old bowel troubles. A. comforted and reassured her, saying that leaving her did not mean she did not love her. When Betty was obviously testing out how far A. would yield, the latter set some limitations which called forth: "You are no longer Mummy but Miss A." She was told Mummies love children even when they do not give them everything and later that Mummies love children even when they are bad. By dint of frequent repetition, often upon request, it was felt that some impression was made because Betty found it less necessary to make demands. She was also told that she was able to give A. her bowel movement when she thought A. loved her, but withheld it when she thought A. did not.

When Betty returned to the Children's Center, P. talked to her about her unhappiness when A. went out. She told her all Mummies had to leave their children at times, that her Peggy-Mummy would too. "No, she wouldn't." When told her Peggy-Mummy would have to go to work, Betty replied, "I'm going to work today." Then she became somewhat aggressive and destructive. That evening she sat on A.'s lap the entire time. She said she wanted Peggy-Mummy to come and see her and immediately added, "My Peggy-Mummy hasn't got a place to keep me."

Betty's mother was able to come and visit the next day. It was a stiff, self-conscious meeting—Betty swaggering in, stiff-legged like a little boy. When A. joined them, Betty looked them both up and down repeatedly. After taking her mother to the door, she came running back freer and happier. During the following day she mentioned several times *loving* A. but *liking* this or that other person.

At Thanksgiving Betty went for several days to A.'s farm. Again she showed concern and had bowel trouble when told about the trip, but calmed down when it got under way. She had an intense reaction to the house; stood before it as though charmed, saying, "What a lovely house." Inside, she jumped up and down with delight. It was *her* closet, *her* bed, "*our* house". She ate a big dinner and went to bed willingly; slept soundly for more than twelve hours. The next day she said, "We are going to live here alone always." All attempts to intrude upon this fantasy with the reality of leaving in a few days were met with, "No, no, no." Visiting neighbors and an afternoon reluctantly spent with another child so upset her that she came home very excited and cried in her sleep all night. House guests who arrived the next day further increased her restlessness and she ate very little. The scene upon departure shows the tenacity with which this child clung to her fantasy. To all attempts to awaken her from her nap because it was time to leave, she responded by rolling over and falling asleep again. When she was finally picked up she flung her arms around A.'s neck, clung to her and sobbed out, "I don't want to go home. I want you and me to live here." When she was carried down despite resistance, she ran back upstairs. It required the help of one of the guests to bring her down. All the way home she sat on A.'s lap, sad, quiet, and unresponsive. Following this visit, Betty became much less demanding and seemed to be making a conscious effort to be a good "big girl". She played by herself for long stretches of time. Again the theme of her being Mama and A.'s being the little girl was very prominent. It remained difficult for her to let A. go out and a weekend visit with A. at the home of friends evoked the old reactions.

At this time her mother informed the agency that she was pregnant and expected to marry the baby's father. We realized then that she had already been pregnant when she refused to remain on the job where she could have had Betty with her. We learned also that she was living with the sister of her fiance, and was accepted by his family. Upon careful review of her history, it now became evident that her period of real social breakdown had been short, as compared with long years of a stable work record. She still wanted Betty as soon as she was married and we now felt that she might really some day take her home.

As she became more secure with A., Betty was better able to accept her therapist whose role it seemed necessary to explain to her. For a long period Betty had certainly felt her as an intruder, but now she began to mention her to A. occasionally. P. consequently explained that it seemed as if Betty were looking everywhere for a Mummy and that she wanted to help her get over that; that she really need not look for a Mummy since she had her Peggy-Mummy. A few days later A. referred Betty to the therapist for answers to her questions about her birth, her birthday in the winter, etc. P. told her that her Peggy-Mummy had had her in a hospital where she had lived with her and taken care of her for a long time, had fed her, bathed her and changed her diapers, etc. At the end of this interview, for the first time, Betty did not want to leave. It was suggested that she play with the other children downstairs and she was asked which one she liked best. She said "you" emphatically, showing that she was still absorbed in the previous conversation and had a sudden wave of affection for the therapist who had aroused old feelings for her real mother. In many interviews during the following weeks she acted like an adolescent with a crush, apparently overwhelmed with feelings she did not know how to express.

The six-week period previously set for Betty's living with A. was now drawing to a close; it now seemed necessary to send Betty to a school. Although this was presented to her in the light of prestige— doing what an older boy in the house was doing—it affected her behavior immediately; demands increased, she was more restless and anxious, she often cried and called out in her sleep. Her baby sounds and gurgling on the toilet during periods of bowel retention were louder and of longer duration than ever before. Once A. saw her draw back a fecal mass that was half out. Smearing was widespread

—over abdomen, genitals and thighs. Betty kept referring to school, wanted A. to be there with her. More than ever she was interested in A.'s buying this or that house on the street for the two of them to live in forever by themselves. Her birthday was approaching and the only present she wanted was a toy house. When she received it, she was absorbed in playing with it; took it off into a corner of the room and sat with her arms around it for almost half an hour. She proclaimed that A. and she lived in it, and finally took it to bed with her.

As a surprise Betty's own mother came to her birthday party. Although still a little timid and ill-at-ease, Betty nevertheless approached her mother very differently from the way she had at the last visit. She smiled at her happily, put her arm around her and spontaneously told her what she had done during the morning, as though to include her mother in her life. However, during the cake and ice-cream ceremony, where Betty was a charming hostess, she kept beaming at A.

We were unable to find any home or school that would take Betty. Her uncle wrote that he was about to be inducted into the Army and could not have her. Her mother was living with her future sister-in-law in very close quarters and expected to be confined in six weeks. Since we were not absolutely certain she would be taking Betty home afterward we did not mention the possibility to the child. The only immediate solution was for A. and Betty to take up residence again at the Children's Center. Staff members, including the therapist, alternated in spending nights and weekends there.

Although Betty was happy about moving to the Children's Center she repeated her old pattern of crying out in her sleep, her temper tantrums and her excitable behavior. When discipline could not be avoided, she became unmanageable—shouted that she was going to find a new Mummy and a new home, wanted to pack her clothes, etc. She was told that she was making it necessary for A. to punish her, so that then she could hate A. and leave her; also that Mummies have to punish their children sometimes. "I want a Mummy who is good!" "A Mummy who gives you everything?" "Yes, my Peggy-Mummy." She soon became affectionate, dramatized moving repeatedly. She pretended to gobble up A., saying, "I eat you because you are good."

Betty's mother sent word that she would be married before the New Year. She wanted Betty home for the Christmas holidays to become acquainted with her new father. The child was told on December 21st. She jumped with joy, became excited, played without

purpose, bumped into things, shouting repeatedly, "I'm never coming
back to you." When A. explained "You think I am sending you
away," Betty answered, "You're a bad Mummy." She was reassured
that A. loved her and was letting her go only because her real Mummy
wanted her. Her behavior was a combination of tenderness and
aggression. She would start to kiss A. gently, then suddenly bite her
lip. Over and over again she needed reassurance about A.'s love and
would say, "I know, we love together." She was happy while packing
her things, wanted to take everything, then again talked about returning that evening. She greeted her mother most affectionately, and
kissed everyone good-by, A. last.

When A. met Betty and her mother after Christmas, Betty dashed
past her wildly and ran the entire length of the station. She looked
pale and tired, moved around nervously, chattering and pulling at
either her mother or A. The latter learned that Betty's mother had
told her about the new baby and sailor-daddy, whereupon Betty announced she was going to live with all three of them after the baby
came. However she seemed anxious to have her mother leave—asked
whether they were going to the farm now. On the train she was
terribly restless, excited and noisy. She asked when A. was going to
have their baby and continued to talk about this for days, even though
she was corrected time and again. At the farm she ran directly to
the bathroom and complained of pain; she ate a huge dinner and
called out in her sleep all night long.

During the few days at the farm, she required constant supervision—she played dangerously with the stove, the lamps, the fire;
on a shopping trip she knocked cans of food off a shelf, ran away in
traffic. It was a striking repetition of her behavior in her third foster
home as above described. Although she was constantly reassured that
A. loved her and only gave her to her own mother because that is
where little girls are happiest, she reiterated that A. and she would
live at the farm forever. On the way home in the train she wanted
to sit with others and said she was going home with them. A. interpreted that she wanted to hurt and leave A. because A. was letting her
go to her own mother.

On their return to the Children's Center, Betty ran through the
house away from A.; in bed she sucked her thumb loudly and cried
out, "When are you going to have the baby?" "Not I, Peggy-Mummy
is going to have a baby." "Oh!" She became affectionate, asked to
kiss A. good night, fondled her hair, face and breasts. This interest
in touching breasts continued—she did it also with her therapist.

Besides licking and sucking A.'s skin, she took a large button on A.'s jacket entirely into her mouth and sucked it. For weeks her play with the therapist repeated itself with few variations. She told P. to be the mother and gave her a baby doll to care for: Betty was the big girl who went off to High School and worked hard at her lessons. After doing the house-work and cooking, the mother was expected to call for her with the baby and they all went home for dinner. Betty sometimes took care of the baby but usually became impatient with her and dumped her back into the mother's lap. Occasionally she threw her out or destroyed her altogether. Her feelings about her mother's coming baby were interpreted. When the sucking or breast fondling occurred, she was told she wanted to be the baby. This was always denied, and playing the big girl was thereupon increased.

Shortly after the mother's marriage Betty's parents came to fetch her for another visit. Betty greeted them with affection and enthusiasm, proudly introducing "my new Mummy and my new Daddy" to everyone.

She returned from this visit with the mumps and A. came down with them a few days later. This necessitated several moves and having various people take care of Betty, all of which the child handled relatively well. The therapist, who among others also cared for her, observed that after a rebellion Betty always came back to assure herself that she was still loved, much in contrast to her behavior of a half year before. She was speaking more maturely, often using one or another of A.'s expressions.

When news came that a baby sister had been born, Betty was very excited. After her mother returned home, Betty was told she was going to visit her family again and asked, "When will I live there forever?" She was told it would be soon. Each day she became more excited and difficult and her bowel trouble started up. A. talked with her about mother's taking care of her previously as she was now caring for the baby. When at the end of this visit her father brought her back he reported that Betty had behaved well at home, and seemed fond of the baby. He was in the process of adopting her. Later that day Betty became excited and shouted that she did not like to live with real mothers, only with make-believe ones; she said she was going to go and live with Mrs. B. (former foster-mother). She compared A.'s food, clothes, bathroom, etc., to her mother's, saying that the latter had "junky" things.

During her last week with A., Betty did a great deal of "gobbling" her up. She kissed her, licked her cheeks, sucked her ear-lobes.

"When I eat you up I can do everything like going out to play by myself." Once coming home from school she said she had a great big bowel movement that didn't fit in the toilet. "Then do you know what I did?" "No." "I made a big bowel movement with clay: a red one, a brown one, a green one, a white one. Then I made a saucer and spoon and put the red one in it and ate it for dessert." "Why did you eat it?" "Then I made a house, a chair, a sled and a baby and ate them all up." "Your baby sister?" "Yes, now she's all gone." That night she had a cold and slight fever. She said she wouldn't go out in the cold to school the next day and could not go out to her Peggy-Mummy's. In bed she clung to A., asked for her baby-doll and went to sleep. The next day she was unusually quiet, solemn and wistful. She asked whether A. would come to see her, was reassured and reminded she would be coming to school twice a week. She was told again that A. would miss her very much, and was unhappy to have her leave but had to let her go to her real mother.

Betty went home to live with her mother and the baby in a small apartment which her "navy-daddy" had furnished for them before he returned to the West Coast. For the first few days she was defiant and stubborn when crossed, telling her mother that she did not have to stay, that she would go and live with Mrs. B. or A. Bed-time was difficult as long as we remained in contact with her, i.e. during the four months after she returned to her mother. When her mother went to bed with her all was well; otherwise she was restless and demanding until late in the evening.

A. made it a point to have a visit with Betty every afternoon before she left school for home. At first she found it difficult to express her longing for A., although her pale face with darkly circled eyes and her strained manner showed it clearly. When encouraged to sit in A.'s lap and told that A. missed her, she again kissed and licked her, as before. Since Betty's remarks indicated that her mother was trying to pull her away from the Children's Center, A. made a home visit and was able to win the mother's cooperation. During the visit A. learned that to her mother's surprise Betty had said at various times that Mummies love their children even when they are bad. Although Betty's own mother was certainly not as tolerant as her previous "Mummy" had been, and there were occasional spankings, A. felt that in general the mother handled Betty with patience, affection and understanding.

Following this visit, Betty was natural and affectionate. Now that she had both her own Mummy and A., the therapist again became an intruder. Betty failed to respond to any comments of a personal nature and occasionally told A. not to pass on this or that information to P. Once when she was destructive during a therapeutic period she was asked whether she was angry that P. was there instead of A., and she nodded. Another time when P. inadvertently came into A.'s room while Betty was there, the latter ran away and refused to come back. This made it impossible to work through with her the deeper meaning of her bowel retention, which was unfortunate.

She had two more episodes of this nature after leaving us. The first occurred when Betty had been home for only three weeks and her mother, suddenly obliged to leave the house, left Betty with her paternal aunt. Several factors seemed to contribute to the development of the second episode. (1) Betty, spying A.'s boots and suitcase in her office, guessed she was going to the farm; her request to go along was evaded (she said the next time she came, "I thought and thought about you all the time"); (2) the mother had spanked Betty that morning for leaning far out of an open window and then refused to kiss her good-by before she went away to Nursery School; (3) her paternal grandfather went on a drinking jag and there was considerable upheaval at home over his behavior. After the first episode Betty came to A. and asked, "My bum hurts again, what did you do for me, Mummy, to help me?" She was told that she need not have that trouble any more since she was now with her own Mummy who would always return as she had this time. Her response was, "I hate that (anal irritation). I don't want it." Although she had previously given evidence of considering these episodes as a disturbance, she had never expressed opposition so strongly.

About six weeks after going home to her mother, Betty began saying "Miss A." as often as she said "Mummy", apparently not realizing it. In a few days it became "Miss A." altogether without any evidence of hostility or withdrawal. She talked a great deal about all she did for the baby and made a show of what her mother bought for her, washed for her, etc.

Although she always spoke of her mother in the highest terms to A., she became quite accusing twice during her therapeutic interviews. Once she suddenly burst out without any immediate provocation, "God damn it, my Mother does naughty things. In the morning she does exercises and the water goes all over the floor. It's dirty." It was impossible to get her to elaborate. Another time when she was making the doll's bed and was asked whether she helped with the beds at home, she said, "No, she won't let me, she isn't feeling well."

"Isn't she? I'm sorry. What's the trouble?" "Oh, she just pretends. She stinks." Shortly afterwards she said, "I call my Mother stinker and she doesn't say anything—you can come to my house and see."

The last time A. visited Betty at home that spring, Betty was very loving with her mother and treated A. affectionately but distinctly as an outsider. Her mother who had first planned to wipe out all of Betty's past prior to the adoption, remarked on the fact that this was impossible since Betty apparently never forgot anything and often spoke of each one of her foster-mothers. She told of Betty's correspondence with her navy-daddy and laughed over her insistence on putting the stamp on his letters and mailing them herself.

The family was then planning to visit the maternal uncle's wife and Betty bade everyone at the Children's Center an affectionate farewell.

The mother has recently reported that Betty had a fine summer with no recurrence of her old bowel difficulties. She was eating enormously. Behavior problems, the mother felt, were not different from those of any other child except for the fact that Betty was so headstrong. The mother had learned to be firm with her and had even overcome the old bed-time difficulties by adhering to certain simple demands. Betty was at this time eagerly awaiting A.'s visit.

Discussion

This child, from the time of her separation from her mother at eighteen months, seems to have been imbued with an implacable longing to return to that mother, whom she mistreated during her brief visits because the child wanted to be with her altogether, not just visited. Gradually this longing led to a fantasy of an all-loving, all-giving mother. In contrast to this fantasy all foster-mothers seemed demanding and punishing people to be got rid of by doing just those things they could least tolerate. It seemed as though Betty's fantasy seemed to be materialized when she found A. She clung tenaciously to her wish to live with A. We undertook to bring this child gradually to an acceptance of reality, to the realization of what she really could expect from a mother. Without this preparatory education, we believe, she could not have adjusted so well to her own mother when she finally went to her.

We have asked ourselves whether such tenacity with real emotional content could have existed had Betty not had a very satisfying early relationship with her own mother—probably a particularly warm one. This is borne out by the mother's certainty that this baby would be a girl because she so wanted her own little Betty; by the fact that she never considered adoption for this child and always planned to have her back some day. The mother's understanding treatment of Betty when she took her back was further evidence of the solidity of this relationship.

We have also raised the question whether Betty's early experience of being lovingly and effusively cared for by her mother every morning, noon, and night, only to be completely deserted by her in the interim— were responsible for sharpening the sense of loss and the demand for reinstatement of the loved mother. We do know that when even this intermittent contact with her mother was interrupted for a week because of illness, Betty reacted with an intense disturbance of elimination, later her characteristic response to feeling abandoned.

Her mother's statement that Betty has apparently never forgotten anything, coincided with our observation. Her wishes and conflicts and fantasies were amazingly close to consciousness; to express them she went no farther afield than to the persons in her immediate environment, with whom she dramatized her struggle or her attachment; she needed no ugly witch, no fairy godmother. She drove hard for immediate gratification of her every wish. We tried to meet this need by giving her a substitute-mother. Her verbal expression and dramatization flourished in this accepting environment and were further stimulated from two sources: (1) At about the time of her birthday she is reminded of her own mother and of the care her mother gave her when she was an infant. Betty's feelings are so vividly aroused that for a time she seems almost to confuse the therapist with this mother of her infancy. (2) As soon as she finds her own mother again, she learns about the coming baby. A., who was at first carefully distinguished from her real Mummy, now becomes fused with her—the child wants *her* to have the coming baby. In this setting she dramatizes with A. all her wishes to be the baby herself—fondles, licks, sucks, is toileted, smears, and talks baby-talk. It was striking how this child seized upon the opportunity to identify herself with A. Heretofore her only good relationship had been the very early one with her mother where she was only tended as a baby. When she was identifying with A., she was usually recreating a mother-child relationship.

We felt that her adjustment to moving in with her mother was accomplished with such relative ease because Betty split off her negative feelings (over her rejection by A.) to the therapist. No doubt she made the latter responsible for the separation. Since she was able to reject her in turn, the pain was less severe.

Those who were first confronted with Betty's severe episode of disordered elimination were so impressed with the picture that they were sure she was suffering from some serious illness. We wondered how often this sort of condition may be the forerunner of intestinal disturbances of a psychosomatic nature. Had she not been under our observation, she would still be labelled simply as having had a tendency to constipation since babyhood. Closer scrutiny of such conditions by pediatricians might yield many interesting observations.

One of us who has had occasion to study delinquent women has felt that many of them are driven by just such a need to have their fantasy of an all-accepting, all-giving mother fulfilled. Their own mothers, when they do return to them, are such bitter disappointments in contrast, that they soon push on restlessly trying to outstrip their discontent. Had not Betty found A. to whom she could form a deep attachment, her emotional relationships might well have remained as superficial as they had been during the summer; she would have had no opportunity for real identification and thence a poorly developed superego. These characteristics, along with her tendency to dramatize her feelings and to demand immediate gratification of her wishes, might in time have developed into the full picture of a psychopathic personality. We tried to save Betty from this fate by giving her a real mother-substitute, to whom she was profoundly attached, with whom she identified at great length, and who gradually was able to show her what she could expect from a loving mother in reality.

Anna Freud has said recently that "apparently spontaneous attachments of the children really arise in answer to a feeling in the adult person of which the adult was not aware in the beginning, or the reasons for which only became apparent after some searching."[3] Such emotional stirrings on the part of the adult when recognized and held under control, as they were here, are of inestimable value. Of recent years there has been an unfortunate tendency in this country to be wary of such emotional identifications and to avoid them.

3. A. Freud and D. T. Burlingham, *Infants without Families*, 1944, p. 63.

THE USE OF DREAMS IN PSYCHIATRIC WORK WITH CHILDREN

By HYMAN S. LIPPMAN, M.D. (St. Paul)[1]

Therapists who are interested in the dynamics of human behavior are acquainted with the significance of dreams, through the publications of the psychoanalytic school. There are many psychiatrists who are not analysts but who know something of the psychoanalytic literature, and use dream material in their work with adults. They have developed skills in understanding dream symbolism and in recognizing latent conflicts in the dreams, working chiefly with the manifest content of the dream.

The literature on the direct psychiatric treatment of children contains few references to the use of dream material unless the child is undergoing psychoanalytic treatment, in which case dream material is used—as in adult analytic work—to get at unconscious material that produces conflict. In our work at the child guidance clinic in St. Paul, as in most other child guidance clinics, there is little opportunity to do very intensive case work. In rare instances it has been possible to offer a child psychoanalytic treatment, seeing him three or four times a week over a period of several months to a year or more. In the main those children who need intensive treatment are seldom seen more than once a week. Many of the children are seen for only one or two interviews in order to establish a diagnosis and recommend indirect treatment. One of our aims has been to increase our treatment program and to this end all of the members of the staff are doing therapeutic work with children. The role of the social worker in direct treatment work with children has recently been discussed by the writer.[2]

Whether the child comes in for diagnostic interviews or for treatment, an attempt is made in the psychiatric interview to get dream material. This has been going on for the past thirteen years in the

1. From the Amherst H. Wilder Child Guidance Clinic.
2. *American Journal of Orthopsychiatry*, Vol. XIV, Oct. 1944, p. 628.

work at the clinic in St. Paul, and this article is being written to present some interesting observations that have come from this material.

In general children enjoy talking about their dreams. Often on awakening in the morning they tell their dreams to each other and to their parents. Many parents tell their dreams to their children, and some consult "dream books" from which they attempt to make interpretations and predictions. When the parents believe that these predictions have value, the child usually does. The young child is rarely surprised when asked by the therapist about his dreams. The older child as he approaches adolescence may wonder why he is being asked to relate his dreams, especially if he has been told that they have no significance. After he is told why the dream material is asked for, ne usually enjoys helping the therapist to understand the material, often accepting it as a puzzle that should be solved.

Usually children attempt to explain why certain material appeared in their dreams. If the dream is of an anxious nature they blame it on a recent frightening movie, or a radio program, or a comic book they read. Children who have had many such dreams may attempt to control the nature of their dreaming by thinking of pleasant things before they go to sleep. This may have resulted from their own observations or from being advised by others to do this. Occasionally a child will say he concentrates on "clean thoughts" to avoid having dreams with sexual content. One boy told of a friend of his who concentrated on ghost stories and frightening experiences so that he would dream about these rather than "dirty stuff". Some of these children may be able to recognize in their dreams that they are dreaming. Occasionally the comment is made, "I wasn't so afraid of that because I knew I was dreaming." One child reported that he was so sure he was dreaming that he jumped from a height in order to end the dream, having learned that he was awakened whenever he fell from high places in a dream.

Occasionally the child when asked to relate a dream will tell a fantasy that he has had but which he believes he dreamed. Sometimes he combines the two. It is a common practice for a child to add to the dream or modify it so that it makes sense to him. If a child feels it is important that he dream, he may make one up to please the therapist. If the "dream" is a very simple one, it may be difficult to determine whether or not it was actually dreamed. In the main, however, children's manifest dreams are distorted and appear to have little meaning in contrast to the fabricated dreams and fantasies that are orderly and whose meanings are readily understood.

Frequently the child denies ever having dreams. Sometimes he admits that he has but says he cannot recall any. It takes little effort to get him to recall especially when he is told that most children dream and that often the dreams are so strange or funny that they don't like to admit having them. The child may be helped to recall by questions such as "What is the scariest dream you ever had", or "What did you dream about your mother or your father", or "Tell me some dream you had about school", etc. One dream may be recalled, then another, and this may be followed by a whole series. Apparently there are some children who do not dream and all efforts made to get them to recall dreams are unavailing.

The most effective way to stop a child from telling his dreams is to try early to explain or interpret their content to him; this applies especially to dreams that reflect hostility or sexual conflict. It becomes apparent to him that dreams reveal secrets and it is therefore dangerous to tell them. He may go away from the interview more anxious and disturbed than when he came, and thus be conditioned against the treatment.

The dream is particularly helpful in disclosing immediate concerns. The child who is in emotional conflict is either currently having anxiety dreams or he tends to recall dreams he has had in the past. When a child says he has been having one frightening dream after another, it is apparent that he is in the midst of conflict and is suffering from anxiety. In the course of a routine interview he may be unwilling to tell what is upsetting him, or he may be unaware of what it is. He will usually have less objection to telling a dream that may readily reveal what is disturbing him, just because it is a dream or, in the case of the distorted dream, because he does not recognize that it is there. Having told it in the form of a dream, he may find it a natural thing to go on discussing the subject. The therapist in recognizing what may be making the child anxious or afraid, may be able to generalize about fears and get the child to feel that there is no stigma attached to being afraid. In some instances children hesitate to tell a dream, through an unconscious awareness that they will be revealing conflicts which they do not wish discussed. The manner in which a child may appreciate the significance of the dream is illustrated in the case of a nine-year-old girl. She related her dream as follows:

"The janitor gave me a gun and told me I had to protect Miss X——, my good teacher. Some man was going to kill her. . . . Then a man who was standing there pointed the gun at the teacher and I screamed. The bullet hit her in the eye (points to her right eye), and killed her."—— She then added, "Oh, I hope Miss X—— doesn't ever hear about this."

When asked why, she said, "She would want to kill *me* instead of her dying like she did in my dream."

The following dreams illustrate the kinds of anxiety material frequently revealed:

An eight-year-old boy complained that in spite of telling his dreams he was still having terrifying ones. He had been told that he probably would be helped in not having so many if he related them and the reasons for his anxiety could be discovered thereby. He said, "You'd think that my dreams were bad if you knew what I dreamed last night,

> "I dreamed I was being chased and was trying to hide. I could hardly move and was terribly scared. I would get away and wherever I'd go I'd find the man who was chasing me. I was afraid he would get me."

The description of the man in the dream resembled his father. He had previously spoken of his negative feelings toward his father but not to the extent that he did on this occasion after telling the dream. He said that many times when his father gets after him he has a wish to get even with him and has promised himself that someday he would. There is of course the possibility that this boy would have discussed his hostility toward his father had he not related this dream, but it seemed particularly easy to discuss it after the dream was told. It was merely the continuation of a theme that he of his own accord had started.

A boy nine years old indicated the source of his anxiety in two dreams he related:

> "I dream we are out walking. Someone takes Bobby (his brother). Then I wake up and go to sleep again and I dream the same thing over again. I see tracks in the snow, and blood."

> "I dreamed that my father was hunting. The gun backfired and he was killed." He was asked if he really dreamed this dream, and said that maybe he just thought that. He added, "But I did dream that my father and mother fell through a trap door."

The two dreams and the fantasy indicate the extent to which this boy is preoccupied with hostility and guilt. He told them quite casually and yet in so doing revealed a great deal of significant conflict. Compare this with the amount of time required in most instances to get a child to speak frankly about his hostility to his parents.

Another instance of hostility expressed in the dream is illustrated in the following dream of a nine-year-old boy:

He was with his father at the newspaper plant where his father works. His father started to reach out and his hand got into a crushing machine. The boy awakened just at this moment.

Questions regarding his father revealed the fact that he is at times very severe with the boy, who becomes very bitter when spanked and feels that he would like to get even with his father someday.

The punishment motif is often clearly seen in the dream. The child, aware of his guilt and concerned because of his behavior, may thus reveal his fear of punishment or his deep need to be punished.

A ten-year-old neurotic whose problem was bedwetting, told the following dream in one of his interviews:

"I dreamed that Mr. and Mrs. H—— were going on a train. I asked them if I could go along with them and they said no. They got on the train but I ran after the train and jumped on. We got to their new place and I saw a crowd of people standing there by the boulevard. I looked around and I saw my sister coming, and I started to cry. I thought I was never going to see her atgain."

It will be observed that there are several themes in this dream. The therapist may choose any one or all of the elements and this will vary according to the amount of time available and the importance of getting information about specific subjects contained in one of the elements. In the case under discussion the boy was first asked about his crying on seeing his sister. He had feared he never would see her again and was very happy when he did—"Maybe I was so happy I cried." This boy had been caught masturbating by his foster mother. She had discussed this behavior at the Clinic and he knew she had. He was asked if he did not think he might have to leave this foster home because of his fear, and then remembered that in the dream he begged them to take him along and said "I won't do it again, auntie". He knew he was referring in the dream to masturbation. The reference to his sister in the dream suggested that she was one of the factors in his masturbation. This was not discussed in this interview but it offered a clue to be worked through later.

Sometimes the anxiety material in the dream reflects conflicts that are so much a part of the child's everyday life that he can discuss them without being concerned or threatened. Since the dream reflects among other things the current experiences of the individual, it may be expected that a child who is living in a state of constant anxiety and tension will have dreams whose content reveals this. It is perhaps safe to say that the closer the anxiety material is to the surface and the stronger the defenses built around it; the less likely will a discussion of it be traumatic to the child. This brings up the question as to why certain children who have had a long series of traumatic experiences, collapse emotionally, whereas others develop more or less an immunity to traumata.

There is danger in getting too much anxiety material early in the treatment. The child stimulated by telling his dream may plunge prematurely into a discussion of facts that he may later regret having disclosed; he may even feel he has been tricked into telling things that he wanted to keep secret. This is more likely to occur in the case of the withdrawn, anxious child. The danger may be averted by the therapist's ability to recognize that the child is being threatened.

One must also avoid making too many inferences from one or two dreams. These dreams may reveal or reflect considerable hostility against a parent, which is merely a part of an ambivalent relationship to that parent. Given sufficient time, positive feelings may be revealed by the same child in a dream or in interviews. There is less danger of coming to a premature conclusion if the child is to be seen several times. It is therefore advisable whenever possible, even in making a diagnostic study, to have an opportunity to see the child several times before attempting to establish a diagnosis. The same reasoning applies to interviews that do not have dream material, and one must guard against coming to a conclusion that a child is deeply hostile to a parent because he has expressed hostility at a time when something has just occurred to have stirred up hostile feelings. Both attitudes toward a parent will be reflected in the pair of dreams told consecutively by a seven-year-old boy:

> "Once I dreamed someone was cutting my dad's neck off and he fell against the garage." A little bit later he added, "Once I saw a white animal in a cage. I think it was a goat. I fell in and went into the cage. It was open. My dad pushed me out and closed the door."

A seven-year-old girl's dream indicates her preoccupation with the subject of pregnancy:

> "I went to visit a place where there were bears. I had a little tiny baby with me. We got to the cage and the baby reached out to give the bear something. He swallowed her and me, too. We were inside the bear's stomach. There was guts there. My mother came, started to pat the bear, and he ate her too. My mamma bit a hole in the bear's guts until she bit a hole right through and then we all jumped out and I woke up."

She was asked why she thought she had a dream like this and said she had been frightened by a big wolf dog the night she had had the dream. This was the factor that precipitated the dream. However, the dream contains also the theme of pregnancy and childbirth. One notes the inclusion of the tiny baby who was with her; the presence of the mother; and eating or biting the way out of the abdomen which was probably her theory of childbirth. The orderliness in the dream suggests that it is a fantasy, and this child had a tendency to fantasy a great deal. Whether or not it was fantasy, it was still a product of her thinking and so was significant.

In the case of oedipus dreams the wish is often obvious in the manifest dream. One of the most frequent dreams of the young girl contains references to illness or death of her mother; in the case of the boy, to the father. It goes without saying that such material is never interpreted to the child.

A clear instance of a dream filled with castration symbolism is the following of an eleven-year-old boy:

"I had a dream last night. I dreamed I had a big loose tooth in the back of my mouth and I pulled it out." He added that he dreamed this because on the night of the dream a cousin who was visiting did pull out a loose tooth.

He continued: "I had another dream. I dreamed a three-legged dog came after me and it talked. I dreamed that *this man* was talking and it seemed funny that a dog should talk." He was unaware that he referred to the dog as a man.

The absence of the tooth and the absence of one leg of the dog are castration symbols.

Aware of the fact that the dream usually expresses as accomplished, something that the individual wishes, one must be on the alert to locate the wish expressed in the dream. This is a relatively simple matter when the wish is obvious in the manifest dream content. When this is not the case the dream must be analyzed to get at the wish, an advantage that is limited to the trained analyst. It would be interesting to determine in what percentage of dreams the wish is discernible in the manifest content. Likewise it would be of interest to know what types of problems in children produce specific types of dreams, or how the dreams of different age periods vary. These and many other questions would require a statistical study that has not as yet been made of the material collected. Such a study is just being begun. A few examples are given where the wish is obvious in the manifest dream.

A twelve-year-old boy had shot and killed his step-father, an abusive alcoholic who had frequently beaten the boy's mother. On the occasion of the killing, his step-father was chasing the mother to beat her. The matter was brought before the court and the boy was exonerated. He was removed from his farm home and placed in a children's home in St. Paul. During the course of the interview he indicated he felt no guilt at all about having killed his step-father because the step-father might have killed his mother. He told the following dream:

"I dreamed that I was home again. My step-father was living. He laughed at me and said, 'I wasn't killed; they just told you I died, to fool you'."

He admitted he felt happy in the dream to know his step-father was not dead. He added that he had frequently hoped at night before he fell asleep that this whole incident was a product of his imagination. It is possible that this would have been learned eventually through interviews but it was disclosed early and simply by means of the dream.

A fourteen-year-old boy who had previously suffered from a tuberculous kidney and bladder reported that he had more than once had the following dream:

He had several penises. There were four alongside each other in a horizontal plane—each about the same size. When urine failed to come out of one, he tried another.

This dreaming occurred about two years before the interview at a time when he had difficulty in urinating and had to be catheterized. At that time he frequently awakened during the night and grabbed the urinal to urinate in order to assure himself that he could. The dream contains the wish that he never need suffer again the discomfort and pain of being catheterized. If one penis did not function he could always use one of the others. Undoubtedly this dream is closely related to castration anxiety but no attempt was made to establish this relationship.

The following dream in a twelve-year-old boy reflects a wish that is obvious and which indicates a state of resistance to coming for the interviews:

"I dreamed you weren't going to be here today. When I woke up this morning my brother told me I was going to have my head examined. I said no, I dreamed he isn't going to be there today."

Resistance to the method of treatment provoked an interesting dream in a fifteen-year-old boy. He was a severe stutterer and was anxious to be helped. He expected to be given exercises that would improve his speech, and was dismayed and unconvinced when told that the treatment would be through interviews in the hope of locating underlying conflicts that were responsible for his stuttering. The following dream occurred on the night after he had had his first interview:

> There was something the matter with the dial of his radio (he had a hobby of building radios). He took it to a repair shop where a Mr. X—— took out almost all the wiring. The patient thought it was stupid of the mechanic to take out all the wires from the machine when the difficulty lay only in the dial. It was a simple mechanical thing which he should have been able to fix without having to tear the machine apart. Mr. X—— explained it was the only way he could tell what was wrong.

These are the words I had used, and I repeated them again as we both laughed.

Children who are failing in school often dream that they have received high grades and are praised for their work. Children who are disturbed by the separation of their parents tend to dream that their parents are living together. Children who are crippled or handicapped rarely suffer from their handicaps in the dream. All of these dreams deny something that is unpleasant and replace it with something pleasant. A passive child's dream may indicate an underlying wish to be aggressive, while a delinquent may indicate through his dream a deep need to be apprehended and punished. This was illustrated in the dream cited of the boy who masturbated.

The discussion thus far has dealt largely with inferences that may be drawn from the manifest dream. All children's dreams are not so readily understood and many of them are as complex and distorted as dreams of adults. To understand the meaning back of the dream—the dream thoughts—one must apply the same psychoanalytic technique used to understand the dream of the adult. The child must associate to the elements of the dream and he quickly can be made to understand what the therapist means through an illustration or two. It is well to explain why the work with the dream is being performed. He will understand the difference between conscious and unconscious thoughts and wishes, and their relationship to emotional conflicts that cause suffering, and will work eagerly with the therapist to find out what his dream "means".

A seven-and-a-half-year-old boy dreamed:

> "I was on a boat and was going to Europe. We got off and stayed on an island for two weeks. There were a lot of horses on the island, with funny big feet like in the Crazy Cat pictures. That was a cock-eyed dream."

When asked what he thought of in connection with "horses'feet" he said he thought of being kicked in the head, and added, "If anyone gets kicked in the temple they either are killed or go nuts." He continued spontaneously by telling about his father who likes to joke and make exaggerated statements. His father told that when he was younger he used to go skiing and wore skis as big as trees. He used to go down hills that were so long that he ate his lunch on the way down. One familiar with dream analysis will recognize the fact that the horse in the dream represents the dreamer's father. Aside from the fact that the horse is a common symbol of the father, the horse in this dream has funny big feet. In his spontaneous associations the boy told of the father wearing skis as big as trees (funny big feet). Since the boy also had associated to horses' feet in another way, namely, he had associated to being kicked in the head the possibility of being killed or becoming insane, one was justified in suspecting that this boy had an underlying fear that his father had hostile intentions toward him.

Actually, this child was referred because of night terrors and fears, and was ambivalent toward his father whom he early had loved, but whom he had grown to distrust through the conscious efforts of his mother to estrange him from his father. Treatment progressed to the point where the boy began to show warmth toward his father, at which time the mother felt further treatment was not needed and suddenly discontinued contacts with the clinic in spite of attempts to prevent the break through work with her.

A dream of a twelve-year-old boy contains a wish not obvious at first sight. A knowledge of the boy's conflicts makes the meaning clear.

> He was riding on his bicycle along a narrow road while his mother and his maternal cousin X——were walking together. . . . They were in the cottage at the lake. Many members of the family were eating—his mother —his mother's father—his two maternal cousins and aunt. He added spontaneously, "My father wasn't there." He, the patient, walked into another room and didn't eat with them.

This boy's mother is Jewish, his father is not. There is considerable religious conflict within the home and the boy is having difficulty in deciding whether or not he will be Jewish. He is disturbed by the hostility shown to Jews and is leaning toward the wish of his paternal relatives that he attend their church. In the dream his mother and his mother's sister's boy are together, while he is by himself. This cousin and he are close friends and he has indicated in previous interviews that he fears his mother and his cousins will reject him unless he decides to be Jewish. When it was pointed out to him after he related this dream that he fears this exclusion, he agreed that it is his weightiest problem. In the dream he is excluded twice, once on the road and then again in the cottage. It will be noted that he and his father are not eating with the family. When this was pointed out to him he said he recalled something which he had omitted in telling the dream, that the maternal relatives were eating bacon and eggs. (This would never happen in reality since his mother's family is orthodox.) He was asked if he wished that they would and could eat bacon and eggs and he agreed at once that this would please him. He said he had wished time after time that his mother's family were gentile.

Two points are of interest in this dream. He left out the fact of their eating bacon and eggs until later when the explanation helped to recall it. Also, when he was asked to associate to the dream his associations were meager and added little to the understanding of the dream. The dream was understandable only through sensing the dream content. This was aided by a familiarity with dream material and an intimate knowledge of the boy's life problems.

The final dream to be presented in this discussion again illustrates the value of ferreting out the hidden meaning back of the manifest dream. The child was a twelve-year-old boy suffering from compulsion neurosis, who had been in analysis at the clinic.

"I dreamed that my brother came back home on a furlough." He paused a minute and then said, "I don't know. It certainly didn't look like him. I was at home with my mother, and she was in bed, and there was a rap at the door. I went to the door and was a little bit excited, and when I opened the door, there was a man standing there. He wore a blue uniform and he had a swastika on the chest. It was hard to see the swastika, it was just barely noticeable, and I think it was because he was ashamed of it or didn't want us to know that he was in the Germany army. His face was awfully funny, too. It looked like a lemon. The lower part of his face around his chin was greenish, and then it just blended into the rest of the face that was yellowish, just like a lemon that isn't ripe and that is getting ripe. I knew it was my brother by the expression around his eyes; that was the only way I knew it was he. He came into the room and then I closed the door. My mother saw him and she got out of bed and started to go towards him, but she wasn't excited at all."

This was the end of the dream. The patient thought it was a peculiar dream. The whole appearance of his brother was different from what it was in real life. He certainly didn't belong to any German army, since he was Jewish. The patient was asked what came to his mind when he thought of a lemon, and he laughed and said, "Sourpuss". This reminded him of his brother's friend, X——, who used to call for him all the time and would not come into the house. He would wait outside in his car and honk. They used to think that he was a sourpuss and wasn't friendly and did not want to come in, but they have gotten to know him much better lately because he has been friendlier. They realize that they made a mistake about that. X—— tried to enlist when the patient's brother did, but he was rejected, and he tried again two or three times after that but they would not accept him, and he tells everybody it is because his finger was injured when he was a child and so he could not get in; but the patient and others suspect that it was something else and that he does not want to talk about it. The patient was asked if he could explain why his mother was not so excited in the dream. Actually, she would be if her son did come back for a visit. He said he didn't know, and the psychiatrist ventured the opinion that perhaps one of the reasons that his brother looked like a lemon and also like an enemy, was that he has been separated from the family quite definitely by a recent marriage. Whereas before he was very close to the

HYMAN S. LIPPMAN

family, the parents have since the marriage felt that he is a stranger. The girl's family, formerly close to the patient's, are now very distant and cool. The patient agreed at once that the family was now much more distant to the brother and that he wished his brother had never gotten married because of the effect that the marriage has had. "However," he added, "I don't feel that way even if the others do feel that way."

He then said spontaneously, "That was a funny suit that he was wearing in that dream. It was blue, like he was in the navy, and he isn't in the navy. But it was a funny blue, it was just like these pants that I'm wearing." The psychiatrist noted that patient's trousers were of a bluish gray material, but more blue, and of a peculiar weave. The patient added, "They were exactly the same weave as this." He was asked if he had thought about that in the dream, and answered, "No, I didn't, but when I got up in the morning and started thinking about that dream I realized right away that it was just like my pants." This led the psychiatrist to the belief that the brother was definitely identified with the patient in this dream, and the patient was told that perhaps it wasn't his brother in the dream entirely, and that maybe *he* was the Nazi, instead of his brother. He laughed when the psychiatrist said this, and said, "You know, W—— and I are the worst Nazis in our room." Asked what he meant, he said, "Well, we always act as Nazis. We get up in front of the room, and salute and say 'Heil, Hitler!' and yell to the students—'Down with the democracies'—'We will inherit the whole world'—'We will conquer everything'." He used other expressions that the psychiatrist did not record, but they were those characteristically used by Hitler and by the Nazis. Several of the other boys in the room carry out this play with the patient and W——, and return the salute and say 'Heil, Hitler'. The patient said that the teacher realizes this saluting is done all in jest, but the patient implied that there was some seriousness in connection with it. He said that one boy has so much gall that after saluting the flag in the morning he says 'Heil, Hitler', and turns around and spits on the floor as if he is spitting on the American flag. The patient added, "I'll bet if anybody really knew about that, that this kid could get into trouble because it's unpatriotic."

He was asked why they carry through this Nazi type of play, and why he did it in particular, and he said, "I don't know, it gives me a feeling somehow of power, because the Nazis have been so successful. They have attacked; they have won out and are stronger than the others," (January, 1943). Psychiatrist asked him if they carried on in any other way. "Yes, every once in a while we'll get together and show some secret plans that we've got of attacking an island belonging to the United Nations. Usually the girls in the room are around us as we tell of our plans, and we have the plans down to a good deal of detail, showing just the way we are going to attack and overpower this island, just like the Germans did it."

He was asked if the United Nations had not made some conquests, and whether it would not be possible for the boys to identify with the United Nations now, "Yah, well, maybe later on we will, but we started this play quite some time ago. The United Nations have only had their victories recently, and maybe the play will change."[3]

The above dream and the discussion that took place is presented in detail to illustrate the way in which the discussion of the elements in the dream provoke significant material. It would have been difficult or impossible to have suspected the patient's identification with the Nazis unless the hidden content in the dream came to light. It is hardly likely that he would spontaneously have told about the play in the school room, because he did not feel that the therapist would be interested, or because of embarrassment, since it reflected an unpatriotic attitude.

It is well to caution the reader again that the manner in which this dream was handled should be confined to the experienced analyst who is doing psychiatric work with children. The word "experienced" is purposely included because the young analyst would do better to confine his treatment to analytic work with patients who are seen daily. The application of psychoanalysis to case work with children or adults should be left to the experienced analyst who is in a better position to do research work in newer techniques. The psychiatric social worker who has been analyzed is in the same position as the non-analyzed therapist with regard to the interpretation of unconscious material in dreams. He does have the advantage of a certain familiarity with dream material through his own analysis and will therefore be more alert to hidden meanings in dreams. He will also have learned the wisdom of staying away from material that will threaten the patient.

For the past year or two some of our social workers in their treatment work with children have asked for their dreams, and have succeeded in obtaining revealing material. Supervision of their work has failed to disclose that the children have been in any way upset by this procedure. Rather, they seem to enjoy relating dreams and discussing them. If the precautions that have been suggested in this paper are observed, many others may enjoy the advantages of the judicious use of children's dreams.

---

3. The important feature of the play apparently is to identify with the stronger group. It is interesting that the patient and his companions have been able to carry on in this way because the patient certainly has been strongly patriotic, has done everything in all of the drives to help the Allied Nations' cause, and stands to gain a great deal more if the United Nations win than if the Nazis win. The fact that he is a deeply neurotic boy is significant in determining the direction of this play, because he has evidenced throughout the treatment a strong feeling of guilt and a deep need for punishment. However, this would not explain the readiness with which the rest of the group has entered into the play.

A CONTRIBUTION TO THE EDUCATION OF A PARENT

By MARGARETE RUBEN (London)

In cases where, for external reasons, child analysis is indicated but not feasible, the child analyst may try to treat the child indirectly through advice to the mother. The first child analysis was conducted in this way by Freud: in interviews with the father of "Little Hans"[1] he advised suitable interpretations of the child's behavior. That early method, which seemed possible only because the father had been analyzed and which has gradually been replaced by direct treatment of the child, is now seldom used because, as Freud made clear, its success depends so largely on the extent to which the parent is able, consciously, to accept and use the analyst's interpretation, and on the relationship that exists between parent and child.

Cooperative work of this kind does have some advantages: the mother's position is easier than it would be if the child were in treatment for she remains in charge of his upbringing. Further, her relationship to him may improve comparatively quickly, i.e., as soon as she begins to gain insight into the reasons for his disturbance.

The following is an account of work with a mother of two daughters, nine and five years old. With the younger she had a good relationship and proved entirely able to follow the process of development and to assimilate and pass on our assistance. With the elder, she failed to do so: as our work proceeded it became increasingly clear that the failure was due to her sado-masochistic relationship to this child. She described Henny, the elder child, as being passionate; Eva, the younger, as cold. The fact was that the mother herself had more passionate feelings for Henny, who for five years had been her only child and who had thus assumed a special importance for the

---

1. "Analysis of a Phobia in a Five-year-old Boy", *Collected Papers*, III.

mother—herself an only child. In the mother's unconscious this had definite negative implications, as she indicated very clearly one day when she told me that Eva masturbated only because she saw Henny do it. She was afraid that Henny might have inherited that practice from her (the mother). Whenever she used my interpretations to torment Henny instead of to help her, it appeared that she unconsciously was punishing herself. When, on the other hand, she had difficulty in accepting my explanations of Eva's fantasies, she generally did so with the remark that *she* never thought of such things as a child. Thus I came to know her own childhood experiences and unconscious conflicts, and was able to make known to her some fundamental analytic principles as well as to relieve her somewhat of her own conflicts.

The consultations were brought about in the following way: the mother came to me for advice about her children and brought me two diaries which she had been keeping since their birth and which she thought might give me some clues as to the causes of their problems. The entries were mostly concerned with intellectual development. The mother had tried to record the phenomena as impersonally as possible, according to the method of William Stern.

Many of the diary entries to which we shall refer show the inevitable limitations in the understanding that the mother can acquire in such consultations as these. However, as long as her own problems do not overshadow the child's they need not disturb the progress of our analytic advisory activity. The detailed description of this case is justified on two counts. First, it illustrates unconscious wishes existing simultaneously in mother and child. One may well ask whether repressed conflicts reemerged in the mind of the mother because the child was now coping with them in the normal course of development, or whether they were communicated to the child because they were constantly present in the unconscious mind of the mother. Second, the case provides an opportunity to observe the same themes and sequences of themes observed in child analysis.

The mother was a warm-hearted, clever woman. Her marriage, the early years of which she and her husband had spent together at a university, was at first childless for economic reasons. Political circumstances brought them to England, where the husband was invited to do scientific work. Here, after the birth of the first child, the mother gave up her professional work as a teacher as well as her private political activities, and devoted all her time and energy to Henny; and later, to both children. This conscious renunciation of all that had until then absorbed her interest was not easy.

The children soon developed well in advance of their chronological age: the home was filled with every kind of constructive toy, books, etc. The father spent the first hour of each evening with the children, telling stories which they or he suggested. These stories ranged from imaginary funny ones to fairy-tales and scriptural tales. These evening gatherings, occasional excursions on Sundays, visits to the theatre, all created a family atmosphere full of warmth and love, limited only by the avoidance of open expressions of tenderness. There was a good deal of mutual banter and affectionate teasing instead.

The conflicts of the children were only partially comprehensible to the observant mother. Apart from the fact that I obtained a few external privileges for Henny, such as the permission to go to bed a little later than her sister, I did not succeed in making the mother understand the unconscious conflicts of the elder child. I had no alternative but to suggest that Henny be analyzed, as she had already developed compulsive symptoms.

Eva, for her part, had developed a series of symptoms that the mother did not recognize as such and that she tried to minimize. At four, Eva was unable to be separated from her mother even for a moment; nor could she go to bed at night without her elder sister. She showed great anxiety in the presence of strangers; in shops she tried to hide behind her mother's skirt whenever any of the clerks spoke to her. As Eva was a particularly attractive little girl with fair curly hair and blue eyes, this was not rare. The anxiety of the child was evident with her father also. Recently, she had not wanted him to see her naked, and had cried when he came to watch her being bathed; nor would she allow him to handle or kiss her. During recent nights she had several times called out in her sleep. It was also noted, within this period, that her toy animals were in general disfavor, and that she had lost interest in her dolls. The mother's main worry was, however, that Eva did not seem able to learn English and there was thus no prospect of her attending the school where her mother had hoped to send her the next year.

Both children were brought to see me. When I asked Eva if she would like to come with me to my room for a little while the mother seemed doubtful. I made the attempt, nevertheless, and Eva followed me obediently rather than because she wanted to. When I showed her my dolls she sat down in a little chair and said with utter contempt, "But none of your dolls can stand up. Mine can all stand up." Then she arose to go, insisting, "But now I must go to my mother." I turned her attention to a box full of odds and ends. She picked up the plasticine at once and started modelling, explaining to me, "Now I'll make a horse." As I saw that she made only the body of the animal I asked if horses had only a body: she answered, with a roguish smile, "No, they have a head, too." When I asked further what else they had, she replied, "Legs," and when I persisted for the third time she hesitated a little and then said hastily, "A tail—but people haven't got one."

In the Bühler tests, Eva was mentally nine months in advance of her age. She failed in one special task that was simpler than many she did pass. This task was to assemble the trunk, limbs, and head of a wooden doll that was given her in separate pieces. She was unable to recognize either legs or arms or to attach them to the body. She fidgetted in her chair, turned red, and finally gave up the attempt. This reaction, considered along with her remarks about the horse she had modelled, seemed to be one key to Eva's main problem, her anxiety as to whether her own body had been damaged.

The consultations about Eva took place about once a week for nearly ten months.

In the first interview the mother spoke mostly about herself. She was very excited by the thought that she might be pregnant. Both she and 'her husband felt they could not afford a third child; but as "fate had apparently decided this" they would manage somehow. She was especially eager to do so as she so much wanted a son; however, being forty years old, she feared she had reached the climacteric. Neither presumption proved correct, and it took several weeks for her to overcome the disappointment about the pregnancy that had not materialized. Her wish for a son was connected with Eva's unconscious wish to be a boy: this became clear, for instance, from the awkward way she set about explaining to Eva her fear of having been damaged. Quite out of the blue she asked Eva one day, "Eva, would you rather be a boy?" whereupon the child almost burst into tears. This first clumsy rendering of my interpretations, which was due, not to the fact that her task was new and unaccustomed but to her own unconscious wishes for masculinity, was in strong contrast to her subsequent explanations, which were sensitive and on the level of the child's understanding.

Entries made in the diary during the period of our consultations show how Eva found her way out of the confusion of her fantasies and anxieties.

I. *The wish for masculinity*

The following material indicated that two topics were open for the mother to discuss with the child: Eva's anxiety and shame at being seen naked, and the death wishes she suddenly felt toward her parents. I decided to tackle first the inhibited exhibitionism and the penis envy, partly because this conflict, to judge from my own brief experience with Eva, was outstanding. Moreover, had I mentioned the death wishes first, the mother might have been expected to feel unconscious disappointment at her daughter's failure to return her love, and this might have impaired her educational skill.

5/25   She is now very interested in the subject of death; she often asks why people live if they've got to die.

5/28   For her big business she is using the pot again. She says she does not like to feel the splash of the water on her.

6/1   She said to me, "I want to keep you with me always, you must never die." She greeted Daddy when he came home tonight with, "It's a good job you didn't let yourself get run over."

6/5   Eva told me: "You aren't old yet, and you won't die for a long time. You mustn't ever grow old." She grasped my hand when a dog ran across the street and a car turned the corner: "He mustn't be run over."

6/6   Eva asked a lady who lives near us whether she had "born" Ginger (the cat).

6/7   She asked whether Henny had been a little boy once. I inquired why she had been so annoyed when I wanted to know the other day if she would rather be a little boy. She replied that boys had to learn English and that all Englishmen went to the office.

6/13   She has got rid of many of her fears. She no longer cries in bed at night or says that she does not want to go to sleep and that I must not darken the room. She allows Henny to watch her having a bath, and doesn't cry when Daddy sees her without her clothes. Today for the first time she allowed me to work upstairs while she was playing downstairs in the living-room.

6/14   At table she asked if Daddy, too, had nipples. I said: Yes, quite little ones, not beautiful big ones such as she would have some day. Then she said: "Am I going to be a man then?"

6/22   She is no longer so terrified by the picture of the spider in the picture-book "Little Miss Muffett".

6/23   This morning, at breakfast she said: "When I have little babies in my tummy, we won't give them away like Ginger's little kittens, will we?"

6/24   She wanted to know from a lady, a friend of ours, if she (like Ginger) had a baby in her tummy. She asked why she had not been made a boy. I inquired if she would like to be one. "I would like to be a man." But she could not say why.

       To-day she said to her father: "Shall I show you what I can do?" The next moment she did a somersault on the carpet. She had practised secretly with Henny.

6/28   Quite of her own accord she painted a spider: "The other animals are afraid of it."

7/1   She dreamt she was on the Heath with us and suddenly we disappeared and she could not find her way home.

       Today she had a real fit of rage when the house which she tried to build of small logs kept collapsing. In her fury she cried and trampled on it and would not accept consolation or advice as to how to make it stand up.

7/2   Father told her the fairy-tale of Mother Carey. She did not want to hear about where the little girl hurts her finger and jumps into the well. She cried: "I'm frightened."

7/6   She complained to me: "Daddy always tells me such horrid stories. I don't like fairy-tales in which there are nasty things." She again has started to run away from all strangers. From the milkman who tried to show her his horses, the gardener who stroked her hair, and our lodger who wanted to chat with her.

7/10   When her father was drinking his coffee this morning, he poured some of it into her milk. She liked it very much. Suddenly she said: "I wish I were a boy." We asked: "Why?" "Then later on when I am a man I could always drink coffee." Since I hardly ever drink coffee, she thought it was a man's privilege.

Eva's anxieties are reduced as she becomes conscious of her wishes for masculinity and proves able to give expression to them herself. She tries to impress her father with her physical flexibility, by doing a somersault. An unusually well-behaved little girl, she now permits herself a real tantrum over her play, giving violent expression to her disappointment with the collapsing tower. She says that the "other animals" are afraid, and so denies her own anxieties. Last and most important she openly declares to her parents that she wants to be a man. She asks whether Henny used to be a little boy once, i.e., whether she too has had the same misfortune to lose her penis. Behind all this is the dread that if she cannot be a little boy she is forever cut off from all manner of desirable things, above all learning English and becoming like her admired father, who goes every day to his office and whose partner and equal she wishes to be. The father, moreover, supports her doubts and disturbs her masculine fantasies by reminding her again and again through his fairy tales of dangerous things that lie in wait to hurt her. It is particularly interesting to see how the new forward groping of her sexual curiosity toward the subjects of conception and childbirth and the dangers involved is directed at first to the neighbor as someone further removed from her—and not to her parents. With them she discusses only her wish to be a man, a subject already entered on by her mother. Still, the new event in the family life of the little girl, the expected arrival of the kitten, gives Eva no rest. She now addresses her question about procreation directly to her mother.

II. *The sadistic conception of sexual intercourse.*

7/15 "When Ginger married her tom-cat, he grabbed her by the neck. Did you do that with Daddy too when you married him?"

   I told her about menstruation. She listened without any particular interest.

8/6 Eva ordered Daddy to tell the story of Big and Little Claus which had frightened her so much a few weeks ago.

8/7 Eva told Daddy, her face beaming with happiness, that it does not hurt the cat at all when the tom-cat makes love to her,—that she likes it very much.

   We were asked out by some people she did not know. She was very friendly, even with the man of the house.

8/16 Eva said Henny had done something naughty—which she hadn't. When we unravelled quite how untrue her story was, she was a bit surprised herself.

8/19 A little girl living opposite, came to play for the first time. When the little girl fell down and cried, Eva came up to me, frightened and said: "I don't like it when she cries." When the child's grandmother asked Eva if she would come and play at their house some time, she said "No" with great determination, but later she said that she would go if Henny would go with her.

8/20. Henny couldn't go with her today to see her friend, because one of her own playmates had come to the house. Eva did not want to go alone. When, however, she saw Monica in the garden opposite, she went over by herself. After an hour she came back, saying Monica had fallen down and was crying.

   She does not want her daddy to "fly" her into her bed any more. Daddy must take no part whatever in her going to bed. She says: "It's because at meals he always orders me about." (When she is too slow.)

8/24 Eva has begun to play with herself and to touch her genitals, imitating Henny.

After the mother has cleared up Eva's fantasies of "sadistic" sexual intercourse in her talk about menstruation, Eva expresses her joy about this comforting state of affairs to her father. Doubtless at the back of her mind is the wish to hear from tim, too, that she has been told the truth.

Eva now asks for the story of Big and Little Claus which only a few weeks earlier made her frightened. In this fairy-tale she can give rein to her own sadistic fantasies undeterred by the fear that "something happens", since Little Claus always comes out on top. The more he loses, the more he gets, and all the fury of Big Claus leaves him quite unscathed.

It looks as if the unfounded accusation that Henny has been doing something naughty is a projection of Eva's own masturbatory activities. Her castration anxieties have shifted to the fear of self-injury. She is in despair when her little girl friend falls and gets hurt.

III. *Eva's pregenital theories of procreation.*

The mother has passed over Eva's unspoken references to self-damage and left the questions they implied unanswered for the time being, but following our discussions, has not forbidden her to masturbate. Now Eva feels free to use the next opportunity of choosing her stories at bedtime to bring out her pregenital, especially her oral-sadistic, fantasies.

8/25   Eva said that the story to-night had to be about a hare. He was to eat something which he was not allowed to eat and Teddy was to fly away with the hare and to drop him.

8/26   Eva wanted a story about a cat, a clock and roses (the clock and the roses stood on the mantelpiece next to each other). Daddy told her about a cuckoo-clock. The cat wanted to eat the cuckoo. Eva thought that quite all right. Then Daddy began to say something about the roses. Eva interrupted at once: "But the cat mustn't get scratched." Her father remarked that after all the cat had meant to eat the cuckoo, and a scratch isn't much; he'd had one himself in the garden today pruning the roses. He showed her his hand. Eva wasn't a bit sorry for him, but kept on repeating: "But the cat mustn't hurt himself." Not unnaturally the cat in the story did get scratched. Eva stopped her ears and could hardly be induced to listen to the end.

8/29   Eva asked for a story about a tower which fell off the house and a cat. When her father spoke of the cat and said: "And then something happened," Eva at once put her hands to her ears and said: "Nothing must happen."

Today again she put one finger into each corner of her mouth and pulled them as wide apart as possible. I scolded: "Why are you always doing that?" "Then more will go in," was her reply.

9/1   Eva told a dream (she made this up as Henny had just told her dream and Eva did not want to be outdone): She went to the letter-box and the neighbor's dog came and tried to bite her.

At the request of the psychologist Daddy told Eva a story about a cat who had bitten her tom-cat and said she wanted to have a baby. The tom-cat did not mind the biting at all and the cat got a lovely kitten. Eva was very satisfied.

9/2   She said that she dreamt we went to the village by bus where, in
      fact, we intended to go today.   There was a cafe there, where we got
      tea and little brown chocolate-balls and little white balls of cream.
      (The mother was surprised at this dream, since Eva had never in her
      life seen either brown chocolate-balls or cream-balls, and so was more
      easily led to understand the significance of the latent dream material.)

9/5   Story: Teddy must again "eat something his mother doesn't want him
      to".

9/8   Story: A cat falls into the water and a dog gets her out.   Daddy asked
      if there should be a boy as well.   "No, I don't like boys."

9/10 I teased her because she is still using her pot.   I asked: "Is it so
      difficult for you to part with your little sausages?"   (It is surprising
      that the teasing request by her mother to part with her sausages is
      apparently considered by Eva as a request to be feminine.   From that
      time she never uses the pot again.)

9/11 Story: about a child that wanted to eat poisonous berries.

9/12 Story: Teddy was to sit in the butter and do ah-ahs and wee-wee in it.

9/13 Story: a loaf of bread tumbling over, a clock from which the hands
      fall off and a camera from which the film reel has been lost.

9/14 Today we tried to get her used again to having Daddy carry her to
      bed.   He got hold of her legs, I of her arms and thus we dragged the
      "little baggage" to bed.   She laughed cheerfully, but then demanded
      that I should restore her to her former position.   I lifted her up
      again, kissed her once more and put her back in bed.

9/15 Although Eva has to play on her own again, now that Henny has
      gone back to school; she does not follow me around all the time, but
      plays quietly in the living-room.
           She asked if Daddy was my baby.

9/16 She was allowed to help with the apple picking.   She was very proud
      of this and said to Daddy: "You are nearly as nice as Mummy."   When
      her father asked at bedtime if he should carry her up to bed, she
      laughed shyly and said I was nicer still and I must put her to bed.
           She remarked about the apples with leaves on their stalks: "They
      will have little babies."
           I pricked my finger sewing today.   Eva asked if it had hurt
      very much.   I said "No" and told her there were quite a lot of beauti-
      ful stories about pricking your finger, but as pricking frightened her,
      we couldn't tell them to her.   She said she would rather not hear them.

9/18 Without being asked, she gave Daddy several kisses in the morning
      when he went out.

9/21 Today again she ran after me everywhere: "I love you so much, I
      don't want to leave you."
           She asked for a story about a little girl who wanted to eat
      poisonous berries.

9/22 I told Eva there are children who believe that a mummy who wants to
      have a baby has to eat something or have something put into her mouth.
      "But I don't believe that," she said.   "What then does she do?" was

the immediate question.   I explained that she had an extra little hole for the purpose down beneath her tummy.   The next question was: "What do you put in there?" She was content with the explanation: "White drops."

She played that Teddy had eaten two poisonous berries.

The essential element throughout is that she must get something without anything happening to her in return; first she demands the penis, then she imagines a bloodless castration, when the penis falls off of its own accord, and finally her wishes are fulfilled with the gift of a child.

As Eva gives expression more freely to her oral fantasies, her attitude towards her father slowly changes.   Although she is still afraid of being put to bed by him and symbolically therefore of the damage she might have to suffer if she brought herself to play a passive part, she is able quite suddenly to take the initiative and love him "actively", spontaneously kissing him good-bye one morning.

The mother's attempt to clear up the fantasies and to tell Eva of the existence of the vagina may appear to have failed as Eva continues her oral and subsequently her urethral fantasy games.

9/23   Story: about a flower pot tumbling over and a house that didn't like to get wet.   She plays quite a lot with her wooden animals; turns her little basket into a sailing boat in which all the animals travel. The small ones go in first, "so that there is no noise".

9/24   This morning she suddenly said to me, "Really, I am *very* fond of Daddy."

9/26   She likes to sit on Daddy's knee in the evenings in her nightdress, but does not want him to carry her to bed.

9/29   Eva painted a cat with four tails.   "She has a little place at the back there and she has four tails so that it doesn't show."   She thought the cat so lovely that I had to cut it out for her.   She showed it to Daddy and said it was the baby cat; tomorrow she would paint the mother. Her father said that strictly speaking it should have been the other way round, as the mother came before the baby.   "No, this little cat is her mummy's mummy."

9/30   She painted a cat with five tails; she said the hole was bigger in this case so she needed more tails to cover it up.   Again she emphasized that the little cat was her mummy's mummy.   I said the cat had only one shoe on.   "She couldn't find it this morning."   Later she painted the missing shoe: "She found her shoe, after all."

10/1   Eva made Daddy tell her "Little Red Riding Hood".   When the wolf was lying in bed Daddy said, referring to the picture, "You can hardly see anything of the wolf there."   "Anything but the tail," said Eva, beaming.

Eva told Daddy that when the wooden animals were lining up the other day the dog bit the little lamb-baby's bottom.

Eva really does accept the vagina, but displaces it to the back, according to her childish knowledge of anatomy and the limits of her bodily exploration. She is able to admit she has a body like her mother's, though still a little ashamedly, as she proposes to cover the place with many tails.   To her mother she gives one more tail, since in her case the hole is larger; and perhaps, too, this is a sop to Cerberus.

IV.   *Emancipation from the mother. Elimination of anxieties after interpretation of her imagined self-damage. The free break-through to the oedipus phase.*

The entries made in the following three weeks show that the child's fear of being injured has increased.   By breaking several cups over a period of several days, she challenges her mother to punish her and so relieve her of her guilt-feelings.   In this period she asks her mother, again and again, before going to bed at night, "Haven't you scolded me today yet?"   This wish is the more incomprehensible to the mother as Eva, at the same time, shows an increased desire for tenderness.   She wants to sit on the mother's lap all the time and play a tickling game, which they have often played before; Eva's special interest in them now undoubtedly shows that they serve to dispel her anxieties about masturbation.   It is as if she wants to achieve both repression and break-through to the impulse by saying, "Punish me for tickling myself and harming myself—but if you, too, tickle me, then it must be allowed and can't be so very bad."   She is told she is old enough to tickle herself if she wants to.

At the same time the content of her fantasies is centered around the bad boys Max and Moritz, whom she would like to imitate, i.e., by harming grown-ups just as she fears she herself may be hurt.   She asks repeatedly to hear the stories about their mischievous pranks, and as she listens, "turns her head away and gives a restrained little laugh".

She hears that the damage she has imagined has befallen her genital organ (her "wound") is not the result of masturbation, and that she has not lost the little tail.

10/18   Eva had a slight cold for a few days, and every night I smeared some cream into her nose as a remedy. When she was better she wanted to continue with the cream and grumbled when she did not get it. This morning she told her Daddy that she dreamt he had bought some new cold cream.

The dream censorship arranges the typical displacement from below upward. The father's new cold cream will cure her, i.e., overcome the disappointment that she is not a boy herself; in the unconscious mind of the little girl the sperma is understood to be a consolation gift, which is to help her have her father's child.

V.   *Conflicts during the oedipus phase.*

10/19   Eva asked for "Cinderella". Both times she accepted quietly the cutting off of the toe and the blood in the shoe. The second time her father said that, of course, it hurt considerably. Then she said without emphasis: "I don't want to hear that." However, she let him go on with the tale. She no longer asks me if I have scolded her yet to-day. She goes to bed very cheerfully at night.

10/20   Eva saw the neighbor's child fall down in the street again. The child screamed, but Eva merely said to me very quietly: 'I don't like to hear her do that."

10/21 She was told a story about someone who hurt his arm chopping wood. She protested she did not want to hear that story. She wants to become an architect and tells me every day of the shops and houses she intends to build. All the houses will have balconies.

10/24 Eva was told the story of "Hansel and Gretel". At first she was afraid on the children's account, then she said: "That poor witch."

10/25 Eva talked about Hansel and Gretel all day long. She is no longer sorry for the witch, but keeps wondering whether the children were right to push her into the stove. On the other hand, she didn't say a word about whether the parents were right to leave the children in the wood.

10/29 Eva was afraid when the story of "Snow White" was told her. She stopped her ears when the hunter took the child into the woods to kill her. Only when she heard that the hunter didn't do it, was she reassured.

10/30 Tonight "Snow White" was told again as her bed-time story. Eva was quite relieved when the queen was dead; she was very excited throughout the story. This time she was not sorry for the villain who got what she deserved as she had been sorry for the witch in "Hansel and Gretel".

11/4 Eva had been playing with her wooden animals; afterwards she declared: "The wicked elephant has killed the bah-sheep mother, but then the dear boo-cow has come and had a new bah-sheep mother for a baby."

11/20. In the morning I went into the nursery, with very cold hands, to dress Eva. "What did Daddy do to you to make your hands so cold?"

11/23 At breakfast Eva suddenly remembered her old baby-spoon. She said she had been too grown-up to use it for a long time. Her Daddy asked me: "What shall we do with the spoon?" Before I was able to answer, Eva cried: "We will keep it for my babies."

12/5 Eva had light flu with a little temperature, but she was quite cheerful. She was angry when the doctor came and didn't utter a word during his visit. She turned her face aside each time he looked at her during the examination.

12/6 She is much better. In the evening she let her Daddy carry her upstairs quite happily. (During the day her bed was in the living-room.)

12/27 For the first time Eva has talked happily at the baker's shop and showed the woman the new little rabbit she got for Christmas. She never cries now when blood is mentioned in the fairy-tales.

1/2 Today we attended a choral recital (German and English Christmas songs). From the start, Eva felt very much at ease among the hundred or so people present.

1/12 She says "Good morning" in the shops and answers when she is spoken to.

1/25 At breakfast this morning we happened to talk about having babies. She said she did not want to have any children. Daddy asked her: "Why not?" "Oh, when you get those drops into your little hole, I am sure it hurts."

In the evening she asked again whether people could have children even if they were not married.

Her favorite color is now red; it used to be brown.

2/13   Eva likes to be told fairy-tales and is no longer afraid when listening to them. Her face looks less babyish.

2/15   Eva is building a house for the wooden cat. She remarks about it: "She is living in all the rooms, but not in one right at the top. A witch is living there, but she is quite nice to the cat."

Eva said to me yesterday: "You must wash my glass today" (a piece of rough glass for tracing pictures which are put underneath). I said I wouldn't do it now, as she had asked in such a nasty voice when she knew that I'd a lot of work to do. This morning she said to me: "My dear little cat, wash the glass. But I will not order you about any more."

Eva shows that she wants to become an architect and all the houses are to have balconies, a well known symbol of pregnancy. The difficulty she experiences in developing her marriage fantasies is created by the unfavorable part her mother has, willy-nilly, to play in these. Note her selection of fairy-tales. It is in "Cinderella" that she first becomes the favorite and it serves the wicked sisters right. With this solution she quickly disposes of her competition with Henny. Now the conflict for Eva increases when her rivalry with her mother comes to the forefront. In "Hansel and Gretel" she is puzzling over whether one can really push the witch into the fire. It is not until "Snow White" that Eva has the courage to be pleased when the stepmother is killed at last. The next day Eva has the fantasy about the elephant and the bad stepmother which enables her to escape responsibility for her death wishes while opening up to her a way of making amends for them. "It is not I at all who wants to kill Mother, it is Father who does; but I will give birth to a new mother for him" and, we may add, "then he will have what he wants and at the same time so will I."

Summary

Various psychoanalytic studies that deal with the phallic phase in the girl, describe the difficulties that may hinder normal development at this period.[2] Before the girl enters into the oedipus situation, the phallic phase has to be overcome; the ego has to give up its

---

2. Abraham, K., "*Manifestations of the Female Castration Complex*", *International Journal of Psychoanalysis*, III, 1922.

Freud, S., "The Infantile Genital Organization of the Libido", *Collected Papers*, II; "Some Psychological Consequences of the Anatomical Distinction between the Sexes" *Internat. J. Psa.*, VIII, 1927; "Female Sexuality", *Internat. J. Psa.*, XIII, 1932.

Deutsch, H., *Psychoanalyse der weiblichen Sexualfunktionen*, Vienna, 1925.

Fenichel, O., "The Pregenital Antecedents of the Oedipus Complex", *Internat. J. Psa.*, XII, 1931.

Bibring-Lehner, G., "Über die phallische Phase und ihre Störungen beim Mädchen" ("The Phallic Phase and its Disturbance in Girls"), *Zeitschrift für psychoanalytische Pädagogik*, VII, 1933.

masculine attitudes and accept the emergence of passive traits, as a necessary prerequisite for future feminine development. The discovery, in this phase, of the lack of a penis, which in the literature receives equal importance with the castration complex of the boy, creates psychological changes of great consequence in the girl's object-relations and in her libido position. In the normal course of events a change occurs in the object-relations, as the girl at first holds the mother, to whom so far all her libidinous inclinations have been addressed, responsible for the damage she feels she has suffered. She directs towards her, therefore, her strong negative feelings. Her interest now turns to the father. Disappointed with her own inferior organ, she abandons her previous actively directed phallic masturbation; and the aggressive tendencies become changed into passive tendencies. The girl wants her father to make up to her for the lost penis by giving her a child, and therefore all her sexual inclinations turn toward him. Her relationship to him becomes intense. The girl has grown into the oedipus situation: she becomes even more hostile to her mother, now her rival.

Eva, who according to her mother has passed through both the oral and anal phases without difficulty, shows her first regressive tendencies and early symptoms after an illness about six months prior to the beginning of the analytic interviews. She has German measles, and her body needs to be inspected for rash. We may assume that in this period she becomes aware of her lack of a penis. Her first reaction is disappointment and intense shame: she tries to hide the imagined defect by refusing to be seen naked by her father or sister. The desire to hide herself is expressed in other ways: she retires behind her mother's skirts; she manages to make her mother thoroughly ashamed of her stubborn inaccessibility, and afraid that the child may not be able to learn the language used at school.

Further regressions occur in Eva's behavior after her unpleasant discovery. She renews the libidinal cathexis of anal functions and products; and just before the beginning of the interviews she reverts to infantile passivity in that she gives up playing with her dolls—a play that affords little girls the chance to live out actually all the ministrations they must endure passively at the hands of the mother,—and also gives up playing with her wooden animals whose symbolic masculinity is prominent (elephant's trunk, long neck of giraffe; baby lions). In proportion to her feeling of helplessness Eva abandons herself to dependence on her mother. Her sadistic wishes against her parents are naturally intensified by all these struggles.

At this point she is brought to see me.

The revival of her hope that her penis—displaced upwards to the nipples—is still going to grow, is shown in her remark to her father, "Look what I've got here." A complete break-through of her wishes for masculinity is brought on by her mother's readiness to discuss them with her. However, the father disturbs her fantasies again and again with his gruesome fairy tales. She now seems to fear that even if her penis does grow she will lose it when she grows up— then she will have to bleed like her mother, whose menstruation she attributes to an act of violence during sexual intercourse. Perhaps, too, the mother has done something violent to the father, gripping him by the neck".

In the ensuing choice of stories she gives expression to the inner riot of her active and passive fantasies. At first she is only concerned with getting a penis; all the oral-sadistic fantasies have in common the aim to incorporate something that is withheld; and in this connection it is essential that nothing is allowed to happen to the little cat, it does not get hurt. Yet the child is so greedy that she has to stretch her mouth to make it wider. After she hears from her father that the tom-cat is not angry with his tabby for biting him, so that she could get a kitten, Eva works this out in her dream of the little chocolate and cream balls which she also gets—introducing a further infantile theory that children are made of excrement and sperma. Thus, at a time when her masculine longing for a penis has not yet died down, she manifests her first "feminine" desire for a child. She begins to let her father handle her again, cautiously, because unconsciously she is afraid to expose herself to a painful passivity. Gradually she adapts herself to her new feelings for him, and he becomes her unique love-object.

After her mother has told her where babies come from and what the little hole is for, Eva forms her first definitely passive fantasies. The flower pot falls down, the sailing-boat harbors many little animals, and the smaller ones come first so that they do not have to fight for their place. There are signs of further advancement into the oedipus situation when she calls attention to her guilt feelings, asking to be scolded. This must surely mean she has permitted herself the first negative feelings against her mother; in which there is, in addition, a strong element of reproach, revealed in the cat pictures: the child seems to say, "If you had been my child and had a little hole that bleeds, then I would have covered it up at once with many tails."

And now Eva becomes more and more confident in her behavior with her father. She tells him that the dog has bitten the bah-sheep baby's bottom. We may add: because the bah-sheep baby is no longer afraid, and has let him do it.

A period follows during which Eva tries to settle the conflict between her wishes and her feelings of guilt. Masturbation and castration anxiety reappear. She seeks escape in a stronger attachment to the mother; she initiates the tickling game, and so avoids responsibility. But at the same time she accuses herself of breaking things. The internal struggle between masculinity and femininity is once more in full force: fearful of passivity, Eva becomes, again in her fantasies, one of the bad boys, Max and Moritz (who saw through the plank on which the tailor is walking—which she fears the tailor may do to her if he were to "cut her out" a lady's dress). By ending the exciting tickling games and again explaining the sex difference, the mother calms down the child's conflicts.

Eva is now free to turn fully to her father. In her dream he buys the cream to heal "the wound": with this acknowledgement she enters into the oedipus phase. Once more he is allowed to tell her fairy tales that previously frightened her. First, in "Cinderella", she disposes of the rival sisters; in "Hansel and Gretel" she is concerned with the lawfulness of harboring death wishes against the witch, whereas in "Snow White" she even enjoys the competitive struggle that ends so well for herself. In the story she invents (11/4), it is not she but the father who kills the mother; she remains the good girl who gives birth to a new bah-sheep mother. At the end of the diary we see how Eva settles the relationship with her mother to the satisfaction of both parties. She has struggled to a decision: she is now willing to live in the same house with the witch, though she only concedes her a small room on the top floor. However, the witch is a dear one who is nice to her.

In real life, Eva now expresses her wishes freely: as an architect, she will always build houses with balconies (unconsciously, everyone is allowed to have babies) ; and she looks forward to giving her baby-spoon to her own children.

The color red has now lost its horror for her, and she prefers it to brown.

Judging from information recently received from her mother, Eva has become a happy school girl, in whose particularly good progress there may be found perhaps the last sublimated vestiges of her former ambitious desires.

THE RELUCTANCE TO GO TO SCHOOL

By EMANUEL KLEIN, M.D. (New York) [1]

Most children have experienced some of the symptoms associated with a reluctance to go to school. All of a child's worries, fears, anxieties, self-consciousness, feelings of inadequacy, his relations to his parents, to his siblings and to himself, tend to gain reflection in the school situation. The symptoms associated with school distress range from the physically expressed anticipatory anxiety symptoms such as morning nausea, vomiting, diarrhea, abdominal cramps, great difficulty in getting up in the morning which often vanishes magically on holidays, to disorders in learning and behavior in the classroom, and finally to the avoidance of school called truancy. Chronic, well-established truancy is a complex phenomenon involving the interaction of social and intrapsychic forces. Secondary gains are promine ʾ, and the original intrapsychic causes tend to become obscured. In acute forms, with which we here deal, the mechanisms involved appear more clearly; and a knowledge of them is helpful in understanding the more chronic forms.

The refusal to go to school can be broken down into three component motives: anxiety, aggression and secondary gain. In varying proportions they combine to form the anticipatory anxiety symptoms, the disturbance in behavior and learning functions in the classroom, and the refusal to go to school. The aggression and secondary gain are most prominent in chronic truancy. Often both the teacher and the pupil see only these motivations and are not aware of the anxiety that is almost invariably present. When the truancy is well established it requires considerable therapeutic work until the child becomes aware of the basic role that anxiety continues to play in his difficulty. In the acute forms of truancy anxiety is quite obviously the chief motivation and requires the greatest attention.

---

1. From the Bureau of Child Guidance, Board of Education.

Surprisingly little seems to have been written on the acute syndromes. Broadwin described some aspects in a paper entitled "A Contribution to the Study of Truancy".[2] A. M. Johnson and his associates discussed eight cases and found the acute fear of school to be brought on by the outbreak of anxiety in the child and the mother.[3]

The anxiety about school can be conveniently separated into a fear of the teacher, a fear of the pupils, and a fear of the school work with expectation of failure. Although these fears intermingle, reinforce each other and shift from one focal point to another, it is helpful to isolate and trace them separately. In different syndromes, varying according to the age and personality of the child, one of them tends to be the prominent factor with the others subsidiary.

In young children fear of the teacher can appear suddenly in striking form, and quickly gain great intensity. It rapidly becomes an overwhelming dread, assuming a primitive, oral character. At first associated with a particular teacher, it soon involves the school as a whole, and then any school. It is greatly fostered both by the child's absence from school, and by the efforts often made by the parents, teachers, and administrators to get the child back to school.

Victoria was a nine-year-old girl in the 4A grade. She was referred for sudden refusal to go to school. She had attended her new class for three days and then would not return, offering illness as an excuse. After a couple of days the parents saw that she was not physically ill and forced her back to school. She remained there for a little while and ran home. For the next few weeks her parents put great pressure on Victoria. The mother, the dominant member of the household, pleaded, coaxed and beat the child severely. In spite of the cruelty of the pressure, the child stubbornly refused to go and she was brought to school by sheer force. She seemed so distressed that the school referred her to the Bureau of Child Guidance.

When first seen Victoria was a very distressed, unhappy child. She sat in the waiting room, immobile, head bowed, fists clenched, staring at the floor. Brought into the office, she would hardly talk and could not be induced to play. She could verbalize little about her intense dread, repeating "I can't go— I can't go." In several interviews, she told of her unpleasant experiences with a stern teacher. Before entering her class, Victoria had heard from other pupils that the teacher was strict; her older sister, who had had this teacher previously, had warned her "Wait until you get into her class—she's a murderer—she will make you work." With this background Victoria met her new teacher. When on the first day the class was asked to write something about the Revolutionary War, the child was so frightened that she

2. *American Journal of Orthopsychiatry* II, 3, 1932.
3. "School Phobia", Ibid., XI, 4, 1941.

wrote very little. The teacher collected the papers and on seeing Victoria's poor performance, made her stand up, scolded her and held her up to ridicule. She insisted that Victoria was lazy and warned her that she would not be able to get away with that kind of stuff in her class. The next morning Victoria had the greatest distress in anticipation of going to school. She was filled with anxiety, felt nauseated, and could hardly make herself go. After several days of similar experience in the classroom, she refused to get out of bed in the morning and said she was sick, and from then on her mother could not force her back to school. The child was reassured by the examiner that she would not have to return to that particular teacher but would be transferred to another one; she could not accept this either. The transfer was arranged, to no avail. Finally she was told that she did not have to go—that she would receive instruction from a tutor and that when the fear of school was over she would again attend. On this basis the child responded very quickly and in a little while she got over her acute distress. She sat at home during the school, spending some of the time with the examiner or the tutor. The rest of the day she spent playing with her friends very much as before.

Victoria was found to be a child closely attached to a strong and energetic mother. The father was a weak, ineffectual person, who had never earned a living for the family and who was looked upon with contempt by all of them. He worked intermittently and spent most of his time at a coffee house, idling and playing cards with his cronies. He played a minor role in the life of the family and was kept on, only on sufferance, by the mother. She worked, took care of the children and the house, and gave both affection and discipline. Victoria was closely tied to her mother by a strong bond of dependence, love, and fear, together with deeply repressed hostility. She had had many experiences of intense fear and anxiety in relation to her mother, when the latter was angry and had punished her severely. Sometimes she resisted her mother in a passive, stubborn, tenacious way, clinging to her point in spite of her mother's great anger. The harsh teacher had quickly assumed the form of the primitive, aggressive mother who might devour the child. Victoria had a large number of fears, many of which were expressions of fear of being bitten. She was afraid of cats and rats, of fish and mosquitoes, of witches and kidnappers. When working out these fears in play, she was able to enact them if she took the role of the aggressor rather than that of the victim. At such times her own strong oral drives came out dramatically; saliva actually drooled from her mouth as she played the part of the witch who steals and eats the child. These oral fears had been projected on to the teacher and then on to the whole school, which became a kind of devouring monster.

Victoria responded well to treatment. After about a year she returned to school and after two years she seemed entirely recovered not only from the school fears but from her underlying neurosis. She conquered her fears of the dark, she went to camp, and learned to swim well without fear of being bitten by the fish. She gained a good deal of independence from her mother, made a good social adjustment and worked up to her capacity at school. During the first six months she was seen three times a week, then twice a week, and eventually once a week.

Although the result was good, there were many difficulties in her treatment that could have been avoided. Victoria was distressed at her inability to go to school, but she accepted the situation and adjusted only too well to the examiner and the tutor. After her neurotic mechanisms had been worked through again and again, and she seemed to be doing quite well, school still remained a very dreaded place. Any mention of it would bring distress. She was told that in the new school she would not have to attend any classes, but would sit in the principal's office, assisting her, and if she liked, participating in such activities with the children as gym or dancing. Even this was very hard for her to face and the examiner accompanied her to school on several occasions before she was finally able to make herself enter the building. However, each of these attempts, although at first unsuccessful, always brought out new material and enabled one to work through some of the previously developed material. Later, Victoria was able to stay at school, although not participating in activities; she slowly increased her participation and finally became a normal pupil. When she completed Grade 6B, she had to return to her previous school because the second school went no further. For a little while there was some distress in anticipation, but it was thoroughly worked through in advance and when the time came she was surprised to find that she was so little frightened of her old school.

Victoria's school history was typical of one kind of acute dread of school. She had had considerable resistance to beginning school, had been fearful for the first few weeks but had finally overcome her fears. For the two terms before the outbreak of her trouble she had a very kind understanding teacher to whom she became greatly attached, and whom she had been unhappy to leave. When she learned that her new teacher had the reputation of being stern, she quickly built up great anticipatory dread. The change to a new stern teacher, to a new school—especially to a larger and more distant one—or moving to a new neighborhood, is often a precipitating factor.

Victoria was the first case of its kind treated by the examiner. Subsequent experience indicated that in spite of the very good result, an important mistake was made in the treatment. The child with acute school dread presents a delicate problem in handling. On the one hand, harsh attempts by the parents and school to get the child back to school greatly increase the child's fear and make the therapeutic task more protracted. Unfortunately, not getting the child back to school promptly has almost equally bad results. If the child remains out of school for a while, there is a quick development of primitive regressive fear, in young children of an oral character, in older ones of a paranoid nature simulating schizophrenia. The child soon is unable to accept any school or any teacher, even the kindliest and most understanding. The school building itself becomes the threatening devouring object. This regression and spread can be prevented by getting the child back to school promptly. If one is convinced of the importance of doing this, it can be done in practically every case, if the school is cooperative. The child is told he must go to school every day, but does not have to stay there, and does not have to attend the classroom. The child can stay in an office, assist the office staff, read or draw, and can leave at any time. At first it seems like a futile or even harsh procedure to have the parent persuade the fearful resistive child to dress himself and accompany him to school if he only stays five or ten minutes, but it actually is of great importance. Some of the most difficult treatment problems have occurred where a sympathetic school principal has put a child on the suspense list and he has remained at home. The treatment is greatly speeded up if the child maintains even a fragmentary daily contact with the school from the start. When he is excused from attendance, he may become fairly happy and able to play with his friends; and the school anxieties may remain quite inaccessible as long as he is not in any contact with the object of his dread.

The importance of maintaining attendance is further brought out by the frequency with which the acute dread breaks out after an illness which keeps the child away from school. Alice was a girl of thirteen in Grade 7B in a Junior High School. She was experiencing some dread of school based on her difficulty with her academic subjects, her dislike of her teachers, and her fears of the aggressive girls, their fights, and their obscene language. She found it hard to go to school but had only an occasional absence until she developed an upper respiratory infection with pleuritic pain. She was in bed for a couple of weeks. When the illness seemed over she continued to complain of pains, in an effort to escape school, and then she refused to return in spite of extreme pressure and beatings by her mother. Another child kept going to school in spite of distress until the week's fuel-saving holiday between terms, and then could not resume attendance.

There are a number of constellations that are often found among children who develop acute dread of the teacher. One of the commonest is that exhibited by John, a seven-year-old boy.

John was very closely attached to his mother. He slept with her until he was four, when his younger brother was born. He strongly resisted his displacement by his sibling and kept coming to his mother's bed at night. The intense oedipal relationship, fostered by his mother's handling of him, naturally resulted in great fear of the father. This was heightened by the father's actual severity. The father was an Italian who followed a rigid cultural pattern of paternal authority over the family. He had been especially restrictive to the older girls. Before John was born the father had a coal and ice business and had made a satisfactory living. With the depression he had lost his business and was unemployed for a long time. The family's standard of living was reduced. He got odd jobs, and eventually was on W.P.A.; he searched in vain for a better job. The social pressures impinging on him were transmitted to his family. He became more tyrannical at home, was irritable to his family, drank more wine than formerly. John was born during this time, a not entirely welcome arrival in a family that already had five children. Both John and his younger brother experienced a considerably more stern and irritable father than had the older boys who apparently had no outstanding neurotic traits. The stream of John's fear of his father was fed by his great attachment to his mother, which would have stimulated neurotic fears even of a gentle father, and by his father's objective harshness.

John's first kind teacher in the small school became a mother substitute. But an unfortunate experience with the custodian on his first day when he got lost in the basement, together with the unwise handling by his teacher of this frightened boy, led to a transfer of his fear of his father on to the teacher and the school. The sex of the teacher had little bearing on the process.

Parallel with his fear of the teacher, was his longing to be with his mother, which he satisfied by staying at home. This longing was reinforced by his anxieties as to what might happen at home while he was at school. John had witnessed the primal scene many times during the years that he slept with his parents. His tendency to regard it as an attack on his mother was reinforced by the occasional scenes of actual violence he witnessed when his father, while intoxicated, had thrown a shoe at his mother, and when he had struck her. John feared these experiences; he was afraid that while he was at school his father might assault his mother sexually and physically. His anxiety was of course intensified by jealousy. On the days when his father had to go to work at noon, John was especially afraid to go to school.

Another source of anxiety about his home, while he was at school, was his fear that his younger brother might get hurt. John had experienced terror dreams in which his brother was kidnapped. This transformed jealousy of his brother assumed great heights, and whenever the brother was ill with a cold, John was worried that his mother was not taking proper care of him, and that the brother might die. John's fear of school pushed him from school; his love for his mother, his anxiety that his father might injure her, his jealousy of the possible sexual relation between his parents and of his mother's relation to his younger brother, and his anxiety about his brother— all pulled him to the home.

Another common constellation, in contrast to the girl with a strong tie to a dominant mother and a weak oedipal tie to the father, as exemplified by Victoria, is that of the young girl with a strong sexual tie to her father.

Mary was a nine-year-old girl whose father was very indulgent. He brought her candy or a present every night. She insisted on eating the candy before supper: her mother protested but was forced by the father to yield to the little girl. Mary suffered from night terrors in which a giant or gorilla attacked her. She refused to sleep alone in her room: although her mother tried to insist on this, she was compelled by the father to put Mary's bed next to theirs, and told to hold the child's hand during the night. When the father was at work the child clung to the mother, accompanying her everywhere. In the first interview, the mother had to come into the playroom and stay with the child. The secondary gain from dominating and thwarting her mother by means of extreme anxiety and tenacious clinging was very apparent. The wish to be with the mother in order to separate the parents was equally evident.

After a few interviews circumstances did not permit further treatment of this child. Her mother placed her in a hospital, and there the picture changed strikingly. Mary tried to get on the doctor's lap to make sexual advances, to expose herself. There was an adult flirtatiousness and provocativeness that one would expect only in an older sex delinquent. This child gave evidence of persistent spying on the parents, watching for a chance to see her father in the nude, much surreptitious use of rouge and nail polish, and a receptivity to sex experiences with an adult. Investigation revealed that the child's provocative behavior was a result of identification with her mother.

Generally the mechanisms are less extreme.

Helen was an attractive girl of seven with acute dread of school and teacher. When forced to attend she vomited; she was publicly called "Miss Vomit" by several of the teachers. After the acute anxiety picture had faded Helen also showed a marked flirtatiousness and a false sophistication during the treatment interviews. She had a simpering manner, and with a great deal of false modesty and affectation told of the boys who were in love with her. Her parents encouraged this attitude. They were pleased to tell their friends of the "dates" that a boy tried to make with her, and of a letter she received from a boy she met in the country. She showed great interest in her nineteen-year-old sister's relation to boys and to the sister's probable engagement, envied the sister, put on her jewels, and kept thinking whether she would accept the engagement ring were she in her sister's place. The mother was a good-looking, well-dressed woman with an extreme interest in clothes, and an affected, flirtatious manner. Helen showed extreme attachment to her father, fostered by his attitude to her. He caressed and petted her a great deal, he bought her many gifts, some relatively expensive and adult, like a bottle of good perfume. He put pressure on the mother to indulge the child. There was fairly open jealousy between mother and daughter for the father. The mother resented the child and was very angry at Helen's extreme attachment to her. In the child's clinging, in addition to her anxiety and her guilt over her hostile wishes toward her mother, the secondary gain of dominating and thwarting her mother plus the unconscious motive of separating her parents, of preventing them from being alone together, was again prominent, as in the case of Mary.

Another common constellation is that of the boy who is strongly tied to an over-critical, rejecting mother.

Joseph was a thirteen-and-a-half-year-old boy in the 8B Rapid Advancement class, in a Junior High School. He had been an honor pupil, quiet, well-behaved, "the nicest boy in the class". The visiting teacher reported that

a month before his referral he had begun to cry in the machine-shop class.
After the period he went home. He was away from school a few days, and
on his return said he didn't like the machine shop. The visiting teacher
arranged for a change in program, but he only attended for a day. His
mother, who was employed, beat him severely to make him go to school but
without success. The boy was home for the next five weeks. His mother
thought he was bluffing and kept beating him, till the visiting teacher made
her stop and told the boy he could stay away from school till the end of the
term. The mother was an uneducated Italian woman who spoke almost no
English in spite of her twenty-five years of residence in the United States.
She was seen only on one occasion and refused to return to the clinic, saying
she did not want to miss her work.

Joseph was a short slight boy, tense, anxious, with a marked startle
reaction. He did not know what made him feel bad in the machine shop.
He had gone home to bed, stayed there crying for three days and then returned
to school. He felt bad again as soon as he arrived, and all during that day.
After this he refused to go. The bad feeling continued, until the visiting
teacher made his mother stop beating him, and until she told him he would
not have to return to school for the rest of the term.

Joseph described his mother as very anxious, restricting and severe. She
would yell if he got sweaty or got his clothes dirty, and beat him with a big
wooden spoon if his clothes were torn at play. When he was four-and-a-half
his mother put him in kindergarten and went to work. There was only a
morning class, so he used to wait in the 1A classroom until his older sister
was released from school and then she looked after him. He was very
closely attached to this sister. A few years ago she suddenly ran away from
home after a quarrel with the mother, and he now missed her very much.

Joseph had slept with his mother until he was nine. In spite of her
harshness he was greatly attached to her, and he strongly repressed his
hostility. He was fearful of losing her. When angry, she often threatened
either to place him in a home, or to leave the family and never return. When
he was a little boy, Joseph was very fond of bonfires. His mother warned
him strongly against them, threatening to burn his fingers if she caught him
with matches. In characteristic phobic fashion he then developed a fear of
fires. Later he became worried that their house might burn down. He was
uneasy when he saw a fire engine, and if there was a fire in the neighborhood
he was worried that it might spread to his house. Once on his way to school
he passed a fire in a house a block away from his house. Throughout that
morning he was very uneasy at school.

During a recent quarrel with the father, the mother had again threatened
to leave home. At about the same time she had also threatened to put Joseph
in a reformatory when he had come home with torn clothes after a fall during
a game. His anxiety about the possible loss of his mother was renewed. This
was certainly fed by his great guilt about masturbation. He feared bodily and
genital harm and developed strong feelings of badness and dirtiness. He had
confessed to his priest and tried hard to conquer the impulse to masturbate.
When he found himself doing it again he developed acute anxiety.

A week before his acute school difficulty he had a bad toothache; two days before he had to have the tooth extracted, which he had dreaded. The tooth removed was a big one (molar) and he felt funny inside when he looked at the empty space. The dentist told him another tooth was bad and probably would require extraction also, with the cutting of a gum flap. The night before his acute anxiety at school he had been thinking about it, had felt frightened and cried. The extraction was connected with castration fear because of masturbation guilt, and the latter connected with his fear of loss of his mother as a punishment for his badness. The sounds of the machine shop, where his fears had broken out, had reminded him of the dentist's drill.

After he had become acutely distressed his father had bought him a puppy for which he had always longed. He had a dream that all of the dog's teeth had fallen out and were lying on the floor. He had awakened frightened and had run to the dog to see if it were true. During his third therapeutic visit, after he had returned to school, he had a dream in which a teacher, an Italian woman, told him to wash his hands. Instead he went to the roof and watched the children playing. She caught him and asked him if he had washed his hands. He admitted he had not, and she threatened him with being sent to the principal. In his associations the hands were dirty because of his masturbation, and connection between the dread of his mother's leaving him and his sexual activity came out clearly.

Joseph's case shows how quickly these children with acute problems can sometimes respond. Joseph was seen ten times between January and June. After the second interview he returned to school. After the fourth the school distress disappeared. Joseph became less dependent on his mother, lost his anxiety about losing her and developed better social relations with other boys. His mother's harshness continued, although she stopped beating him, but he was able to tolerate it. During the treatment he had to face the trauma of losing his beloved puppy. His mother did not like its barking in the morning and told him she would get rid of it. When the dog barked early in the morning Joseph would jump out of bed and hold its mouth, or beat it in his eagerness to get it quiet. The mother kept insisting the dog must go and finally Joseph was able to accept this. He gave the dog to a friend so that he could continue to see and play with it, and although he missed it, he did not react neurotically to the loss. It seems very likely, on the basis of experience with other children, that had Joseph been allowed to stay out of school for a few months while under treatment, the treatment would have had to be very protracted.

The cases thus far presented make it evident that in addition to the fear of the teacher and the school, these children have a fear of separation from the mother, which going to school involves. The child may fear that his mother may go away forever because of his badness. This occurs most often where the mother has threatened to leave home because of the child's behavior or where there has been conflict between the parents. The child may fear sexual or physical assault on the mother by the father. This occurs most often where the boy has a strong oedipal attachment to his mother, is jealous of his father and wants him out of the way, and has a fear of retaliation which the father reinforces by harshness toward mother and child. The girl may fear that while she is at school her mother may be killed in some accident. This occurs most often in girls with strong repressed hostility to a thwarting mother on whom they are dependent. The fear represents a return from the unconscious of the formerly repressed hostility; it is strengthened by the oedipal attachment to the father, jealousy of the mother, and the wish to have this rival out of the way. The child may be jealous of the relation between the mother and a younger sibling who remains at home, and may experience this directly, as a fear of being displaced by the sibling as a love object while he or she is away at school; or, in inverted form, as a fear that the sibling may be injured. In spite of these anxieties about the mother, the child often can separate himself from her to go out to play, but cannot do so to go to the feared school. In addition to the fears, the child has the secondary gains from staying home, of being with the beloved mother, of separating the parents, of thwarting and dominating a hated mother, or of defying a hated father. In the secondary gains the libidinal pleasures of being with the mother, or the ego gains of dominating and defying a parent, intermingle.

Among the fears of school, the fear of other children usually plays a reinforcing rather than a dominating role. The timid boy is often fearful of being hit, teased or bullied by his companions. This occurs most often in poor neighborhoods where many of the children are relatively unrestrained in their social relations. The lot of the neurotic boy in a delinquent area is in reality a very difficult one. The social life of the children is marred by violence, gang formation, exploitation of the weak by the strong, seizure of playthings, extortion, and extreme threats. The timid boy meets the situation early in life by clinging to home and mother. At school age he must have further contact with his fellows through school attendance, and he shrinks from it. Often he tries to solve his problem by attaching himself to the gang, denying his own weakness by his delinquent acts, and borrowing the strength of the gang. Most of the members of the delinquent gang have gone through this cycle to some degree, and represent in part over-compensated neurotic children who have been forced into this pattern in an effort to escape the harsh fate of the neurotic child in the slums.

As one would anticipate, the children who develop the most acute fear of their companions are those whom circumstances have transplanted from a gentler neighborhood to an impoverished one. Following the protracted unemployment, sickness or death of the father, the family is forced to move to a slum area and the children must try to adjust to a much harsher social environment, a difficult task even for a well-adjusted child. The fear of the tough companions is heightened by the feeling of loss of security and protection when the father dies, becomes chronically ill, or even when he becomes unemployed for a long time.

In some cases fear of schoolmates suddenly mounts acutely and becomes the primary source of the fear of going to school.

Seymour, a Jewish boy of fourteen, attending a Junior High School in a slum area, suddenly began to truant, without the knowledge of his family. He got up at the usual time, took his books as though going to school, waited for the postman so he could intercept the notice of his absence that the school sent his parents, and left the neighborhood. He spent the school day in a movie or a distant park, in constant fear of encountering a policeman or truant officer, and came home when school was over. His family were orthodox Jews; they had reacted with extreme distress to the elopement and marriage of their daughter to an Italian. At home the boy kept hearing about the bad habits of Italians, of their readiness to use knives and stilettos. He and an older sister had secretly been visiting the excommunicated sister and had been in great dread of detection. At school two aggressive Italian boys had bullied him, and taken his comic books. Seymour's castration fear about his masturbation and his guilt and fear about his secret visits to his sister coalesced with his fear of the Italian boys, and he stayed away from school to avoid them. He responded quickly to treatment and interpretation, returned to school after one interview and after three interviews seemed to be getting along better than before his acute outbreak. Circumstances did not permit more protracted treatment of his underlying difficulties but follow-up indicated that he, his family and his school were well satisfied with his adjustment.

In adolescent children with school dread, a factor sometimes involved in the fear of other children is the acute discomfort aroused by the obscene language of schoolmates. The precarious success of the adolescent child struggling to master his own sexuality is threatened by the verbal sexual activity of his companions. In children with obsessional traits, in whom words and language often assume disproportionate importance, the obscene words carry unique significance. This is particularly true of the child who earlier in life has grappled with the problem of the return of repressed sexuality from his unconscious, in the form of obscene words. In the passive boy with a strong unconscious homosexual component, the use of the words by his companions arouses these most threatening feelings and presents a grave problem to him. In general the dread of obscene words as a strong factor in the fear of companions is a grave prognostic sign, and tends to point to an obsessional neurosis, a seriously neurotic character formation, or a pre-psychotic or even beginning psychotic state.

Fear of classmates more often expresses itself in chronic symptoms within the classroom, frequently in clowning. Because this symptom expresses aggression toward the teacher, the anxieties generating it are often overlooked.

Michael was a fourteen-and-a-half-year-old boy who came to see the examiner of his own accord because his closest companion was being treated here, and he decided to seek help for himself also. He said he had been truanting from school for many years, and was far behind in his grades, but now wanted to prepare himself for serious study of music; and because he had moved recently, he wanted the examiner's help in getting into a school that had a good orchestra.

Michael gave a long history of school difficulty. When he was a child in his early classes, he used to be teased a lot because of his big nose and because of his timidity. Some of the teasing, especially about the nose, which was in fact quite large, had continued down to the present time. He said he started making the other boys laugh to show them that he was somebody, and then he became the clown of the class. He used to imitate the teacher, and laugh at her, and then found that he was having fits of laughter. At first he did not want to stop these attacks because they made him feel good, everybody got excited, and the whole class talked about him. Then to his great distress, he found that he could not stop laughing, even though he wanted to, and he laughed uncontrollably for long periods of time. Shortly after this he completed Grade 6B and went to Junior High School. There he was still more fearful of the aggressive boys but he began to solve his difficulties in a new way. He came under the domination of a friend who liked to pretend that he was a gangster and a big shot. This friend quelled Michael's fear of truancy by telling him that no harm could come to you if you truanted provided that when they caught you, you would say that you really liked school and wanted to go but you did not go because they did not treat you fairly there. Under the influence of this friend, he would truant for long periods of time, once for forty days in a row. He, his domineering friend, and a couple of other boys, would spend the evenings playing musical instruments in small beer gardens and stay up until three or four in the morning. The next day they would all meet in the park, sleep on the benches until noon, play in the afternoon, come home at three o'clock, practise their instruments, and at night would go looking for places where they could entertain and make some money. His father, whom he described as a domineering, and sometimes brutal man, learned of the truancy and beat him with great violence. The frequency and severity of the beatings finally made Michael attend school but with marked resistance to the learning process and with the development of sly ways of disrupting the classroom.

The child who clowns in the classroom very commonly is found to have a history of teasing by his companions because of his timidity. They call him sissy, ridicule him and torment him. The boy tries to meet the painful situation by actively bringing on the laughter of his companions rather than waiting to endure it passively. He clowns and in this way determines the time when the other boys laugh at him. The clowning still brings him a good deal of ridicule but it is tempered by some admiration and therefore is more acceptable to him. At the same time making other boys laugh has as its motive disarming them, making them laugh at him instead of beating him; it is a kind of plea for mercy and a self-degradation, in relation to the other boys. In Michael's case, the anxiety behind the clowning would come in severe attacks and result in his fits of uncontrollable laughter. The realization that he lost control again terrified him because it was the wish to command the situation that had led to the clowning.

The fear of failure in school work is a very complex symptom, deriving its energy from many sources, and found to a greater or less degree in every type of school difficulty. In adolescents, it often is the central thread in an acute school difficulty. A fairly frequent clinical picture is that in which the adolescent pupil in Junior or Senior High School develops increasing difficulty with the work, generates a fear of failure, and then refuses to go to school. Often, a schizo-phrenic-like picture develops. The pupil is very self-conscious about not going to school, avoids his companions, sits alone at home and gradually withdraws from most activities. There develops a good deal of projection with ideas of reference; the pupil feels that the boys in the neighborhood are all talking about his failure to attend school and ridiculing him for it. The withdrawal can become quite pronounced and the diagnosis of schizophrenia is often erroneously made. The syndrome differs from adolescent schizophrenia in that it is more responsive to psychotherapy; sometimes the acute picture will vanish in a relatively short time, and one is left instead with the ordinary neurotic difficulties of the adolescent.

Martin was a fourteen-and-a-half-year-old boy in the second term of high school. He had not attended school for a month. From the beginning of the term on he was increasingly resistant, exaggerating small illnesses and offering many somatic complaints such as headaches and faintness. His father had put a great deal of pressure on him to make him go but had thus only increased the boy's resistance. Martin then spent his entire time at home, sitting in a room by himself, reading and making wood-carvings. At other times he would spend the whole day in the movies seeing the show over and over again. He said he wanted to go to work. His father took him to a well-known psychiatrist who said that the boy was unapproachable therapeutically and suggested that he be excused from further school attendances and permitted to go to work. The father came to the examiner to arrange for this.

Martin was an over-sized obese boy, very acutely distressed and anxious. He told how he had done pretty well at grammar school until the eighth grade when he began to experience trouble with some of his subjects. In high school he had increasing difficulty, especially with Spanish. At the end of the first term his teacher gave him a grade of 65 but Martin felt that this was just a favor to him and that he really deserved to fail. In the second term, he found he could not do the Spanish at all and also had a great deal of trouble with mathematics. He was very much ashamed of his failure in school and felt that it was evidence of his total inadequacy.

Martin's father was a successful business man. He had been a poor boy and worked his way up in the world and now owned a factory. He was aggressive, domineering, and had had high hopes for Martin; he had set aside money for Martin's college education and had hoped that Martin would become a doctor or dentist. The father had been bitterly disappointed at Martin's school failure and had made his disappointment very clear to the boy.

Martin brought out that he had been a disappointment to his father as far back as he could remember. As a child, he had suffered from a glandular dysfunction, had a small genital, and been very obese. He had been treated with endocrine injections. He was always clumsy, inept at sports, and fearful of the other boys. They picked on him and he could not fight back. They called him sissy and cry-baby. The father was very disgusted with his timidity, often taunted him for it, and tried to make him fight his own battles.

Martin's mother had died of pneumonia two years previously. She had been a very tense, nervous woman, worrisome about the children. Martin had often been told as a child that he was making the mother sick by his bad behavior at home. After her death he had severe guilt feelings, believing he had contributed to it. His bad behavior had consisted largely of feeding difficulties: refusal to eat, or vomiting when forced to eat. On the advice of a physician, the father had warned Martin that he would "strap" him hard if he vomited again. This stopped the vomiting. The mother fed him forcibly up to the age of six, and was made frantic by his resistance. She was quite severe about cleanliness, and scolded him a great deal for being dirty. Martin clung closely to her in spite of his father's efforts to get him away from his "mother's skirt". There was intense rivalry with the eight-year-old sister, who was much more competent than Martin.

After the mother's death the family went to live with a married aunt and her grown-up children, who had done well at school and who had always been held up to Martin as good examples.

Martin told of his extreme fear of ridicule by the other boys, the fear of the fellows around his block talking about his school failure, and about his unwillingness to go to school. He was ashamed to be seen in the street. He did not go out until five or six o'clock and would invent various tales to account for his absence from the school and the street.

Martin was very unhappy living in his aunt's home. His aunt was very strict about neatness. She and her husband both tried to ridicule him into attending school, and he hated them. He felt desperate and thought that the only solution was to run away. He knew of an abandoned cabin in the country near where they had once spent the summer. His plan was to get some money, buy a lot of canned food, go up there and hide away until the school term was over and then work during the summer. In the fall, with the money he had earned he would make his way to some distant part of the country, keep on working, and not come home until he had made a success of his life. Martin hoped that when he grew up he would become a famous doctor and show everyone that he could really be something; or he dreamed of becoming a rich stock broker.

The psychological examination showed the boy to have an I.Q. of 112, which was actually adequate for good performance at high school level though not for his ambition to become a doctor. The Rorschach examination was suggestive of schizophrenia.

Martin was first seen near the end of the school term and before the summer vacation. An attempt was made to get him to go back to school on a very light program. Martin came to the school building, spoke to the principal and then ran out. By this time the vacation period had started. Because of the need for immediate therapy, Martin was referred to a psychiatrist who could work with him during the summer. In the fall he was encouraged to register in a small private high school and in a short time was again taking a full program. Martin is still under treatment and is doing very well at school. His father puts many obstacles in the way of therapy, often reminding the boy that he is spending twenty dollars a week for the treatment and schooling. In spite of this Martin continues to attend and to make progress.

A very characteristic feature that Martin presented was his exaggerated ambition. The syndrome of acute dread of school failure often develops in children of average intelligence whose parents plan to have them go to college and achieve a great deal. The child clings strongly to his unrealistic ambition even when it is clear that it cannot be realized and when he is at the same time totally avoiding school. One of the objectives in the treatment is to bring the ambition more closely in accord with the realistic possibilities, but this is a difficult therapeutic task. In another similar case, a girl who had been attending college for a year but who had failed in almost all of her subjects for lack of attendance, clung to her skill in drawing because when she would study medicine she would need it to make anatomical drawings. Traces of the old ambition tend to remain for a long time after it is apparently given up. In such cases the ambition is closely related to pleasing one of the parents and winning their love. Frequently one of the parents has greatly over-praised the child for school success, and heaped rewards on him for school achievement; and through this excessive praise has created a situation as bad as that created by excessive criticism and lack of encouragement.

Adolescents with the syndrome of acute dread of school failure and a generalized withdrawal from activity are not infrequently given shock thereapy on the ground that they are schizophrenic. This has very unfortunate results; it interferes greatly with subsequent therapeutic possibilities and should clearly be avoided in these cases.

Of seven cases of acute refusal to go to school treated by the examiner, all but two returned to school in a short time and made satisfactory adjustments at various levels, depending in large part on the amount of time available for their treatment. The two (Victoria and John) were treated before the examiner was fully aware of the great importance of bringing about a return to school at the earliest moment, at *any level of school participation that the child can tolerate*. They responded eventually, and one of them (Victoria) who was treated intensively can now be regarded as cured of her underlying neurosis.

Of three cases being treated currently by the examiner, one, a boy of five-and-a-half years, has dramatically overcome a very intense acute anxiety phase in five contacts and is attending school without distress. His mother feels that the problem is solved, and she may become reluctant to continue to bring him for treatment.

The second case is of an eight-year-old boy with strong, overt oedipal attachment to his mother, and great fear of his father, which was transferred to an aggressive classmate. This boy had to be weaned gradually from his mother by having her sit in the classroom for the first two days. She then sat in the hallway adjoining the classroom for three days, and finally in an office in the school for a week, until the boy could remain in school without her. This case was complicated by a large amount of secondary gain, due to the family pattern of bribing the boy with gifts to get him to conform to their demands. The boy's school fears have subsided but there is continuation of his outbursts of rage in which he strikes his mother and calls her obscene names when she does not yield to him.

The third case is of an eight-year-old girl who has had strong death fears about a very aggressive and rejecting mother. She had to be weaned from her mother even more gradually, and it took six weeks before the mother could stay at home while the child was at school. This case was likewise complicated by a good deal of secondary gain, as well as by a marked obesity.

Summary

Acute dread of going to school occurs in children with strong castration anxiety, great masturbation guilt, and repressed aggressive impulses toward a parent on whom they are greatly dependent. These children are fixated at the oedipal or pre-oedipal level. An increase of tension in the school reactivates a regressive dread of the primitive punitive parent, projected on to the teacher and school, which frightens the child away from the school. An increase in sexual longing, fear or guilt toward the parents, reactivates the oedipal or pre-oedipal fear of sexual injury of the mother, injury to the mother by a projected aspect of the child's oral-sadistic impulse, or desertion by the mother: these anxieties draw the child to the mother. School failure becomes tied to masturbation guilt and fear of loss of love; shame about school failure reactivates a paranoid shame at inability to control one's sexual impulse.

Brief psychotherapy based on psychoanalytic insight usually can bring about a quick recession of the acute phase, and more protracted psychotherapy can modify or overcome the underlying neurosis.

THE MEANS OF EDUCATION

By OTTO FENICHEL, M.D. (Los Angeles)

In considering any educational influence, it is necessary to distinguish three factors:

(1) that which is being influenced, i.e., the mental structure of the child;

(2) the influencing stimuli, which converge upon this structure;

(3) the influencing process, i.e., the alterations that occur in the child's mind in response to these stimuli.

The first of these factors is, in the final analysis, determined by human biology, the second by the cultural environment in which the child is reared. Hence, it is appropriate to assume that the first factor is a subject for study by biologists, the second for sociologists, whereas the third would be in the realm of psychoanalytic research. In a science of education all three disciplines would have to be employed.

Any such schematic division is, to be sure, only relatively valid. The mental structure, to begin with, is not identical with the hereditary biological constitution which can be investigated by biology; it is actually composed of both this constitution and all previous external influences. It is not possible to disregard these external influences in any single respect. Already in utero, environmental formative influences are at work, and even developmental tendencies, which are certainly innate, need precipitating external stimuli to materialize. Strangely enough, even in the realm of the biologic needs—which in their relative force and specific form are necessarily influenced by environment—the decisive contribution was not made by a biologist, but rather by psychoanalysts. Certain primitive needs, such as hunger and the need for warmth or for excretion have, of course, been studied thoroughly by biologists. But for a considerable number of other needs and impulses—and precisely for those whose modification through education forms character—it is not a biological treatise, but rather Freud's *Three Contributions to the Theory of Sex,* that is the basic textbook; in other words, the very existence and operation of infantile sexuality had to be reconstructed from the psychoanalyses of adults.

The influencing stimuli are of course manifold. Those of interest in a discussion of "education" are the systematic and institutionalized ones. They are not quite so varied as other external stimuli, inasmuch as traditional ways of child rearing are usually relatively characteristic for a given cultural sphere, or for a given society, or a given sector of a society. The study of the history and social function of these traditional ways certainly belongs in the field of sociology. Both history and social function are very complicated. All educational procedures contain conservative elements reflecting the history of the society in question, as well as tendencies toward reform, corresponding to current social ideology which, for its part, is determined by social and political conditions and changes.

In any event, the objective social function of educational institutions differs greatly from the thoughts entertained by individual educators as to their educational goals. The institutions aim at the production of certain character structures which not only induce "sociality" within the next generation, but also the development of certain ways of thinking, feeling and reacting in general, which effect adjustment to the existing order. Those individuals, whose mental structure has been molded by traditional educational procedures to conformity with the existing order, present the chief obstacles to necessary changes within this order; on the other hand, attempts to reform educational systems will be unsuccessful, or at least greatly limited in their effectiveness, as long as the existing social order requires maintenance of the old educational institution in its own interest.

In spite of the divergence of educational stimuli, certain general, basic educational tasks connected with the small child are identical in all societies, namely the furtherance of certain developments in the mind of the child. Before we consider the third factor, the processes within the child's mind, let us first examine these general developmental tendencies. Infants and small children live mainly according to the so-called "pleasure principle". They obey every impulse, have no interest except that of getting rid of their tensions; their continual attempt to do whatever they feel like doing at the moment is restricted only by the inhibiting force of their physical limitations. Unquestionably it would be impossible to have a society composed of individuals who live according to the pleasure principle. Uncontrolled instinctual impulses are uncontrolled natural forces.

However, no two-year-old child, even without the benefit of "education", would retain his original, primitive kind of behavior. Cumulative experience forces him to take into consideration the prospective reaction of his surroundings to his actions. "Reason" develops, and opposes unreasonable behavior. He who eats as many sweets as he pleases may expect a tummy ache. He who grabs at the beautiful fire gets burned. He who tortures his environment will be tortured in return. Life governed by the impulse of the moment is gradually (although never completely) transformed into life governed by the "reality principle", a situation wherein reality and the probable consequence of intended actions is subjected to judgment. Pleasure is renounced in order to avoid subsequent pain, or to attain subsequent, more intense pleasure. As the ego of the child gains in strength, it learns to bear tensions by postponing the reaction, and to interpolate between stimulus and reaction a kind of "trial action" in fantasy, which affords insight into the prospective consequences.

Education certainly can and should help in this development. It is not necessary for every child to burn himself; education can anticipate the pain of burning through warning or threatening. This holds true especially for the experience: "he who tortures his environment will be tortured in return".

We do not know how a child would behave without any "education". We do not know to what extent the natural encounters with reality would suffice in the development of reasonableness. But we do know that in actual practice more is demanded of every child than pure reasonableness, that educational procedure everywhere is not merely help in the development of the "reality principle", but frankly of an emphasized and exaggerated reality principle. How the parents react to instinctual acts becomes the child's main "encounter with reality", and serves as the motivating force for the child to change his instinctual behavior.

This affords a key to the basic principles of all education, principles which are obvious in the training of small children, but which become more involved as the problems of the more subtle guidance of older children arise.

The development of judgment is created by the production of instinctual conflicts brought about by external forces, that is, a remodel-

ing of certain instincts in such manner as to connect their goal with
the repression of other instinctual impulses. In the case of the burned
child this is obvious. It is the instinct of self-preservation that, after
the experience, appears to be stronger than the original desire to play
with fire. Crude child training works in the same manner. It con-
nects pain with certain pleasures, until the fear of pain becomes
stronger than the desire for pleasure. The underlying principle in more
subtle education is no different. Only, however, the pain that becomes
connected with the pleasure to be suppressed is a more subtle one.

It is characteristic of children that they very deeply need love and
affection from the persons of their environment. This is a psychic
component of the biological helplessness of the human infant. The
infant is wholly dependent on external care and would perish without
it. Its concepts of objects and of reality are formed in connection
with experiences of hunger and satiety (attained through external supplies), or, to state it more generally, through the alternation of states
of need and satisfaction. In the course of this process, the child
becomes aware of his actual weakness and is obliged to relinquish what
is probably the initial feeling state, omnipotence. Instead he now
develops the feeling that grown-ups, who can either give or withhold
satisfaction, are omnipotent. The child's longing for love and affection from these persons is simultaneously a longing for participation
in their omnipotence. The self-esteem of the child is dependent on
the flow of these supplies. When the child is loved, he feels powerful;
when neglected, he feels helpless and in danger of becoming "nothing
at all". This dependence of self-esteem on external supplies (food or
love) can be understood through observation in later life of the type
of person who has remained fixated on this level. For many persons,
their fellow-beings are mere instruments for obtaining supplies or
approbation; if they fail to receive such external supplies, they have
no adequate sense of identity. The normal person gradually learns
to achieve relative independence of the environment in the matter
of self-esteem, which is measured rather by comparison between his
actual behavior and his ideals; however, the primitive type of external
regulation of self-esteem remains operative in everyone to some extent.
It is this emotional dependence of self-esteem that becomes the vehicle
of all "more subtle" ways of education. If the possibility of receiving
this vitally needed affection becomes dependent, because of educational
measures, upon the suppression of certain original instinctual demands,
the situation is similar to that of the child who grabs at the fire. Again
a conflict arises between the impulse in question and the interest of

self-preservation, the latter here making its appearance in the form of the need to be loved. The child acquires a readiness to sacrifice certain of his interests in order to secure the supply of necessary affection. In general, this is the psychology of sacrifice which is always a lesser evil accepted voluntarily in order to avoid a greater one.

And now it seems clear we have identified the three basic means of all education, namely, direct threat, mobilization of the fear of losing love, and the promise of special rewards. The second means can be applied effectively only if the child has previously experienced the fear of losing love.

Fear of punishment and fear of losing the parents' affection differ from other frightening experiences that impel the child to defend himself against the demands of his primitive pleasure principle. Other dangers require unconditional cessation of the dangerous activity, but in the case of these fears the activity may be continued in secret, or the child may pretend he feels "bad" in circumstances where he actually feels "good". (Ferenczi once remarked in a lecture on this subject: "Out of this lie, morality came into existence.")

Objection will probably be taken to the statement that threats and rewards are the sole tools of education. The application of these principles, it may be said, can perhaps achieve some sort of training, but not that which education fundamentally desires: good behavior not only through fear of opposition to the grown-ups (who can, after all, be deceived), but good behavior for its own sake.

Actually, an internal acceptance of suggested ideals or anti-instinctual standards is developed only after a period during which the child has a two-fold ethics, one operative when he feels himself watched by grown-ups, and another one effective when he is alone or with other children.

It is an important step in maturation when prohibitions set up by the parents remain effective even in their absence. There has then been instituted in the mind a constant watchman who signals the approach of possible situations or behavior that might result in the loss of the mother's affection, or the approach of an occasion to earn the reward of mother's affection. This "watchman" completely fulfills the essential function of reason described earlier: the anticipation of the probable reactions of the external world to one's behavior. A part of the child's ego has become an "inner mother", threatening potential withdrawal of affection.

The fact that the need for the parents' affection arises as a longing to be united with their omnipotence makes it understandable that every child wants to be like his parents, to "identify" himself with them. Of course the original wish is to identify with the parents' activities, not with their prohibitions. The ideals established by the parents are, of course, an essential part of their personality, and the child in striving for rewards does not want merely to suppress certain undesired impulses, but also to fulfill positive ideals. This general striving to be like the parents may make it easier for the child to accept prohibitions also. The actual identification with the parents' prohibitions is rather a displaced substitute for the intended identification with their activities, forced upon the child by external necessity.

The first "internalized parental prohibitions" are very strong in so far as they are connected with the threat of terrible punishments, whose origin will be discussed later. But they are weak in so far as they may be easily disobeyed or circumvented when no one is looking, or when other circumstances seem to permit something previously forbidden. The internalization of the prohibitions is not yet a final one; it is still easy to shift them back to persons in the external world, like policemen or bogeymen. The child still fluctuates between yielding to his impulses and suppressing them; there is, as yet, no unified, organized character in the prohibitions. It is a situation where, under educational influence, one part of the child's own instinctual interests is utilized for suppressing other instinctual interests.

A next step in development is taken when such a "unified organized character" enters into the prohibitions, ideals and standards acquired through education. Under our cultural conditions, this occurs between the child's fourth and seventh year, and in the following way:

The child loves his parents, and he does so with a real, that is, sexual love. The parents do not satisfy these sexual desires. The child remains unsatisfied and tends to look for compensation. People who are disappointed in their wishes react by fleeing into the past, by reactivating earlier wishes that once did find satisfaction. The disappointed child, too, reactivates a very archaic aim, the very oldest form of love, if it is permissible to call such a thing love at all: the aim of incorporation of the loved object, of taking it into one's own body, of becoming fully united with it. We can also put it in the following way: "If I cannot love my parents, I want to be like my parents." The early wish for identification with the parents, which has been mentioned before and which was present before any other kind of love, is remobilized when the child realizes that certain sexual longings of his have no hope of fulfillment. When the parents forbid the child expression of his sexual desires, he psychically takes the parents into his own person. A part of his ego, changed through this incorporation, then speaks in his mind in the same way as the parents have hitherto spoken. The fact that this change within the ego, which promotes the final incorporation of both parental ideals and prohibitions, is the successor of and the substitute for the child's sexual interest in his parents, the so-called Oedipus Complex, accounts for the fact that anti-instinctual attitudes often have attributes characteristic of instincts: they are impulsive and irrational. Think, for instance, of the ascetic passion of an ascetic. The reason for this is that through educational influences, instinctual impulses have been transformed into anti-instinctual impulses. Many a modern person has some of the attributes of an ascetic, that is, he represses instinctual demands not because reason requires it, but rigidly, instinctively, blindly. The incorporation of the parents' standards and prohibitions is called the "superego" because, though it is a part of the ego, it has a power over the rest of the ego similar to the earlier power of the parents over the child. The mode of mastering impulses by a rigid and instinct-like superego is, in a normal person, subsequently replaced by the mastering of impulses by a reasonable ego.

The erection of the superego creates a multiplicity of new problems, some of which are extremely complicated, others of which still remain unsolved. They need not be considered in this discussion. ·

The principal change brought about by the creation of a superego is that the child has become emotionally more independent of external affection, because his superego now decides whether or not he is worthy of being loved. Anxiety as a regulator of the primitive impulses has been partly supplanted by guilt feeling. However, conflicts may arise between the child's ego and superego, which again make him seek the helping intervention of the adults around him. Often the child is seeking external "forgivers" or "condemners" to defend himself against an unreasonable superego. Such needs, again, are used by educators who in the last analysis have no other means at their disposal than threats and rewards,—although threats and rewards become more and more subtle, the more highly developed the child's ego becomes, and the more lofty the ideas that are at stake. However, educational influences after the sixth or seventh year are by no means limited to the child's superego. It is not only the superego that is

influenced by satisfying and frustrating experiences, and more particularly by suggestions as to how to react to satisfactions and frustrations (presenting examples of different ways of reaction, or blocking
other possibilities of reaction). What is commonly called "ego"
or a person's "character", i.e., his habitual ways of reacting to external
as well as to internal demands, is created by experiences of this kind.
Even the so-called "id", i.e., the instinctual impulses, is dependent on
educational influences to the extent that external experiences determine the relative strength of the various impulses, in other words, the
distribution of the available energy among them. Thus we see that
"education" not only induces a person, by means of threat and reward,
to suppress his original pleasure-seeking impulses. It does much more
in a positive sense by determining what happens to the energy of the
repressed impulses, through changing the ego by the very act of
suppression, as shown in the example of the creation of the superego.
Blocking off certain types of reaction to frustrating experiences,
facilitating others, especially through direct examples or through
the creation of ideals, are ways of achieving such change within the
ego. Examples and ideals are, of course, socially prescribed and
limited.

And now a formulation of the hidden dangers of "bad" education can be undertaken. Whereas the reality principle says: "Do not
yield to your impulses where such impulses are dangerous", a given education may artificially picture too many impulses as "dangerous".
The child may be forced to repress his impulses to such a degree that
severe damage may result. That is to say, the repressed instincts still
exist in his unconscious, a circumstance that has a two-fold consequence: first, they may reappear in an undesired form as neurotic
symptoms or character disturbances; second, the energies needed in the
constant struggle of repression are not available for other purposes.

There are two characteristic features of childhood that augment
this danger. The first is the child's magical orientation, which causes
the child to feel that everybody and everything, including the inanimate,
feels and acts as he himself does. The fantastic nature of some of his
impulses gives rise to fantastic expectations of punishment. This
"retaliation fear" makes him overestimate slight threats and regard
them as severe ones, and thus makes him the readier to accept educational prohibitions. As the carrier of the retaliative power, the superego is not only as strict toward the ego as the parents previously were,
but it also endangers the child's ego in the manner he had earlier
wished to endanger his parents.

A second consequence of the biological helplessness of the human infant is that every man takes into his later life a memory of the time when omnipotent outsiders set everything right when he himself was too weak to do so. This memory becomes the basis for a yearning which may be mobilized whenever the individual encounters a situation of helplessness. An active and independent attempt to master the world will be adopted when there is a possibility of succeeding. A frustrating and suppressing "authoritative" upbringing, inducing a lack of self-confidence, creates a passive longing for external omnipotent helpers. There are many ways in which various societies have abused this "yearning back".

What, then, causes education in some circumstances too relentlessly to hammer into children the conception, "Your impulses are dangerous", and where is the borderline between that which is necessary and that which is harmful?

To be sure, it is not necessary for every child to burn himself; education can and should anticipate the pain of burning by warning or threat. It is necessary to teach a child to take into consideration the interests of other people, because this taking-into-consideration is objectively the condition that governs the supply of love needed by the child. But it is also true that occasional satisfaction facilitates the relinquishment of perpetual satisfaction; definitive repression, however, results in the disturbance of all activities through the return from the repression of the unsatisfied impulses.

One sometimes hears the statement that infantile sexuality might become dangerous if it were not repressed. Precisely the psychoanalyst, it is said, knows best that man is an instinct-driven being, that "the beast in man" is still alive, and that man would only kill and seek sexual enjoyment had he not learned to control himself. Actually this danger is not so grave. Experience shows that unsatisfied instincts are much more difficult to master than occasionally satisfied instincts. Sexual instincts are periodic phenomena that disappear after being satisfied and reappear only after a lapse of time. Economic instinct regulation by means of periodic discharge is possible. If the analyst today so often finds sexuality asocial and therefore dangerous, analysis shows that this is the consequence of a previous sexual repression, which hinders full periodic psychological discharge. Some people fear that unless a child represses his sexuality, he may become useless to society; he will expend all his energy in the sexual field, and nothing will be left for sublimation. Such a deduction is not justified. Sublimations are, it is true, produced by sexual energy (without explaining in detail, it may be added, by pregenital and not genital energy), but a voluntary suppression of sexuality does not bring about sublimation, but rather repression. The result is that the unsatisfied sexual impulse remains in the unconscious unchanged, and, from there, disturbs the intended sublimated activity.

If one remembers that prior to Freud science did not even know of the existence of infantile sexuality, one realizes how intensely mankind must have wished that it actually did not exist. Awareness of this wish should warn us against subscribing to the idea that infantile sexuality is dangerous, since this idea may be the product of the same tendency.

Thus the question arises as to the source of this tendency against accepting the existence of infantile sexuality. Of course, the anti-instinctual orientation of traditional education is an outgrowth of both present and past social situations, and must be criticized in the light of these social situations. The social limitations are perhaps best seen in the failure of too quick and simple attempts at reform. "Progressive education", in trying to avoid the errors of the preceding period and in order to prevent frustrations, has sometimes gone to the opposite extreme. It has, thereby, become no less dependent on social forces than "authoritarian" education. "Avoidance of frustration" is certainly impossible. Reality necessarily brings frustrations, and an artificially protected childhood is therefore a very poor preparation for it; the avoidance of early frustrations has the same effect as intense ones on persons brought up normally. The tendency of educators "always to be lenient" has the further consequence that (1) the child gains the impression that aggressiveness is terribly forbidden; when he feels aggression, he must repress it; the external leniency makes the superego (at least in its attitude toward aggressiveness) stricter, until the child may even long for an external strict authority as a relief; (2) the parents have to repress their own aggressiveness, which certainly will eventually make its unvoluntary appearance in an undesired manner and to an undesired degree.

There is no doubt that an artificial change in the education of a few individual children cannot spare these children severe conflicts. Actually, it is just the opposite. Sooner or later such children will be driven into even more severe conflict, because they will hear on all sides the contrary of what they are taught at home or at their special school.

The temptation is great to digress, to investigate the present day situation in the light of a critical sociology of education. However, not much is yet known about this. The way to do it would be to compare the relations between educational procedures and prevalent character structures (and their social functions) in different societies. Modern anthropology has just begun to attack these questions; its work is, of course, seriously hampered by the lack of recorded history of most primitive societies. To return to modern conditions, I want to present two examples to give a general glimpse of the complexity of the problem.

A person's self-esteem, as well as the content and extent of his defenses, depends upon his "ideals". Ideals are developed less by direct teaching than by the general spirit that surrounds the growing child.

An authoritarian society must promote readiness to subsequent submission in its members by drumming into them the idea of all authority: conditional promises. "If you obey and submit, you will attain (real or imaginary) participation in power and protection." A democratic society favors the ideals of independence, self-reliance and active mastery. Societies in which "authoritarian" and "democratic" elements are engaged in active struggle will be contradictory in their ideals as well. The child learns that he must submit and obey in order to get the supplies he needs; and at the same time he learns: "Stand on your own feet." Historically the "authoritarian" type of ideal was unopposed in feudalism; the subjects actually were provided for if they renounced their independence, and the psychic readiness of the majority of the people to accept such dependence was necessary to preserve society. Rising capitalism brought the opposite ideal. Free competition required the new ideals of equality and fraternity. The subsequent development of capitalism, however, not only created anew a majority of people who had to be kept contented in relative frustration and dependence, but economic contradictions gave rise to such instability in the social structure that, with the disappearance of free competition, there was a resurgence of authoritarian necessities. Simultaneously every member of society feels endangered in any attempt to become solidly established, and even in his very existence; hence the individual's activities are hopeless, and thus regressive longings for passive-receptive regulation come to the fore again. Old feudalistic ideals are revived and even intensified; and the result is a mixture of ideals, conflicts and, later, neuroses. Differences in economic conditions as well as in the history are responsible for the enormous variations in the mixture of "authority" and "democracy" encountered today in different countries. In general, all capitalistic society, by preparing the children for the role that money and competition will play in their life, favors the intensification of anal-sadistic strivings. This is the more unfavorable because, simultaneously, genital sexuality is discouraged and thwarted.

A second, even more general example: It is characteristic of present day society that many people are unable to satisfy their needs, despite the fact that the means of satisfaction are present. Textbooks of psychopathology discuss at length the deficiencies of the superego in persons who steal. But actually it seems that the problem should be formulated in another way: Why is it that so many people do *not* steal? It is true that in the first place they abstain because they are prevented by force. But the majority are not prevented merely by force and fear of punishment. Social reality has succeeded in awakening, in a special kind of conscience, an intra-psychic force that opposes the needs that ask for satisfaction. One does not steal because "it is not right" Thus special social institutions bring about the development of special counter-instinctual forces in the members of that society. This same necessity must likewise be the decisive factor in the anti-sexual orientation of certain civilizations.

These problems cannot, of course, be discussed in detail here. I shall be content if I have succeeded in making it clear that science (psychoanalysis among others) cannot do more than study the psychic characteristics of human beings, the mechanisms of pedagogical influences, and the actual use that has been made of these influences in various societies. It cannot set goals. What actually will be done with the knowledge compiled by science is dependent on social factors. Lest these conclusions sound too pessimistic, I hasten to add that latent within all scientific knowledge is the possibility of practical application and improvement.

PSYCHOANALYTIC EDUCATION

By WILLIE HOFFER, M.D., Ph.D., L.R.C.P. (London)

Since psychoanalysis has come into being its data and theory have influenced educational doctrine and methods increasingly. This is because it has always focussed interest on individual history, and especially on childhood development. Thus certain behavior disorders which in pre-analytic days were considered evidence of simulation or naughtiness are now considered manifestations of neurotic conflicts or fairly normal accompaniments of growth. However, it would be a mistake to assume that the relation between psychoanalysis and education has developed beyond its infancy. Even the most optimistic can only say that during the forty years that have elapsed since the inception of psychoanalysis there have been some remarkable instances of its successful application to education.

Three facts have now been realized: first, that the teachings of psychoanalysis in regard to childhood and adolescence can in the future hardly be confined to a chapter or two of general instruction but must become a subject for postgraduate study; second, that child analysts and educators must work together; and third, that though the main demand for psychoanalytic instruction now comes from social workers, clinical psychologists, teachers, and workers in special institutions (like the Southard School, Menninger Clinic, Topeka), the interest of all kinds of educators in its preventive possibilities will gradually be enlisted.

Some plans have already been considered. In its Five-year Report (1932-37) the Chicago Institute for Psychoanalysis(1)[1] states:

"During the past year the demand on the part of teachers and schools for psychoanalytic instruction and consultations has definitely increased. Although our children's department is now restricted to complementing our research work on adults, the Institute has been conscious since its foundation of the great importance of instructing educators and parents in the principles

---

1. Numbers in parentheses refer to the bibliography at the end of the paper.

of personality development. This represents the future field of preventive work. We are equally convinced of the importance of a large scale consultation service for educators and parents. Yet we feel as we did at the time of the publication of our last annual report, that this important task should not be undertaken in a haphazard way but requires careful organization. Although its social importance is beyond question, the Institute, in its present form, devoted as it is primarily to teaching and research in psychoanalysis, cannot undertake ths complex task. Such an undertaking would require a number of additional analysts on our staff, child analysts, and specially trained social workers, indeed a separate division."[2]

Logical as these plans for collaboration may be from the point of view of the professional psychoanalyst, scepticism is aroused when one realizes how hard it is to put them into practice. During the past thirty years whole series of lectures have been arranged for educators but with a few exceptions, among which social workers have played an important part, they have not led to the desired results. On one hand, the psychological interest of the educator must be profound, to begin with, if he is successfully to undertake an intensive study of psychoanalysis; besides, many educators need not only a "training analysis" but a personal character or therapeutic analysis. And still the most promising experiments with the most talented collaborators may be frustrated by the limitations imposed on them by school authorities. On the other hand, psychoanalysts deterred by such adverse experiences often do not realize the immense changes that have occurred in the educational profession, and the heightened qualification of the average modern educator. As a matter of fact, the history of "psychoanalytic education" does include two experiments with selected groups of educators, which were unfortunately terminated by external interference. One of these is credited to the Psychoanalytic Institute in Berlin at the peak of its activities after the first world war; and the other, to the Vienna Institute during the ten years before the Anschluss (1938). Both were possible only because the psychoanalysts conducting them had themselves been actively engaged in educational work for many years. They were well aware of the basic differences between a therapeutic-analytic approach and an educational-analytic approach to the child. It was clear to them that a catalyzer was necessary.

This catalyzer, child analysis, has brought about an ever closer and more fruitful exchange of functions between education and therapy. Now that psychoanalysis has been enriched by its method,

2. A separate division of this type existed from 1932-38 in the Vienna Institute for Psychoanalysis; a short report of its experience was presented at the International Psycho-Analytical Congress, Paris, 1938 (2).

and in turn by the knowledge of forces and mechanisms at work in the child, what actually can it offer to education? Can it do more than remedy the failures, i.e., supplement customary methods in education? Can it make a direct contribution by teaching how failures may be reduced or even avoided? Or can psychoanalysis go beyond this reformative work and offer new concepts, techniques and aims to educators? These questions are not merely speculative; yet they can be answered only after educators and psychoanalysts will have met and worked together experimentally for a considerable number of years, and, if possible, concerned themselves with all branches of education.

The Therapeutic Application

Charcot subjected children suffering from hysterical fits to exploration under hypnosis; Freud, however, stated in the earlier years of his work (1898) that his own method "demands a certain measure of clear-sightedness and maturity in the patient and is therefore not suited for youthful persons and for adults who are feeble-minded or uneducated". But he thought "it very probable that supplementary methods may be arrived at for treating young persons"(3). The account of the first experimental treatment was published eleven years later in the well-known "Analysis of the Phobia of a Five-year-old Boy"(4). The prerequisites for this analysis were Freud's doctrines of infantile sexuality (with the oedipus complex) and of the unconscious, and the slightly modified technique of free association and interpretation; it was conducted only because of the father's active interest in psychoanalysis. But when one thinks of the specific difficulties encountered in subsequent attempts at child analysis one wonders whether it was really mere chance that the first analysis of a child's neurosis was carried out by a person so closely related to the patient. Implications for the function of parents and of the whole environment are involved here; and the problem has no little bearing on the relationship of psychoanalysis to education.

There were several other early attempts to bring psychoanalytic help to neurotic children. Simultaneous with the publication of "Little Hans" a Swiss minister, Oskar Pfister, started work along similar lines with young members of his religious community(5). Activities like these appealed to many persons and teachers (e.g. Hans Zulliger) in spite of the generally strong opposition they met from psychologists, physicians and educators. Pfister's approach to the child's neurosis and character abnormalities, though now considered obsolete, was certainly not ineffective(6). A comparison with the analysis of Little Hans suggests that again the role of paternal, family, or social authority cannot be neglected. In adult analysis the cure is carried forward by the patient's suffering, his will to recover and his transference; social resistances are thus overcome. In child analysis, however, one had to take into account, beside the child's immaturity, his ever-present fear of punishment, fear of lack of loyalty to parents, God, or the social code—powers which at that time no outsider dared challenge. The child's resistance was not of a psychological nature, as we understand it, but of a social nature; therefore the question of technique did not obtain until the social resistance had been overcome. This could only be achieved if the child's father or father-substitute, such as the head of the religious or school community, became directly involved in the analytic activity.

The next major contributor, Hermine Hug-Hellmuth(7), was eager to disentangle analytic and educational processes from each other. She intended to be the first psychoanalyst to establish child analysis as a special branch of education in cases where the child was unmanageable within his family and in urgent need of treatment. Her primary concern therefore was to harmonize psychoanalytic aims with those of the family, school and society. No doubt most of the children she had to deal with showed not only the usual signs of neuroses and unsuccessfully concealed anxiety, but also a certain degree of social deterioration, which because of psychological neglect by the family overshadowed the basic psychoneurotic conflicts. Hug-Hellmuth's first step was to practise child analysis in the child's home or in a children's ward. Thus she made herself to some extent independent of the parents' and the child's will to cooperate, and confined child analysis to a mere buffer function in an environment interested not in her method but only in the final result of her work. From personal experience I can say that Hug-Hellmuth spent most of her effort in finding out secrets that the child had intentionally withheld from educators— and thus she opened the door to the child's fantasy life. As she did so, the child tended more and more to act out his conflicts, to the great bewilderment of his family. This of course often endangered the continuation of the treatment; where, however, it did continue, improvement often followed and sublimation took place. In other words: these attempts were mainly characterized by the treatment of symptoms in children of latency and pre-puberty, and were aimed at a better adaptation in these children to the environment by alleviating superego demands and by encouraging the sublimation of instinctual drives. It was not desired that personality changes should be effected through the release of instinctual drives. This does not mean that repression was not occasionally resolved nor instinctual impulses tolerated; sexual curiosity was certainly noted and satisfied through enlightenment, and parental prohibition of masturbation was lifted. But as a whole the tendency was to release only as much of the instinctual tension and of the anxiety, both under repression, as could be diverted into "sublimation" immediately and not into conscious fantasies and acts. The concept of renunciation played little part, if any, because analysis did not proceed to the points of fixation of the specific fantasies.

Thus psychoanalytic education at the end of the first World War meant almost exclusively the application of certain principles of analytic therapy. To become a psychoanalytic educator meant to become a therapist, to "cure neurotic children". The ensuing development was largely determined by two reactions to the advancing insight into Freud's work: one came from the group of educators who doubted whether therapy could serve as a preventive measure in a changed educational system, the other came from the group of professional psychoanalysts who insisted that all the conditions of analytic treatment be observed. It was not claimed that psychoanalytic therapy was the only means of dealing with behavior or personality disorders in the immature, but that its applicability to children had first of all to be evaluated under strictly therapeutic conditions; other practical considerations should be postponed until principles of child analysis should have been established.

The outstanding names in modern child analysis, Anna Freud(8) and Melanie Klein(9), are now widely known. The bearing of their concepts upon education is naturally of interest. The educational implications of the Kleinian concept are almost entirely negative. "Deep psychology" is considered to be solely the realm of the professional psychoanalyst, and the antithesis of educational psychology. Accordingly, it follows that observations made by parents in the home are irrelevant for the task of the child analyst.[3] Anna Freud's work, however, has opened new, positive and promising channels for the development of educational doctrine.

What is the relationship of Anna Freud's technique to the child's education in home and school during its analysis? Briefly, it is determined by the degree of the child's immaturity. When the immaturity

3. The Kleinian concept of the development of the child's mind is fully discussed by Edward Glover in this Annual. See also 10, 11, 12, 13.

is high, yet does not amount to contraindication, analyst and educator must cooperate intensively; with children less immature, as in advanced prepuberty or adolescence, the analysis will gradually resemble that of adults. The psychoanalytic procedure itself is not educational. Analysis is retrospective, concerned with the past, but it is of course not merely that: when it associates itself with the patient's ego, however immature, to alleviate superego demands, to correct fantasies concerning the parents, or to release sexual and aggressive drives, the attitude of family and school may become of some importance. When, for instance, fantasies become active, they result in instinctual eruptions like indulgence in autoerotic activities, aggressiveness, hypochondriasis, eating and excretory disturbances, and, most of all, anxiety states. In this respect child analysis will periodically have an anti-educational effect and will put a greater strain on educators than would a full-blown, untreated disorder that had been controlled by purely educational measures.

During a child analysis, the emotional involvements of the environment come into play also. The mother's difficulties have been clearly described by Dorothy Burlingham(14). Teachers, social workers, pediatricians may show similar reactions, not entirely attributable to irrational motives. I am not thinking here of unanalyzed educators, whose motives may be mere curiosity and professional envy, but of those who work with children most rationally and devotedly.

On the basis of her experience Anna Freud demands close cooperation between child analyst and educator. The inference is that child analysis can be carried out only in an analytic milieu (just as surgery, epidemiology and pediatrics can be successful only under favorable conditions). This point of view should have a far-reaching influence on the organization of educational facilities where prevention of neuroses and early treatment are desired.

Now that child analysis has been freed of its earlier limitations it will certainly contribute more and more to our knowledge of psychological disorders. But it will probably not achieve broad social range for many years to come. To overcome this inherent handicap, its educational implications should be fostered and not rejected as troublesome, unworthy, or fantastic.

Furthermore, child analysis is an invaluable instrument for psychoanalytic research, but its future is in no way secured; there are now only a few experienced child analysts and the temptation is strong among some to change over to full-time adult analysis. This is understandable; but the danger for the future is that child analysis will be taught by analysts less experienced in it than is desirable. Even more serious is the likelihood that if the manifestations of infantile neuroses will be dealt with by strictly educational methods (naturally without effectively touching basic conflicts), the need for adult analysis will later be greatly increased. Educators should be helped to understand these facts. A basis for collaboration with them must be provided. Until it has, we cannot tell what far-reaching effects child analysis may have on educational method and doctrine.

The Preventive Application

The shadows caused by pathology lead scientists to look for the lights of prevention. Yet in psychological prevention, on which much thought and effort has been spent, one still feels rather in the dark. One envies the physiologist and pathologist who can give definite although limited advice as to how to control such evils as dental caries, for instance, or the more common infectious diseases, postural abnormalities, or flatfoot. It is useless to blame social organization for the lack of psychological prevention as long as so little is known of its real nature. The experiences of the past thirty to forty years suggest that for a better understanding one should try to think in terms of generations rather than in terms of years, and of large groups of people rather than of single cases. Psychoanalytic prevention, however, only aims to establish the psychological basis of mental disorders and to find techniques of avoiding them. It certainly cannot attempt to direct behavior in surroundings alien or hostile to psychological ways of thought. It must therefore be the domain of the educator. Freud himself, from the very beginning, encouraged us to think not only of cure but of how to minimize or prevent the "traumatic effects of education on children". We shall consider presently a series of suggestions that have emerged during the rapid development of psychoanalysis. A synthesis was suggested by Freud in his later papers, but it has thus far not proceeded to the necessary experimental state because the precursors of prevention, i.e., child analysis and the training of educators, have themselves not yet passed their trial stage.

The scope of prevention, here as in medicine, is conditioned by clinical experience, and not by preconceived ideas as to how a human being should look or how he should behave. It began with "the sexual traumas of childhood", the effect of the seduction of children by playmates or adults, which was thought to lead to "premature sexual excitation"; and, in turn, to either hysterical or obsessional neurosis(15). But before clinical experience could begin to supersede the ancient moral attitude, the whole complex of infantile sexuality as a regular phenomenon in the evolution of human sexuality had to be described(16). This caused a complete change in the clinical conception of neuroses and perversions. Clearly, it appeared that education played a double role in the evolution of neuroses: on one hand, by stimulation of infantile sexuality during the normal processes of growth, and on the other, by suppression of their most direct manifestations; the former possibly leading to the formation of fixations, the latter to repression and other mechanisms of shutting out instinctual demands from consciousness. The Scylla and Charibdis of all education, over-indulgence and over-frustration, were established(17).

The basis of psychoanalytic education has now become far more complicated, but for our present purpose of studying methods of preventive education this description may be sufficient. For a long period subsequent developments centered around the question of how to avoid "pathogenic repression" of instincts. Thus educators turned the course of preventive education towards the Scylla of giving way to the natural drives. Results were largely dependent upon the social and religious milieu from which the children came. Two groups of infantile sex drives had to be faced: the autoerotic pleasures, which are practically inaccessible to direct educational method; and those pleasures that demand an object. Educators can affect only the latter. It is thus hardly surprising that sexual curiosity became the first sphere for the application of preventive measures(18). From adult analysis it had been known that early repression of sexual curiosity played an important part in the fixation of infantile sex theories, common to neurotics and perverts. But what does "satisfaction of sexual curiosity" in children mean? To some it meant giving the child complete information about the facts of adult sex life in order to end once for all the child's craving for sexual knowledge. This may have been correct in cases where the child's manifest curiosity expressed a need for permission to know and to share in fantasy the relationship between the parents. But sexual curiosity sets in before the oedipus situation reaches its height; and very early it shows a pleasure-seeking character, like the normal curiosity of adults. Moreover, it is independent of direct educational interference. The child's own body and bodily functions (or those of other children or animals) can be used for gratification. These facts ought to have been taken into account by psychoanalytically-influenced sex reformers, as Freud very early drew attention to infantile sex theories(19). Erik Homburger Erikson(20), and, more recently, Anna Freud(21) have again tried to impress on educators the broader implications of sexual curiosity in intellectual development.

Just after the first World War emphasis was shifted from the problem of sex enlightenment to that of sex education. Attention was now to be directed to the pleasure-seeking sexual interests as a whole, and not merely to sex curiosity. The object was to minimize the frustration of instinctual demands, and to avoid castration fear and the condemnation of sexual activities. The child's right to enjoy his instincts was to be actively encouraged. It was thought that the child needs to be hardened against unavoidable interference from people who do not share his parents' views; and that if natural development were to proceed unhampered, gradual progress would follow automatically according to the stages described by Freud. Thumbsucking, pleasure in dirt, smearing, exhibitionism and scoptophilia, masturbation, and attempts at intercourse were expected to give way step by step to the normal processes of the latency period. Such experiments, spread over a number of years, could only be carried out by parents who themselves had a fair knowledge of the development of the instincts. When the child reached school age his sex education, free from the usual traumatic interferences, would be completed: he would settle down to normal activities, less hampered by repression and more inclined to sublimation. Furthermore, it was hoped that with the relaxing of conventional education, neuroses would be prevented. Children brought up in this way were also expected to feel safer when exposed to sexual experiences at school or in the street.

Much stress was naturally laid on the management of the oedipus situation. Masturbation was not restricted; expressions of jealousy were encouraged; the parents' bodies were not hidden from the child's sight; curiosity, which we now believe was excitement, was satisfied, and information willingly given; expressions of hate and discontent were never disapproved of. Special care was taken when a younger child was about to be born; the changes in the mother's body were no secret, the child was permitted to take part in the preparations for the newcomer, and his reactions after the birth were carefully watched. In general, there was also a tendency to avoid any form of prohibition. The mother did not threaten to withdraw her love when her own and the child's wishes were antagonistic. Paternal authority was replaced by the explanation of all demands and the constant appeal to the child's insight and affection. Authoritative demands were condemned as they were considered sadistic and likely to cause castration fear.

Some experiments with psychoanalytic group education were based on similar concepts. Vera Schmidt(22) in Moscow ran a home for children under five entirely according to these principles; she reported very favorable results in sexual and personality development. She also stressed the untoward effect of this form of education on the emotional life of nurses and nursery teachers who had not been analyzed. Most of them broke down after a few months. Similar results were reported by Bernfeld(23) in a home for war orphans, opened shortly after the first World War. Both experiments were short-lived and do not allow definite conclusions about group education. Aichhorn's experiences(24) with socially and psychologically neglected adolescents were more favorable. His individual work with juvenile delinquents was even then based on concepts different from those of the postwar period (1918-1924). Some of the experiences Hans Zulliger(25) reported were based on similar ideas.

To the surprise of those who had advocated it, psychoanalytically-based sex education did not yield satisfactory results; many cases of character disturbance and behavior disorder in children brought up along these lines, became known. It is true that in comparison with children reared in the conventional way, these children appeared less inhibited (i.e., they had less respect for the needs of adults). They were brighter, and showed a variety of interests and talents; but they were often less curious about the more complicated world of objects, they had no perseverance, and they easily relapsed into daydreaming, which made them appear introverted. They clung to many infantile habits, which gave them cheap consolation in the face of disappointments. Periodically some showed lack of control of bodily functions, in enuresis or encopresis. They very readily gave vent to emotions that vanished as quickly as they appeared. Thus the expected changes during the latency period did not occur: only a limited reduction of instinctual expression could be observed. Normal school life put a great strain on children and teachers. Even in modern schools these children showed comparatively little spontaneity, and their concentration was disturbed. They seemed egocentric; group demands affected them little. They were extremely intolerant of the demands of adults: time tables, meal times, table manners, routine hygienic measures, even if leniently handled, became sources of conflict. Traffic policemen and park keepers were regarded as main public enemies. The children were involved in a constant struggle against a world full of demands and duties. It became clear that their education did not harmonize with the restraints of city life.

To the psychoanalytically-trained observer these children showed an unexpected degree of irritability, a tendency to obsessions and depression, and certain peculiarities which during subsequent analytic treatment usually proved to be concealed anxiety. When these children reached the period of latency, development could not be revoked; psychoanalysis had to be called in to deal with the threatened deterioration of character.

How could the drawbacks of psychoanalytic sex education be explained? They had been caused not by an erroneous but by an incomplete application of analytic principles. The results of adult analysis had been applied too rigidly to sex education. After the first World War psychoanalysis progressed from a psychology of instincts to one of personality; but it was still too early to make use of the newer views on ego and superego development. The paramount importance of the lack of early sex education in the elaboration of neurotic conflict had indeed been demonstrated; but the alternative to the old-fashioned neglect or denial of infantile sexuality is not to admit its existence and then leave the child alone with his various drives. This is merely another way of neglecting the immature organism. Beside the child's power and desire to enjoy pleasure from his own body, there is the desire to be like an adult. This desire is anchored in the depth of the oedipal wishes, which are prone to frustration even without any external influence. To excite castration fear in the boy and penis envy in the girl no other stimulation from the outside is necessary than the unavoidable sight of the other sex's genitals. Psychoanalytic education now must do more than protect the child's right to elaborate on his instincts. The child's poorly-developed ego faces powerful instinctual sensations and tensions, which we call "internal dangers". In the human race instincts are controlled first by the ego and then by the superego. Considerations for both made necessary the next steps in the application of psychoanalysis to education.

The Educational Application

Modern concepts in psychoanalytic education are based on a knowledge of the qualities the immature ego displays during the first five years of life. General experience suggests that the child's ego is weak, that the instincts constantly demand gratification from it, and that it needs care and support from outside. It grows in strength and expands its activities in proportion to its ability to control component instincts and object-relationships. For this a strong narcissistic cathexis of the ego is necessary. Experience in psychopathology shows how the instinctual demands from inside, and stimulation (frustration) from outside interfere with ego development—as for instance, exaggerated maternal care may inhibit it by replacing ego functions. It is a commonplace that most children up to five, and certainly all who later struggle with life neurotically, pass through periods of upheaval in which subsequent disturbances are rooted. Thus clinical considerations play an important part in psychoanalytical education in the same way that somatic pathology does in the physical care of young children: this fact distinguishes our line of thought from that of other schools in educational psychology(26).

In the understanding of the "minor" neurotic disturbances of early childhood emphasis has now been shifted from the role of the instincts to the role of the immature ego. Whereas during the period of purely preventive application education was thought to act directly on the instincts—in consequence of which anxiety was aroused and the ego was impoverished and restricted in its activity, today we believe that education acts on the ego itself, making use of its constant endeavor to harmonize instincts and functions. This is demonstrated, for instance, in the young child's continual attempt to strike a balance between autoerotic drives and drives directed toward the mother-object. Left to himself, the child of about fourteen months, as described long ago by Freud, regularly shows a liking for his bowel products. Playing with feces and enjoying their smell is a necessary stage in instinctual development. But in our culture it is opposed to the child's need to feel safe and in full possession of his mother or nurse. She does not actively share in these pleasures. The child's ego has to face two instinctual demands, and the mother's active attitude definitely helps him to come to a decision. In these days the struggle usually ends in a compromise, the mother offering the child some substitute material to play with and smear. But if the anal component instinct is constitutionally strong and if the child feels compelled to succumb to it, adaptation is more difficult: the ego may easily show reactions of anxiety and may need educational help, which, as psychopathology shows, often miscarries.

Any failure of this integrating and harmonizing function may result in a split of the immature ego, part of which may remain at a primitive level for many years or even for a lifetime. A tendency to anxiety may follow. The eventual outcome of this split will be decided by the constitutional disposition, the strength of other component instincts, the oedipus situation, and new identifications.

Clinical experience suggests that beside the tendency to anxiety, the sequel to the split in the ego is the formation of a specific, primitive fantasy that "solves" the original conflict in a pleasurable way. Meanwhile, in its general development, the rest of the ego tends to follow the reality principle. Modern pre-school education does much toward strengthening that part of the ego that turns toward reality, and thus supports, though often in vain, its effort to keep instinctual demands outside of its organization. From the psychopathological point of view anxiety is therefore a helpful sign that the integrating function of the ego has failed.

The oedipus situation and the subsequent formation of the superego puts the highest strain on the ego's ability to synthesize. The most pleasurable and therefore the least tractable of all the instincts, the genital instinct, and the strongest object-relationships have to be dealt with.[4] By the time the child enters the latency period his personality has assumed definite form. Superego demands will deepen the gulf between the integrated personality and the unconscious fantasies, which will take advantage of any weakening of the ego in sleep, illness, or any other contingency. Emotional disturbances, anxiety states and neurotic symptoms may now become obvious and of social importance.

The problem of antisocial behavior and delinquency deserves special consideration. The manifestations of faulty integration naturally change with growth and with a changing environment; hence antisocial behavior that has not developed in an antisocial environment has almost always a neurotic background dating from early childhood. In such children, too, it appears that a specific fantasy is the fundamental psychological structure, which during latency stimulates the delinquent trends. Aichhorn holds the view (not yet published) that some types of delinquents who have not been socially neglected, notably the imposter type, need treatment in two stages, spread over a number of years: the first stage aims at transforming the antisocial character traits into neurotic symptoms; the second deals with the neurotic-perverted personality, which in its emotional regression approximates patterns of early childhood. This is not to imply that the first stage should not bring about socially desirable changes.

The educator cannot reach the child's basic neurotic conflicts during latency or puberty. The appropriate treatment of all conditions that involve the superego is child analysis. Other methods, though they may be of high social importance, can only rarely reach etiological

4. Apart from the reports of the Hampstead Nurseries(27) little is known about the child's normal handling of this strenuous and most complicated period. The child of today seems little prepared to express emotions and fantasies verbally; and one may wonder whether the modern educator does not rely too confidently on play and abreaction.

levels. All further progress, however, will be dependent on further scientific data.

There is a "crying need for the results of longitudinal research on personality development"(28). No amount of successful child analyses and no miracles that well-trained educators and parents may report, can replace a prolonged experiment with children and adolescents from birth to maturity. Only after the experience of such research shall we be able to assess whether or not it is possible to prevent or modify early traumas, and to what extent the ego's faculty to integrate id tendencies can be developed and utilized.

BIBLIOGRAPHY

1. *Five-Year Report,* Chicago Institute for Psychoanalysis, 1932-37, p. 26.
2. Report of Proceedings, Paris Congress, *International Journal of Psycho-Analysis,* XX, 1939, p. 212.
3. Freud, S., "Sexuality and Etiology of the Neuroses", *Collected Papers,* I.
4. Freud, S., "Analysis of a Phobia in a Five-year-old Boy", *Collected Papers,* III.
5. Pfister, O., "Anwendung der Psychoanalyse in der Pädagogik und Seelsorge", *Imago,* I, 1912.
6. Pfister, O., *Psychoanalysis in the Service of Education,* London, 1922.
7. Hug-Hellmuth, H., "On the Technique of Child Analysis", *International Journal of Psycho-Analysis,* II, 1921.
8. Freud, A., *Introduction to the Technique of Child Analysis,* Nervous and Mental Disease Monograph, 48, 1929.
9. Klein, M., *The Psycho-Analysis of Children,* International Psycho-Analytic Library, No. 22, 1932.
10. Rogers, C. H., *Play Therapy in Childhood,* Oxford University Press, London, 1939. Offers an excellent critical historical summary from the child guidance clinic's point of view. The author finds Melanie Klein's work "essentially therapeutic in basis" (p. 15).
11. Symposium on Child Analysis, *International Journal of Psycho-Analysis,* VIII, 1927.
12. Searl, M. N., "Some Contrasted Aspects of Psycho-Analysis and Education", *British Journal of Educational Psychology,* II, 1932.
13. Rickman, J. (ed.), *On the Bringing-up of Children: by Five Psycho-Analysts,* Kegan Paul, London, 1936.
14. Burlingham, D. T., "Child Analysis and the Mother", *Psychoanalytic Quarterly,* IV, 1935.
15. Freud, S., "Further Remarks on the Defence Neuro-psychoses" (1896), *Collected Papers,* I, p. 155.
16. Freud, S., *Three Contributions to the Theory of Sex,* Nervous and Mental Disease Monograph, 7, 1916.
17. Freud, S., *New Introductory Lectures,* Norton, New York, 1933, p. 204.
18. Freud, S., "The Sexual Enlightenment of Children" (1907), *Collected Papers,* II.

19. Freud, S., "On the Sexual Theories of Children" (1908), *Collected Papers*, II.
20. Erikson, E. H., "Psychoanalysis and the Future of Education", *Psychoanalytic Quarterly*, IV, 1935.
21. Freud, A., "Sex in Childhood", *Health Education Journal*, II, 1944.
22. Schmidt, V., *Psychoanalytische Erziehung in Sowjetrussland*, Internaionaler Psychoanalytischer Verlag, Wien.
23. Bernfeld, S., Kinderheim Baumgarten, 1922.
24. Aichhorn, A., "über die Erziehung in Besserungsanstalten", *Imago*, IX, 1923.
25. Zulliger, H., "Psychoanalytic Experiences in Public School Practice", *American Journal of Orthopsychiatry*, XI, 1941.
26. Hollingworth, L., "Education", in *The Problem of Mental Disorder*, National Research Council, Committee on Psychiatric Investigations, 1934, p. 370.
27. Freud, A. and Burlingham, D., *Infants Without Families*, International University Press, New York, 1944.
28. Sears, R., "Survey of Objective Studies of Psychoanalytical Concepts", *Social Science Research Council*, LI, 1944, p. 141.

INTERPRETATION AND EDUCATION[1]

By EDITHA STERBA, Ph. D. (Detroit)

Publications dealing with education based on psychoanalytic insight frequently discuss the part played by interpretations given to the
child, without either clearly stating what "interpretation" may mean
in their context or fully realizing that the child's reaction to a psychoanalytic interpretation may be vastly different from an adult's. In
recent years a change has gradually taken place, the implications of
which I here attempt to discuss.[2]

The application of psychoanalytic principles in education in its
first and primitive stage was based on the following assumption:
neurosis results from repression of instinctual drives; the prevention of
neurosis, as one essential aim of education, must therefore avoid or
abolish these repressions. The child was to be spared traumata and
prevented from developing anxiety. In order to avoid incorrect ideas
concerning the sexual life of the adult—the role of which in the
neuroses of the child was being confirmed by a steady flow of clinical
observations—complete information on the facts of life was to be given
as early as possible. In order to avoid the repression of instinctual
drives, all manifestations of sexual or aggressive tendencies were to be
interpreted thoroughly. All the contents of the id were to be interpreted and made conscious, without consideration for the infantile ego.
No thought was given to the question of how these instinctual tendencies were to be mastered, or to the fact that a weak and immature ego
would need a great deal of help in controlling them. The ego was to
be spared the necessity of repression; it was thought that through interpretation the energy of the id would be put entirely at the disposal of
the ego.

1. Read at the Forty-fifth Meeting of the American Psychoanalytic Association,
Detroit, May, 1943.
2. See also Steff Bornstein, "Missverständnisse in der psychoanalytischen Pädagogik
("Misunderstandings in the Application of Psychoanalysis to Pedagogy"), *Zeitschrift
für psychoanalytische Pädagogik*, XI, 1937, 2.

Interpretation at this stage of the development of psychoanalytic education aimed at giving assent to the instincts, and education consisted in allowing them freedom, not in mastering them. However, since neither the inner pre-formed tendency to repression nor external necessity permit the satisfaction of all instinctual impulses, but of only a small part of them, education with the assistance of this kind of interpretation must sooner or later come into conflict with the outside world. Such conflicts lead in turn to rejections, disappointments, frustration and traumata in one area or another—frequently from another direction than that of the educator.

A case which I once treated will demonstrate these points.

Henry was a four-and-a-half-year-old boy who came for analysis because the mother could do nothing with him. He came from an open-minded and analytically-versed environment, and was brought up according to the educational principles I have described. The parents tried to spare their intelligent and precocious child every kind of trauma; they avoided restriction and frustration, inquired into every one of the boy's questions and ideas, and treated him like an adult. They had of course explained the facts of life to him in great detail. They attempted to understand the underlying causes of each of Henry's impulses and felt it incumbent upon themselves to tell him immediately "the meaning" of anything he made or did. Thus Henry, apart from enjoying the autocratic position of the only child, had hardly ever experienced any kind of restriction and had not learned to be considerate of other people. His arrogance and impudence as well as the way he demanded everything for himself without any regard for his environment was looked upon as being particularly attractive and charming so that his opinion that he was an exceptional child was continually confirmed. Though he was really clever and alert for his age, his domineering and arrogant manner was extremely unpleasant. The older Henry grew the more disagreeable became his lack of consideration for his environment.

Eventually it became necessary to criticize Henry's actions or to refuse him something, if matters became too bad. However, Henry did not react to criticism; at most he would interpret the criticism of the adults as the expression of their anger, jealousy, or death wishes, just as his own actions had been interpreted to him. "Go away, you idiot," he said to his mother when she felt compelled to threaten him with the withdrawal of her love; "I'll kill you. You are horrible. I'll be glad when you are dead." Once when a relative locked him in a room because she could no longer stand his aggressions, he was quite cheerful. "I'll have a house to myself," he said, "everyone else must die. I want to live quite alone and cook for myself."

The parents did not tell Henry why he was brought to me: they were afraid he would construe the treatment as punishment for his naughtiness and as a threat of castration. His visits were explained to him by another of his symptoms, his eating difficulties. When he came he immediately began to talk about the latter problem with that unpleasant air of superiority he always exhibited in speaking about himself. "I know exactly why I won't eat," he told me. "It's because I want to be dead, to lie in a coffin and to be buried." Then he would begin a favorite game, which he repeated time and again compulsively and in which either his own or his mother's burial was represented. At the end big blocks were laid on the grave, which he trampled down so that, as he said, his mother would be sure to stay there.

But Henry understood that he had been brought to treatment not only because of his eating problems. Though the people in his environment maintained that he was free from anxiety, during his first hour he told me of his own accord a dream that illustrates the failure of this education to "freedom from anxiety". "I often dream of fluttering," he said. "At night there is always fluttering; it wakes me up, and then I see a big butterfly on my pillow, looking at me with glowing eyes and I'm so frightened I can't even call for help." He had told this dream to no one, but he rightly assumed that I would be interested in it. Given a candy or something to nibble, he would say, "I see, I'm getting that so I'll tell you about the fluttering." However, he was not at all disinclined to talk to me about his real problems. He knew not only how naughty and aggressive he was, but also the meaning of these tendencies mainly from former interpretations given to him by his parents. He said, "I have to smash and destroy things. I can't help it. Something inside me always wants it. . . . Do you know what I do with people I like? First I kill them, cut them up in little pieces, roast them, and then eat them up." At the end of such conversations he would attack either me or my things in the room. "Do you need this?" he would ask; and if I did not reply immediately he would say, "You must say you need it, and then you must say to me quickly, 'I know you don't want to smash the *things*, but *me*, the *person*.' Say it quickly, or else I'll get so angry that I'll kill you. I'm not afraid of you but you must be afraid of my anger because I want you to be!" Henry was repeating to me all the explanations that had been given to him.

He became more and more insufferable to the people around him and though his relationship to me was positive no progress could be made because I could explain nothing to him that he did not already know. The only thing was for the parents to change their method of education. Fortunately just at this time the father, who had always been indulgent, was away on business. The mother was to join him with the little boy for the Christmas vacation. Upon my advice the mother for the first time took drastic action, telling Henry that such a naughty, inconsiderate child could not be taken to visit his father but would have to stay alone with relatives in his home town. The effect of the mother's departure exceeded all expectations. From one day to the next Henry was transformed. He became silent and straitened, renounced his aggressions, and was suddenly so good that the people around him were greatly worried. Thoughtfully he asked me a question which for the first time showed a changed attitude. "I'm always thinking now, 'Does a person live only for himself or do the other people mean something too?'" During the mother's absence Henry occupied himself with such thoughts as, "The better I grow, the sadder I am. I can't do anything anymore, only think, and nothing makes me happy now."

After the mother's return the eating disturbance grew worse and a new symptom appeared. He would swallow, choke, and say, "I have to be sick," and then would vomit. It was quite obvious that he made himself vomit. The mother was in despair because he became visibly emaciated. As he would not eat anything while with me either I advised the mother to buy him some sweet chestnuts which he liked very much. He tried to eat some during his analytic hour, choked, grew quite pale and said tearfully, "I must go out and throw up." I asked him insistently why he had to: reluctantly he admitted the reason, "Well, there's a kind of big bloody ball that is always coming up into my throat. Inside it is a little black thing made of skin and I can't swallow anything and have to vomit to get rid of it because it's so big and presses my throat." The next day he regretted his frankness. He felt he had told me more than he wanted to. "That was only a joke about the ball in my throat. I said it for fun. You mustn't believe it. I'm not going to vomit, I'll only cough!" After a little while he stood up, came quite close to me, laid his hand on my abdomen and asked, "Isn't there really a baby inside?" After he had asked me several times if there wasn't a baby in me, when I would have one and why I hadn't one yet, I said, "You're very much afraid there might be a baby inside there, aren't you? Perhaps you are frightened that the same thing might happen to another woman?" "Who could that be?" he asked laughingly; "do you mean my mother?"

In this connection I reminded him of a fantasy he had once told me: "A chimney sweep had made a big gun, all black; the chimney sweep was covered with blood. Then from out of his stomach came a bloody ball that was a child; then the child became a cannon, too, and shot everyone dead." I now interpreted his symptom to him, to wit, that he believed his mother had left him behind when she went to visit his father so that she and the father could make a child, and that the child was now in the mother's belly. He was acting as if the father had made the child with *him*, and as if the ball in his throat were actually this child in *his* body. In this way he would have the same thing as his mother and would also have been with his father. I added that he should realize that the reason he was not taken to visit his father was that he had been naughty and inconsiderate and had had to be punished. In any case, I explained, it was not possible for a little boy to get a child from his father, as he well knew. (I did not at this point go into the question of the defense against the passive fantasies.)

Henry's psychic situation at the beginning of the treatment showed clearly the effect of misdirected interpretation of each of his sexual or aggressive tendencies. These interpretations had brought his immature ego more and more under the mastery of the craving for satisfaction and of aggressions. The deeper the interpretations were, the more they emphasized the libidinal demands that stood behind his aggressions against his mother, the greater the instinctual energy that was liberated from the barriers of the normal restrictions of the oedipal situation and that demanded satisfactions. The parents familiarized Henry with the content of his oedipus wishes without regard for the fact that those wishes could not be gratified but must be renounced. However, in spite of the instinctual freedom that they wanted to give him he actually hated his mother and wanted to kill her. Henry felt this way about his mother because she gave him an unrestricted interpretation of his wishes to spare him frustration, and because Henry was only a little boy and could not take his father's place with his mother. When the mother, toward whom he was very ambivalent, refused or forbade anything, she was hated rather than loved.

It is evident that the child's ego could defend itself against instinctual demands which the interpretations and the attitude of the people around him had so greatly increased, only by developing anxiety. In spite of the interpretation and the parents' affirmative attitude toward his drives, or rather *because* of these two influences, the child's relationship toward the parents was obviously neurotic. This came to light with the first important frustration: when the mother made the trip alone to visit the father, Henry reacted with a symptom that indicated a passive-feminine attitude toward the father, and that was founded on an oral theory of impregnation which should have been discarded at the age of four-and-a-half years.

It seems essential to distinguish between the interpretations given by the parents and those given by the analyst. Even in analysis there was nothing else to do but bring to consciousness the id content of the vomiting symptom, in other words, the unconscious wish to have a child by the father; but in the interpretation of the analyst the ego was confronted with the demands of reality.[3]

We must also differentiate between the use of interpretation in child analysis and in adult analysis. In the latter, interpretation brings to consciousness unconscious processes belonging to the past, adjusts displacements, confronts the adult ego with the infantile dangers and shows many of the defense mechanisms to be superfluous. With the child everything is current and has to do with present processes; the frustration has to be accepted while the infantile instinctual striving is still in force and linked to its original objects. The adult has to learn this only later; he then has the advantage of a strong and mature ego, which usually makes the renunciation easier to bear than it is for the child.

I now turn to an example illustrating what I believe to be the correct use made of interpretation in the analytically-directed education of a normal child. My report concerns that period of development in

3. Such confrontation with reality, which is implied in every interpretation, brings about the partial devaluation of one of the most important sources of infantile pleasure, that of magical thinking. Persistence in magical thinking over too long a period plays a great part in neurotic symptomatology and must be abandoned in childhood if there is to be a healthy adjustment to reality.

a little girl in which penis-envy and the oedipal wishes are in the foreground.

Three-year-old Jane attended a nursery school where there was also a little two-and-a-half year old girl, Mary. Mary had an older, very naughty brother of almost six who went to the same nursery school. At first it seemed that Mary did not envy her brother and that she had the best relationship to him, until one day in school she began to cry and to complain loudly that she wanted to be just like her brother: she wanted to be a boy, and she began to copy her brother's naughtiness. At this point three little girls, all only children who had known the difference between the sexes for some time, joined Mary's complaints without any apparent reason. Among these children was Jane. She suddenly developed a great friendship for Mary, mothered her and took care of her, but at the same time her even and sunny disposition changed. She became cross and naughty if any of her things were damaged and was inconsolable when she could not find things that she herself had long ago lost or destroyed. She behaved, in short, as if any disturbance or damage of her possessions was equivalent to a threat or injury to her person. She also began systematically to take toys or books to the nursery school which she supposed the other children would not know or not have. She achieved her purpose at once. When the other children demanded these particular toys Jane declared with authority, "They belong to me alone. Nobody is to take them away from me." When the children tried to pull the things away from her she resisted and there was so much quarreling that the nursery school teacher finally asked the mother not to let the child bring any more of her things to school. The mother took this opportunity to explain to Jane the reason for her behavior; she told her that she took the toys with her only so that she would have something which the other little girls in the nursery school did not have. At the same time she made it clear that she could never get what she wanted, she could never become a boy, and must realize this fact.

Soon after this interpretation was given the little girl began to imitate everything that Mary's naughty brother did. Until this time she had always been polite and agreeable with visitors. Now, instead of saying, "How do you do?" she would puff in their faces, make grimaces and refuse to obey. If anyone said, "You are just like a naughty little boy!" she would cry radiantly, "That is just what I am!"

Again the mother intervened with an interpretation, and told Jane that by copying the naughty boy she thought that she could become a boy herself, but that the fact that she was a girl could not be altered. At the same time the mother talked often and in detail of the difference between the sexes, telling Jane that she, too, had an advantage, because eventually she would be able to have children. This second interpretation, like the first, implied a frustration. It made identification with the naughty boy impossible; however, Jane was offered two-fold assistance in overcoming the penis-wish. An attempt was made to show her that the female genitals have advantages of their own; and the identification with the dearly loved mother who in her turn had had to give up the same wish was a help to the child in her own renunciation.

The effect of this interpretation can be followed best in Jane's subsequent behavior. Her naughtiness stopped soon after the interpretation, and only in her fantasy play could one still detect attempts to deny the unpleasant reality. Thus Jane invented a characteristic variation of her favorite fairy-tale, that of Mother Holle, the gold-Marie, and the pitch-Marie. Jane entered the story herself; comforted the poor pitch-Marie, took alcohol and gasoline with which she rubbed off the pitch, so that pitch-Marie became just as white and clean as she had been before. Jane at this time had the opportunity to see older girls who already attended school present a play that they had written them-selves; some of the girls took the parts of good pupils and some those of naughty ones. A school inspector visits the school and is mocked by the children as a funny old maid. First the children let a wasp fly into her eye so that she is almost blinded; then, dressed as ghosts, they visit her at night and frighten her terribly. Jane repeated this play over and over again. Her mother had to play the inspector, dolls were the school children, and Jane herself appeared as the Savior who caught the wasp, made compresses for the eye of the inspector and comforted her in her fear of ghosts. No inter-pretation was advanced for this fantasy since it did not disturb the relationship to reality and since it constituted a harmless consolation for a loss which the little girl felt so deeply.

Further developments showed that it was not difficult for Jane to transfer her object-love to her father and to arrive at a far-reaching identification with the mother. The arrival of a baby sister gave the external impetus to this progress.

The very fact that interpretation brings about frustration often makes it necessary to refrain from interpretation, in spite of a clear understanding of the situation and the fact that the instinctual ten-dencies may be seen very clearly in the child's attitude. Every child must be granted a little of the instinctual gratification which is gained in fantasies. Interpretation should not make such fantasies impossible if it seems that the child has in this way found a non-neurotic way out of an ego-instinctual conflict, thus sparing himself stronger, eventually neurotic mechanisms.

In the phase of her most intense oedipal tie Jane found a substitute for the father in the equestrian statue of a general which she saw on her daily walks. She spoke a great deal about the general, demanded that one sing her songs in which his name appeared, and kept a picture of the statue as a treasure. She made no secret of her feelings and announced that she loved the general better than anyone else. "The first time that I saw him I fell in love with him." She was fully conscious of the fact that he had been dead a long time and that this was only a kind of play. In the meantime, she achieved a displacement back to the original object: her father had to play the general, to speak with a deep voice of command while she said to him, "Daddy, be the general, really be him so that I can show you how much I love him." Jane was not disturbed in this play because her parents had the impression that her attitude toward the beloved warrior was that of a wife and protective mother, and that this method of handling oedipus wishes was a harmless one.

Once when the father went walking with Jane she put her arm in his and said, "Do you know, Daddy, this is the way married people walk together?" The father then said, "Do you know that all little girls would like to marry their fathers, but they can't do it, and later they marry someone else and are very happy about it." The child answered promptly, "Now what could we do with Mother? We'd have to send her away. I want to marry someone else when I grow up and have babies and then you would be the grand-parents."

This was an opportunity to observe that Jane had supported the frustration of her undisguised oedipus wishes very well. Soon afterwards she took a walk with her father, mother, and a little friend of her own. The father wanted to take her arm, but she turned away from him and said, "You go with Mother. I'll go with Tony." One could see here how she had been able to divert her oedipus wishes to another object, in a form well-adapted to reality. Finally she developed out of her infatuation for the equestrian statue a fondness for horses and riding. When she was allowed by an unmarried officer who owned some horses himself, to ride horseback, she transferred all her love to him, pretended that she was cooking for him, that she lived with him, and, briefly, that she fulfilled all the duties of a real wife.

We have contrasted interpretation in two types of educational situations: one in which it was misdirected, and one in which it was sensibly applied. The essential function of interpretation was identical in both. In every case interpretation must find a hidden meaning and make what is unconscious conscious. The difference between the methods we have described lies in the attitude of the person who interprets. Through misdirected interpretation the ego was pushed up against a wall; it had no other recourse in its helplessness than to take refuge in pathological defense mechanisms, chiefly in the form of aggression towards the educating and interpreting person, and in anxiety reactions.

In contrast to this, in psychoanalysis id contents are confronted with reality. Since interpretation operates as a frustration of the instinctual strivings and demands a renunciation of magical thinking the ego requires strengthening in order for the interpretation to be effective. This kind of interpretation is nothing more than an educational act, a demand for progress from the pleasure to the reality principle. In the process of education interpretation is of great assistance, even though it is more frustrating in its effect than mere forbidding or suppressing. The recognition of unconscious contents and the communication of these to the child makes it easier for the educator to help the child's ego in the struggle against the instincts and to offer him other possibilities of discharge and sublimation. However, in education, interpretation should be applied sparingly, only where it is assumed that the child would not overcome his instinctual difficulties without their being brought to consciousness, and that he would be forced to have recourse to pathological outlets. In such cases interpretation will operate as a prophylaxis of neurosis. Interpretation is also advisable when unconscious instinctual wishes are manifested in the form of reality-disturbing behavior. Analytically-trained educators will refrain from interpreting many of the things they know, realizing that interpreting means frustrating and that forces of the id are pressing toward discharge; if such discharge will not cause too much disturbance in the outside world or be too damaging to the ego, it should be granted.

CHILDHOOD AND TRADITION IN TWO AMERICAN INDIAN TRIBES

A Comparative Abstract, with Conclusions

By ERIK HOMBURGER ERIKSON (San Francisco)

I.

Some years ago the writer, a psychoanalyst then studying infantile neuroses, had the double good fortune of accompanying the anthropologist H. Scudder Mekeel to a Sioux reservation on the Plains, and of visiting with A. L. Kroeber some Yurok Indians on the Pacific coast.

The original conditions and cultural systems of these two tribes differed strikingly. The Sioux were belligerent nomads, roaming the North Central plains in loosely organized groups, pursuing "dark masses of buffalo". Their economic life was dominated by the conviction that "you can't take it with you"—either here or there. Their possessions were few and changed hands readily. Generosity and fortitude were their cardinal virtues. The Yurok, on the other hand, lived in a narrow, densely wooded river valley which steeply descends into the Pacific. They were peaceful and sedentary, gathering acorns, fishing, and preparing themselves spiritually for the annual miracle of the salmon run, when an abundance of fish enters and ascends their river, coming like a gift from nowhere beyond the ocean. They owned real estate along the river, considered that to be virtuous which led to the storage of wealth, and gave monetary value to every named item in their small world.

A. L. Kroeber has written of the anthropology of the Yurok, H. S. Mekeel and others, that of the Sioux. It was the purpose of the writer's trips to collect additional data concerning the rapidly disintegrating systems of child training in both tribes; and this, in order to throw further light on present-day difficulties of reeducation among the Sioux, and for the Yurok, to interpret some of the compulsive

319

weirdness of their ancient tradition. This he did in two impression-
istic and speculative papers[1] a comparative abstract of which follows.

II.

Today Indian tribes are American minorities. Remnants of their
old concepts of childhood are compromised by attempts at accultura-
tion, whether successful or not. But these remnants, whether still
practised or hardly remembered, are all that will ever be known.
For in the past child-training was an anthropological no-man's land.
Even discerning white observers preferred to assume—with contempt
or with elation—that Indian children were untrained "little animals".
The Indians in the meantime have silently clung to items of child training which, as questioning quickly discloses, are of great emotional
importance to them. In discussing "mental hygiene" problems in
Indian reeducation, white educators, too, reveal unofficial observations
and private prejudices of great potency. In order to understand the
cultural equation in his data the author found it necessary to review
some of the successive images of themselves and of one another which
the two groups had developed since they had first met.

The original image of the Sioux is that of the warrior and the
hunter, endowed with manliness and mobility, cunning and cruelty.
The very image of the Plains Indian with feather trophies in his bon-
net now adorns the American "nickel" (as trophy or as ideal?). But
since the olden days the Sioux has been beset by an apocalyptic sequence
of catastrophes, as if nature and history had united to declare total
war on their all-too-manly offspring. Only a few centuries before
the whites settled among them, the Sioux had left their original home
territory further East and had adjusted their lives to one creature:
the buffalo.

It is said that when the buffalo died, the Sioux died, ethnically and spiritually.
The buffalo's body had provided not only food and material for clothing, covering and
shelter, but such utilities as bags and boats, strings for bows and for sewing, cups and
spoons. Medicine and ornaments were made of buffalo parts; his droppings, sun-dried,
served as fuel in winter. Societies and seasons, ceremonies and dances, mythology and
children's play extolled his name and image. (S. p. 106.)

The whites, eager for trade routes and territory, upset the hunting
grounds and slaughtered buffalo by the hundred thousands. Eager for
gold, they stampeded into the Black Hills, the Sioux' holy mountains,

---

1. "Observations on Sioux Education", *Journal of Psychology*, 1939, 7, 101-156; and
"Observations on the Yurok: Childhood and World Image", *University of California
Press*, Berkeley and Los Angeles, 1943.
In the following, S, after a quotation refers to the first paper, Y, to the second.

game reservoir, and winter refuge. The Sioux tried to deal with the U. S. generals, warrior to warrior, but found that the frontier knew neither federal nor Indian law. Forced to become cowboys, the Sioux soon found their grasslands destroyed by erosion, their herds decimated by selling booms and depressions. Finally there was nothing left but abhorred homesteading within the confines of reservations—on some of the poorest land in all the states. No wonder, then, that some missionaries convinced the older Sioux that they were the lost tribe of Israel.

During this historical period the Sioux encountered successive waves of white men who typified the restless search for space, power and new ethnic identity. The roaming trappers and fur traders seemed acceptable enough to the nomadic Sioux; certain American generals were almost deified for the very reason that they had fought them well; the Negro cavalry, because of its impressive charges, was given the precious name "Black Buffaloes". The consecrated belief in man demonstrated by the Quakers and missionaries did not fail to impress the dignified and religious leaders of the Sioux. But as they looked for fitting images to connect the past with the future, the Sioux found least acceptable the class of white man who was destined to teach them the blessing of civilization, namely, the government employee.

The young American democracy lost a battle with the Indian when it could not decide whether it was conquering, colonizing, converting, or liberating, and sent successive representatives who had one or another of these objectives in mind—a historical doubt which the Indians interpreted as insecurity, much as children do when faced with their parents' vacillations. The discrepancy between democratic ideology and practice, furthermore, is especially pronounced in the hierarchy of a centralized bureaucracy, for which fact the older Indian, who had been reared in the spirit of a hunter democracy leveling every potential dictator and every potential capitalist, had a good, if not malicious eye. (S. p. 123-124).

The destitute, malnourished, disease-ridden Indian of today has little similarity to his original image. Life on the reservation seems depressively arrested, like a slow-motion picture. While conversations with older individuals restore the impression of ancient decency and dignity, the tribe as a whole behaves in a fashion analogous to an oral-dependent compensation neurotic: the victim of a one-time catastrophe has adjusted to "government rations" and refuses to feed himself.

It seems only yesterday, especially for the older Indians, that the three inseparable horsemen of their history's apocalypse appeared on their horizon; the migration of foreign people, the death of the buffalo, and soil erosion. Somehow they still seem to expect that tomorrow the bad dream will be over . . . They have asked the United States Supreme Court to give back the Black Hills, the buffalos, the gold—or to pay for them. Some day, they expect, there will be a notice on the bulletin board at the agency announcing that the court has heard them and has made them rich. In the meantime, why learn to farm? (S. p. 103-104.)

Thus the Indians' detailed problems of today are seen against a historical background:

Time for the older Indian, one gathers in talking with him, is empty waiting except for those vivid bits of the present in which he can be his old self, exchanging memories, gossiping, joking, or dancing, and in which he again feels connected with the boundless past wherein there was no one but himself, the game, and the enemy (the not-himself who could be fought). The space where he can feel at home is still without borders, allows for voluntary gatherings, and at the same time for sudden expansion and dispersion. He was glad to accept centrifugal items of white culture such as the horse and the gun . . . But so far he has shown little eagerness for the centers of centripetal existence and accumulation: the fireplace, the homestead, the bank account. For these the educator encourages him to strive; they represent what the educator wants most for himself in life— although preferably far away from Pine Ridge. (S. p. 104.)

As for the younger Sioux of today:

In their *early childhood* they were educated by members of the two older groups for whom the future is empty except for dreams of *restoration*. In their *later childhood* they were set an example of *reform* by the white man's educational system which was increasing in vitality and in perfection of organization. But the promise of vocational perfection, since it had a place neither in the individual's early impressions and childhood play nor among the virtues extolled in tales, cannot easily become generally meaningful. (S. p. 115-116.)

Therefore: Our curiosity in regard to the educational difficulties in the Indian Service was focused first on those psychological realities in both groups in the light of which they characterize persons of the same or the other groups as difficult, disturbed, or abnormal. (S. p. 116.)

The Sioux lack any sense of property, whites say: and indeed, to the original Sioux, a "hoarder" was the poorest kind of a man because, apparently, irrational anxiety caused him to mistrust the abundance of the game and the generosity of his fellow men. The remnants of the old virtues of generosity, however, obviously represent not only a hindrance to federal indoctrination but also most practically interfere with attempts to help the Indian by special rations and subsidies. Recipients of relief are often beset by neighbors and relatives who good-naturedly and with the best of cultural conscience, demand that he provide for them as long as the supplies last. The Sioux are unclean, others complain: hygiene on the prairie was based on the principle that sand, wind and sun take care of the contaminating waste products of the body. Child-birth took place on a sand pile, excrements were deposited in the sunny outdoors, and corpses were left on scaffolds for the sun to dry. Mekeel knew of old Indians who when sick insisted on living in "draughty" tepees behind their new "hygienic" frame houses. The little Indian girl, however, who, on entering a white school, is made to feel that she is dirty, and who learned to start the day with a shower, on returning home during late adolescence, is found to be "dirty" by her elders because she has not learned to observe certain avoidances during menstruation. One of the outstanding complaints brought against Indian children is that they withdraw into themselves or become truant: in the nomadic days, families not only moved from place to place but children also moved from family to family, calling all their aunts "Mother" and all their uncles "Father", thus having at their disposal the welcome of a wide and generous family system. The tendency to pack up and leave when things get tense seems so "natural" to Indian parents that the truant officer finds them utterly indifferent to his complaints.

Every expressed white complaint has a silent counterpart in what the Indians consider the white man's immoral, lazy and dirty nature. The Indian feels that the white man is tense and thus a bad advertisement for his principles of conduct. Above all he beats his own children and is rude to them: an obvious sign of utter lack of "civilization". The Sioux used never to threaten their children with corporal punishment or abandonment. They told them that somebody was going to "come and get them", maybe the owl—and maybe "the white man". This judgment has its counterpart in the opinion of an experienced white educator who claimed that Indian parents "love their children less than animals do". He based his opinion on the fact that the notoriously shy and reticent Sioux parents, after not having seen their children for years, neither kiss them nor cry when they come to get them.

The more confidential a conversation with white or Indian, the more irrational became the accusations concerning the harm which each group assumed the other was deliberately planning to do to children on both sides. Representative is the Indian opinion that white people *teach* their newborn babies to cry, because they do not want them to enjoy life; and the opinion voiced by several whites, that Indians *teach* their children to masturbate, because they do not want them to crave higher things.

Thus, in trying to understand the grievances of both races, the author encountered "resistances" which, he believes, are not based on malice nor entirely on ignorance, but rather, on anachronistic *fears of extinction,* and *fear of loss of group identity;* for the Indian is unwilling to part with the past that provided him with the last cultural synthesis he was able to achieve.

But necessities change more suddenly than true virtues; and it is one of the most paradoxical problems of human evolution that virtues which originally were designed to safeguard an individual's or a group's self-preservation become rigid under pressure of anachronistic fears of extinction and thus can render a people unable to adapt to changed necessities. (S. p. 117-118.)

Most whites, on the other hand, find it difficult to face a minority problem that endangers what synthesis their hardly-won status seems to promise.

Every group, of whatever nature, demands sacrifices of its members which they can bear only in the firm belief that they are based on unquestionable absolutes of conduct. Thus the training of an effective and dependable government employee naturally tends to exclude automatically the ability to tolerate certain classes of people, their standards and habits. (S. p. 119.)

Such resistances—as the Office of Indian Affairs well knows—can not be overcome by administrative and moral coercion but only by gradual enlightenment and by planned historical change.   Otherwise,

Plains tribes (not privileged as are the Pueblos to seclude themselves on self-sustained islands of archaic culture) will probably at best join the racial minorities in the poorer American population. Unavoidably, the psychological effects of unemployment and neurosis will be added to tuberculosis, syphilis, and alcoholism which the Indians have acquired so readily. In the long run, therefore, only a design which humanizes modern existence in general can deal adequately with the problems of Indian education. (S. p. 152.)

As for the "mental hygiene" problems encountered, the author suggests

. . . that it is necessary to confront a possible list of problems as the educator sees them with two other lists, namely those vices which can be traced to old virtues, and new virtues which, if adopted by Indian children, become behavior problems in the eyes of their elders. (S. p. 118.)

This, it seems, is the most astonishing single fact to be investigated: Indian children can live for years, without open rebellion or any signs of inner conflict, between two standards which are incomparably further apart than are those of any two generations or two classes in our culture.

We have been led to consider such discrepancies to be among the strongest factors in individual maladjustment. However, as far as the latent psychological prerequisites are concerned, it seems that at the moment there is more inclination towards delinquency, both in the narrower sense of actual juvenile delinquency and in the form of a general and intangible passive resistance against any further and more final impact of the white standards on the Indian conscience than toward neurotic tension, such as self-blame in the service of the white standards. In any event the Indian child of today does not seem to find himself confronted with a "bad conscience" when, in passive defiance of the white teacher, he retreats into himself; nor is he met by unsympathetic relatives when he chooses to run home. (S. p. 124.)

III

In introducing the data on Sioux childhood, the author points to the various resistances which stand in the way of conceptualizing a child as a gradually conditioned rather than a ready made member of his tribe, race, or nation.   Pre-scientific narcissism caused man to project himself—in the form of Adam—into the beginning of the world; and made him assume the fetus in its beginning to be a tiny, but complete man: these images have given way to the insight into evolution, and into epigenetic development.   We now want to learn how a child *develops* into a white or an Indian, a member of a clan or of a class.

In a recent article I found it helpful to base what we have learned from Freud about the critical periods in early childhood on an analogy between the effects of environmental interference with the first extrauterine impulse manifestations and those of experimental or accidental interference with fetal development. In both, modification or damage affected in the (epigenetically created) organization depends on the developmental time of interference. Any accidental or experimental interference in a given period of growth will change the rate of growth of the system "just budding up", and in doing so will rob this system of its potential supremacy over "its" period, thus endangering the whole hierarchy of developing systems. Furthermore, the whole organism as well as any of its systems is most deeply affected by interference so timed as to hit its first unfolding; at a later stage it might be restricted in its expression, but could not be destroyed as a potentiality (C. R. Stockard.).

Educational environment, by choosing a focus for its interference with the unfolding set of given human elements, by timing this interference, and by regulating its intensity, accelerates and inhibits the child's impulse systems in such a way that the final outcome represents what is felt to be—and often is temporarily—the optimum configuration of given human impulses under certain natural and historic conditions. In thus creating "anthropological" variations of man, instinctive education apparently uses, systematically although unconsciously, the same possibilities for modification which become more spectacularly obvious in the abnormal deviations brought about by deficiency or accident. (S. p. 132-133.)

In making this statement, however, the author, to say the least, falls prey to semantic inertia. For environment cannot be said to "interfere with unfolding human elements". There is no social vacuum in which human elements could for a little while develop all by themselves, in order then—as similar phrases go—to be molded or "channelized" by society.

The libido-theory delineates the quality, the range of potentialities and the limitations of the psychological energy available at a given state of development. To be transformed into expressive and adaptive behavior, however, this energy needs a cultural medium; to develop human elements, i.e. to survive, a baby needs the seductive qualities of human organization. The same acts which help the baby to survive, help the culture to survive in him; and as he lives to grow, his first bodily sensations are also his first social experiences.

The initial "vocabulary" of social experience, in turn, is dictated by epigenetic facts: the successive erogeneity of orifices and peripheral systems, and the step for step expansion of mastery over space. The ready receptivity of mouth and senses (including the skin) establishes the organ-mode of incorporation. The muscle system (including the sphincters) expresses the discrimination between retention and elimination. The locomotor system and the genital organs serve the establishment of intrusion and (in girls) inception.[2]

---

2. For a diagrammatic representation of the interrelation of zones and modes see the author's contribution to Margaret Mead's chapter in the forthcoming edition of the *Handbook of Child Psychology*.

Incorporation and assimilation, retention and elimination, intrusion and inception, are some of the basic problems of organismic existence. Emotional and intellectual, as well as physical, self-preservation demand that one accept, keep, digest, and eliminate; give and receive; take and be taken in *fair ratio*. This ratio is the firm foundation for the later development of the infinite variability and specialization of human existence.

IV

Before the Sioux child was born his mother's relatives and friends for many months gathered the best berries and herbs the prairie produced and prepared a juice in a buffalo bladder which served as the baby's first nursing bottle. A carefully selected woman stimulated his mouth with her finger and fed him the juice while two other selected women sucked the mother's breast till it was ready to give the real stuff of life in generous quantities. Thus the baby was saved the exertion of stimulating his mother's breasts and of digesting the colostrum which precedes the generous flow of milk. Once the baby had begun to enjoy the mother's breast, he was nursed whenever he whimpered and was permitted to play freely with the greast. The Sioux Indians did not believe that helpless crying would make a baby strong, although, as we shall see, they considered temper tantrums in the older child beneficial. Boys in particular, and especially the first boy, were breast-fed generously for a period of from three to five years, during which time the father was supposed not to interfere by making sexual advances to the mother; intercourse was said to spoil the milk. The author points out that if the "length" of the breast-feeding period is a questionable concept if applied to a people like the Sioux, where the advent of a new baby often only temporarily interfered with the first child's breast-feeding: Even where a child had already learned to depend upon other food, he still was permitted to draw an occasional sip from his mother's or (for that matter) any other woman's breasts.

However, this paradise of a long and generous feeding history contained a forbidden fruit. Sioux grandmothers recount what trouble they had with these indulged babies when they began to bite with habitual abandon; how they would "thump" the baby's head and how he, in turn, would fly into infantile rage. The mother's apparent amusement with these tantrums was justified by the explanation that rage makes a child strong. They apparently fostered it. The author makes two observations in this connection. He wonders how well the

Sioux infant was able to abreact rage in muscular movement while still strapped in the traditional cradle board. While it is undoubtedly true that this tight container permitted the newborn to find a comfortable approximation of the fetal state, the author considers the possibility that inhibited expressions of provoked rage established a lasting reservoir of biting and muscular aggression which may well have contributed to the much described "trait" of anger and cruelty in Sioux character. The frustration of the biting period was also reflected in the most common nervous habit, the existence of which was admitted by the older Indians and was still observable in the younger ones:

> At any time, anywhere, one sees children (and adults, usually women) playing with their teeth, clicking or hitting something against them, snapping chewing gum or indulging in some play which involves teeth and finger nails on one or both hands. This seems rarely combined with thumb-sucking; the lips, even if both hands are as far inside the mouth as is at all possible, do not participate in this Sioux habit par excellence." (S. p. 139.)

The author sees in the history of the Sioux child's pre-verbal conditioning an ingenious arrangement which would secure in the Sioux personality that combination of undiminished self-confidence, trust in the availability of food supply, and ready anger in the face of interference, the co-existence of which was necessary for the functioning of a hunter democracy. We shall come back to this point in connection with the conditioning of the Yurok child, the child of "capitalist" fishermen. As will be seen then, in both tribes, the first trauma in relationship to the mother is dramatized in the rituals considered to be of highest spiritual meaning.

> It seems to me that it is this unchannelized energy of frustrated impulses to bite and kick which is the contribution of the Sioux's child training to his cultural personality; it contributes to the urge for communal temper outbursts such as endless centrifugal "parties" setting out to hunt, kill, steal, and rape; to the Sioux Indian's proverbial cruelty both against enemies and against himself; and it finds its most exalted expression in the scene during the Sun dance when "little sticks driven through the breasts of the dancers and connected by strings to the Sun Pole, were pulled free so that the flesh was ripped open": a sacred turning against himself of suppressed—and long forgotten—wishes. (Y. p. 291.)[3]

The generosity manifested in the mother's initial handling of the child was continued in the family's respect for his property and the renunciation of adult claims wherever a conflict arose.

While a Sioux could not refuse a request for a gift, he could refuse to give away his child's possessions; the emphasis, however, was on the honor that would come to the child when he, of his own

---

3. The author also considers the possibility that the remnants of such conditioning and its reflection in historical traits may contribute to the oral-depressive way in which the Sioux accept their—admittedly almost hopeless—lot.

accord, would relinquish his property. The child was not taught that property was "bad", but given an example of extreme generosity by the parents, who even today, to the traders' horror, are willing to let the child waste money that should buy needed supplies.

The first strict *taboos* expressed verbally and made inescapable by a tight net of ridiculing gossip did not concern the body and physical habits, but were of a social nature and first applied to the relationship of brother and sister: When a certain age after the sixth year was reached, brother and sister were not to speak with one another any more, and parents as well as the older siblings would urge the girl to confine herself to female play and to stay near the mother and tepee while the boy was encouraged to join the older boys in cowboy and hunter games. (S. p. 142.)

From then on, the daily patterns for boys and for girls differed radically. The boy was to become restless, brave and reckless; the girl, reticent, industrious and chaste. Boys used miniature bows and arrows and later ropes for an initial imitation and, as soon as possible, the real activation of a hunter's or cowboy's existence. Of interest are the "bone horses", small bones of phallic shape taken from killed animals and called "horses", "buffaloes", "cows", "bulls", etc. The author believes that the constant fingering of these dolls by small boys tended to connect the masturbatory tendencies of the phallic-locomotor stage with fantasies of becoming great hunters or cowboys. While thus sadistic, intrusive tendencies are cultivated in the boy, in the girl, corresponding inhibitions are used to teach her "an extreme state of passivity and fearfulness". Girls were taught to sit modestly, to walk in small, measured steps, later to sleep with their thighs tied together, and not to go beyond a certain radius around the tepee or the camp. It was understood by both sexes that any girls who habitually overstepped such restrictions could be raped by boys without their incurring punishment. The girl, however, who learned to conform could connect fantasies of the brother's greatness as a hunter with the skills she learned. She knew that the brother, as an adult, would be obliged to bring to her the best of what he could rob or hunt; she would butcher the buffalo and, on occasion, the enemy killed by him; her skill in embroidery would come to full display when she would be called upon to ornament the cradles and layettes of his wife's children. Moreover, at certain ceremonies, she would sing of his bravery, and in the Sun Dance she would assist him during his tortures. This is an example of the way in which homogeneous cultures pay in the currency of prestige for whatever restrictions they feel they have to impose. The girl was taught to serve hunters, to be on guard against them, but also to become a mother who would be willing and able to instil into her boys the fundamental traits of the plains hunter. The first basic avoidance between brother and sister thus used the energies of the phallic-locomotor stage and of potential incestuous tendencies to establish a model of mutual respect and generosity among all the "brothers and sisters" of the extended kinship.

The author notes that such relationships were established without that estrangement between body and self which is effected by the idea of sin, and without that estrangement between parents and children which is caused where parents are the sole arbiters of seemingly arbitrary rules. Instead, older children would with ridiculing comment, enforce rules basic to the whole pattern of Sioux existence.

V

The psychopathologist will be especially interested in the way individuals were treated who for one reason or another were unable to conform to these clear-cut differentiations between masculinity or femininity. It seems that conformance, wherever humanly possible, was urged by ridicule. However, for the sincere nonconformer there was a ritual way out—right through the ridicule. The disturbed boy would seek a vision quest in lonesomeness and self-torture. The inventory of such visions were standardized and yet his vision had to be personally convincing to secure the deviant public recognition. One such role was the "Heyoka". A boy would dream that he had seen the Thunderbird, whereupon his father would tell him that he "must go through with it" or be struck by lightning. He was then obliged to behave as absurdly and clownishly as possible until his elders felt that he had cured himself of the curse. Descriptions of such activities make it plain that they are analogous to the involuntary self-debasing exhibitionism in neurotic men in our society. However, in further analogy to the more or less voluntary and conscious role played by great comedians in our culture, a Heyoka, in spite of the contempt freely bestowed upon him, could prove himself so victoriously funny that he would end up a leader among his people. Correspondingly a girl might dream that she must choose between certain objects that are typical for men's and women's activities. After that, it would be recognized that she must be "Witko", which means "crazy". She then would throw to the winds all feminine restraint and probably become a prostitute, sometimes a famous one. A boy may dream that the moon has two hands and tries to make him choose between certain objects, but that suddenly the hands cross and try to force the burden strap of a woman upon him (T. S. Lincoln). If the dreamer fails in his resistance, he is doomed to be like a woman. Such a man is called a "berdache"; he dresses like a woman and does woman's work. He is not necessarily a homosexual (although warriors before going on the war path are said to have visited such men in order to increase their own ferocity). Sometimes, because of his position between the sexes, a berdache could excel in the arts of companionship, cooking and embroidery.

Thus the dreamer's deepest urges present themselves to him as a prophecy and as a command from a spiritual source. The abnormal was not permitted to escape the elastic net of cultural meaning.

VI

The author's first anthropological impressions thus seemed to confirm Roheim's classical thesis that there is a "correlation between the habitual infancy situation" and . . . "the dominant ideas of a group". However, he cannot conceive of the second as being "derived" from the first nor of primitive societies as being solutions of specific infantile conflicts. Such quasi-causal formulations lead, it is true, to the hen-or-egg question,—what came first, the culture or the individual, specific infancy situation or dominant ideas. History, however, has beginnings only in myths; in reality it fuses into prehistory. And whatever the pre-human may have looked like, human beings always have attempted to derive a condensed design of group living that guarded against the *combined* dangers of physical harm (hunger, pain), group disintegration (panic), and individual anxiety; and had as their further goal: survival, accomplishment, self-expression. The treatment of children and other manifestations of a primitive culture evolve from an increasing synthetic tendency in the group-ego, situated as it is in its constituent individual egos. This tendency can be demonstrated somewhat more clearly in primitive societies because they represent condensed and homogeneous ways of dealing directly with one segment of nature. As we shall see later, the synthetic cultural tendency becomes less transparent where (1) tradition, i.e. previous syntheses, become a complicated "environment" that resists resynthesis; (2) the means of production as a whole lose their concreteness to the individual, and only segments of the economic system are immediate enough to permit practical and magic adaptation; (3) where consequently antagonistic social entities are created within the total group—with some entities in their particular segment bent on making other entities subservient to their syntheses.

For a member of such a complicated society it is, therefore, instructive to see how a homogeneous group like the American Indian tribes dealt with human existence. Let us compare the Sioux concepts of childhood with those among the Yurok. These two tribes stand in opposition in almost all the basic configurations of existence. The Sioux roamed the plains and cultivated spatial concepts of centrifugal mobility, the horizons of their existence coinciding with the limits of the buffalo's roaming and the beginnings of enemy hunting grounds. The Yurok not only lived largely in or at the mouth of a narrow, mountainous, densely-forested valley, but, in addition limited themselves within arbitrary borders. They considered a disc of about 150 miles in diameter, cut in half by the course of the Klamath river, to include all there was to this world. They ignored the rest and ostracized as "of ignoble birth" anyone who showed a marked tendency to venture into territories beyond. Instead they cried and prayed to their horizons which they thought contained the supernatural "homes" from which generous spirits sent the stuff of life to them: above all, salmon. The limitation of this world was manifested in its cardinal directions: there was an "upstream" and a "downstream", a "towards the river", and an "away from the river", and then, at the end of the world, an elliptic "in back and around".

Within this restricted radius of existence, extreme localization took place. Old Yuroks proudly point to hardly noticeable pits in the ground as their ancestors' home. Such pits retain the family name. The whole environment exists only in as far as human history has named certain locations. Their myths do not mention the gigantic redwoods which impress white travelers so much; yet the Yurok will point to certain insignificant looking rocks and trees as being the "origin" of the most far-reaching events. This localization finds its economic counterpart in a monetarization of values. Every person, relationship or act can be exactly valued and becomes the object of pride or ceaseless bickering. The acquisition and retention of possessions is and was what the Yurok thinks about, talks about and prays for.

This little well-defined world had, in the author's words, its "mouth open" towards the ocean and lived both in its practical and its magical pursuits for the yearly, mysterious appearance of tremendous numbers of salmon which came out of the ocean, climbed up the river, and usually having left an abundance of food supply in the Yurok's nets, disappeared up the river. The author debates the question as to whether the Yurok knew the complicated life history of the salmon, which, on reaching the spawning territory up river, procreates and dies; while some months later its diminutive progeny descends the river, disappears out in the ocean and two years later, as mature salmon, driven by a "homing instinct", returns to its very birthplace to fulfill its life cycle. The salmon, before entering the river, stops eating and therefore when caught has an empty stomach. As he ascends the river, his sexual organs develop and his fat content diminishes; at the optimum of his physical prowess and nutritional value, then, the salmon has ceased eating and has not commenced procreating. When the Yurok goes to catch him, he purifies hiself, as we shall see, from contact with procreation and abstains from food.

It is the author's thesis that the Yurok show one extreme type of conceptual integration:

Our preconception is this: Yurok thinking, so far as it is magic, tends to assimilate concepts derived from (1) observations of the geographic and biological environment, that is, (a) the lower part of a river valley with a mysterious periodical supply of fish, (b) a prey (salmon) with a particularly dramatic biolcgy; and (2) experiences of the human body as a slowly maturing organism with periodical needs. In the non-magical sphere, of course, the Yurok reaches a certain degree of logic and technique, as do all human beings; but wherever magic behavior seems indicated——that is, wherever mysterious food sources beyond the Yurok's territory, technology, and causal comprehension need to be influenced, or whenever vague human impulses and fears need to be alleviated —the Yurok tries to understand nature around and within him by blending bodily and geographic configurations, both of which become parts of one geographic-anatomical environment. In this environment the periodical affluence of the waterway has a functional interrelation with the periodicity of vital juices in the body's nutritional, circulatory, and procreative systems. Therefore, the Yurok's main magic concern is that vital channels be kept open and that antagonistic fluids be kept apart from one another. (Y. p. 259.)

. . . Every item of Yurok ethnology on which our demonstration can be based is shared by the Yurok's ethnic neighbors where it may have the same, a similar, a transformed, or a different meaning. Here, too, our attitude is clinical: we would expect an individual ego to synthesize individually experience typical for many; similarly, we assume that a group ego (or whatever we choose to name the organized and organizing core of a culture situated as it is in its constituent individual egos) tends to take stock of and to synthesize what has been selected, accepted, and preserved. It is this *synthetic tendency* which in the following pages is to be demonstrated *within one culture*. (Y. p. 259.)

One example of such primitive synthesis is the pervading importance of the "tube" configuration in Yurok thinking. According to Yurok mythology, the Klamath in prehistoric times flowed up on one side and down on the other. Now, it flows only in the downward direction and salmon ascend upward. To be sure that the river is open on both sides and thus an inviting waterway for the energetic salmon, the Yurok, magically concerned, attempts to keep all tube-like things within and around him unobstructed and all fluid-ways uncontaminated. He abhors the double-vector, i.e. a sac-like configuration which is entered and left through the same opening. Points in question are Yurok architecture and the Yurok concept of the human body.

The Yurok have two kinds of houses, the living house and the sweat house. Both are subterranean with a roof a few feet about the ground. The "doors" consist of oval openings just above the ground which admit one creeping human being at a time. The living house, however, has only one such opening (sac) while the sweat house has two (tube). The living house is a very crowded affair:

> Underneath the roof is a huge criss-cross of poles on which salmon is hanging in all possible states of age and eatenness, while a shelf bench between the dugout and the side walls is loaded with enormous baskets full of acorns and utensils in various states of use. The total impression is that of darkness, crowdedness, and endless accumulation. This is where women and children live; the man who comes to visit his home is careful not to sit on the floor, but on a block or stool of the form of a cylinder or mushroom. Otherwise, his place is in the sweat house, where he takes the older boys; there is one sweat house to six or seven living houses. . . .
>
> These two house forms not only serve woman and man, respectively, but also symbolize what the man's and woman's insides mean in Yurok culture: the family house, dark, unclean, full of food and utensils, and crowded with babies, the place from which a man emerges contaminated; the sweat house, lighter, cleaner, more orderly, with selectivity over who and what may enter, a place from which one emerges purified. (Y. p. 268.)

Living house and female anatomy are associated. After contact with either, the man has to pass the "test" of the sweat house. This he enters through the normal-sized door. However, he can leave it only through a very small opening which will permit only a man moderate in his eating habits and supple with the perspiration caused by the sacred fire to slip through. He is required to conclude the purification by swimming in the river. The conscientious fisherman passes this test every morning thus denying his contact with women and as it were, giving daily rebirth to himself through a tube-like womb.

What the Yurok calls "clean" living is an attempt to keep vectors clear, channels unobstructed, and to avoid the wombs of multiplication: woman; the lake upriver from which he thinks the waters of the Klamath flow; the place across the ocean where salmon originate; the origin of his shell money up the coast. The author describes an old Indian woman's melancholic apprehension when she saw a whale enter, play around in, and leave the mouth of the Klamath; the river should serve only one vector; that of ascending salmon. For that which flows in one channel of life, is said to be most eager not to come in contaminating contact with the objects of other channels or with "sac-like" configurations. Salmon and the river dislike it if food is eaten on a boat. Deer will stay away from the snare if deer meat has been brought in contact with water—even posthumously by washing the eating bowls. Salmon demands that women on their trip up or down river, at specified places, leave the boat and walk around a rock. Salmon also dislikes the man who is full of food, or, as we saw, has been in contact with the "woman's inside", and money will leave the house if intercourse took place while it was there. (Shell money is strung on thongs and carried in oblong tube-like purses.)

Only once a year, after the salmon run, these avoidances are set aside. At that time, following complicated ceremonies, a strong dam is built which obstructs the ascent of the salmon and permits the Yurok to catch a rich winter supply. The dam building is "the largest mechanical enterprise undertaken by the Yurok or, for that matter, by any California Indians, and the most communal attempt". After ten days of collective fishing, orgies of ridicule and of sexual freedom take place alongside the river, reminiscent of the ancient Satires of European spring ceremonials.

The author finds indications that these ceremonials dramatize the return, the ridicule, and the re-banishment of a "primal father" figure. For the Yurok's centripetal world was created by a most centrifugal and irresponsible father: The old man Wohpekumeu (the "widower from across the ocean") stood in the middle of the river which went up on one side and down on the other, and cried and claimed that he was lonely. Land appeared on both sides of him. He cried more. A water spout was rising in front of him, slowly coming up to the height of his breast. He cried again. The water came up to his brow. Upon further crying, the spout slowly developed into a woman, first her upper half and then, upon his further tearful insistence ("I want a whole woman") the lower part as well. After having created the rest of the world, the widower gave this woman to his son together with plenty of food, under the condition (which seems habitual with creators) that he must work. Later, however, he seduced his daughter-in-law and became so girl-crazy that he had to be banished. His sons decided that they would also overcome all centrifugal tendencies among themselves, henceforth love clean in their restricted, compulsive and phobic world.

This hysterical God, nostalgic but sly, powerful but inhibited, God-like but unreliable, is the originator across the ocean of the yearly salmon supply. In contrast to him, there is a more compulsive character, a "clean" God, who smoked but never ate, who never desired a woman, and accomplished the great historical deed of banning women from the sweat house. He represents all that the Yurok call "clean". And yet they know that they need a continuous, cautious, well-ritualized contact with the widower who provides food. The author interprets the rejuvenation ceremonial connected with the annual fish dam as dramatizing an early return of the primal father, who, having brought all the salmon (on a deeper level he is the salmon) is ceremoniously defeated by the dam chief, and after much ridicule, banned again. Whereupon the world for a short while is free of phobic restriction, sexual and otherwise. But then the Yurok again begins the "clean" life which helps him to be a conscientious warden of his segment of nature.

This interesting version of the primal father myth suggests some speculation concerning historical elements in its variations.

Let us assume that the Yurok came from somewhere else; with no chance or wish to turn back, they found their way blocked by the Pacific. They settled along the river, and, noticing the periodical salmon run, became fishermen—in technique and in magic.

The human mind is likely to feel guilty and, if necessary, to construct a guilt when it finds itself faced with sudden environmental limitation; adapting, it learns to see a virtue in the necessity imposed by the limitation; but it continues to look into the future for potential recurrences or intensifications of the trauma of limitation, anticipating punishment for not being virtuous enough. In this sense to the restricted Yurok, centrifugality may have become a vice in the past, centripetality a virtue; and the ocean's disfavor, anticipated punishment for centrifugal "mental sins" which Yurok ethics tries to avoid. (Y. p. 276.)

Thus an ontogenetic trauma (the banishment from the mother's body and house) and a historical task would appear synthesized, analogous to the spatial synthesis of geography and anatomy.

VII

In his attempts to gather information on the Yurok's ancient child training system, the author, in some areas, found himself among hostile, contemptuous and resistive people who apparently suspected him of trying to get information on their property rights. He thus not only met some of the old money-mindedness and suspicion; he also was quite aware that the inner distance between Yurok and whites is not so great as that between whites and Sioux. For there was much in the A. B. C. of Yurok life that did not have to be relearned when the whites came. The Yurok lived in frame houses and in fact now lives in super-terranean structures next to pits in the ground which once contained his ancestors' subterranean dwellings. Unlike the Sioux, who, in the buffalo, lost overnight the focus of his economic and spiritual life, the Yurok still sees, catches, talks and eats salmon. When the Yurok man today steers a raft of logs, or the Yurok woman grows vegetables, their occupations are not too far removed from the original manufacture of dugouts, the gathering of acorns and the planting of tobacco. Above all, the Yurok concerned his life with property. "He schemed constantly to lodge a claim or to evade an obligation." According to the author, the Yurok need not forget this "primitive" tendency in the white world, and therefore his grievances with the United States find other than the inarticulate, smoldering expression of the prairie man's passive resistance. In fact, upriver,

only twenty miles from a major U. S. highway, the author found himself treated (and saw visiting white officials treated) as definitely
unwelcome white minority.

VIII

From a few wise old informants, however, the author gathered
this information: The birth of a baby is surrounded with oral prohibitions.   Father and mother eat neither deer meat nor salmon until the
child's navel heals.   Disregard of this taboo causes convulsions in
the child.   (The more "genital" Sioux thinks that a child's convulsions
are caused by the parents' intercourse during pregnancy).   During the
birth, the mother must shut her mouth.   The newborn is not breast-fed
for ten days, but given a nut soup from a tiny shell. The breast-feeding
begins with Indian generosity.   However, there is a definite weaning
time around the sixth month, that is, around the teething period.
Yurok breast-feeding thus is maintained for a minimum period among
American Indians.   Weaning is called "forgetting the mother" and
is enforced, if necessary, by the mother's going away for a few days.
This relative acceleration of weaning seems to be part of a general
tendency to encourage the baby to leave the mother and her support
as soon as this is possible and bearable—and not to return.   From his
twentieth day on, the baby's legs, which are left uncovered in the
Yurok version of the cradle board, are massaged by the grandmother.
Early creeping is encouraged.   The first postnatal crisis for the Yurok
child, therefore, occurs much earlier than that of the Sioux, and consists of a relationship in time of enforced weaning, teething, and
encouraged creeping.   The shorter nursing period, of course, accelerates
the advent of a second crisis, namely, the mother's next pregnancy.

We have referred to the contribution made by the Sioux baby's
oral training to Sioux character structure.   The Yurok child, as we
saw, is weaned early and abruptly, before the full development of the
biting stage, and after having been discouraged from feeling too comfortable with his mother.   The author suggests that this expulsion—
in its relation to other items—contributes to the Yurok character, a
residue of potential nostalgia which consequently find its institutionalized form in the Yurok's ability to cry while he prays in order to
gain influence over the food-sending powers behind the visible world.
There is something of an early oral "hallucinatory wish fulfillment"
implied in the adult Yurok's conviction that tearful words, such as
"I see a salmon" will cause a salmon to come.   It is as if he had to

pretend that he had no teeth so that his food supply would not be cut off. In the meantime, however, he does not forget to build nets.

This concentration on the sources of food is not accomplished without a second oral training at the "sense" stage, i.e. when the child can repeat what he has been told. He is admonished to eat slowly, not to grab food, never to take it without asking for it, never to eat between meals and never to ask for a second helping—an oral puritanism hardly equaled among other primitives. During meals, a strict order of placement is maintained and the children are taught to eat in prescribed ways; for example, to put only a little food on the spoons, to take the spoons up to their mouths slowly, to put the spoon down while chewing the food—and above all, to think of becoming rich during the whole process. Nobody speaks during meals so that everybody can keep his own thoughts on money and salmon. Thus a maximum of preverbal avarice and need for intake, which may have been evoked by the combination of early weaning, not only from the breast but also from contact with the mother and from babyish ways in general is "tamed" and used for the development of those attitudes, which to the Yurok mind, will in the end assure the salmon's favor. The Yurok makes himself see money hanging from trees and salmon swimming in the river during off season. He learns to subordinate genital drives to the pursuit of money. In the sweat house the boy will learn the strange feat of thinking of money and at the same time *not* thinking of women.

These fables told to children in an interesting way underline the ugliness of lack of restraint. They isolate one outstanding item in the physiognomy of animals and use it as an argument for "clean behavior". The buzzard's baldness is the result of his having put his whole head into a dish of hot soup. The eel gambled his bones away. The hood of the angry bluejay is her clitoris which she tore off in "masculine protest". One fable which concerns itself with feces also emphasizes the need for cautious intake and incidentally illustrates the tube concept.

> The bear was always hungry. He was married to the blue jay. One day they made a fire and the bear sent the blue jay to get some food. She brought back only one acorn. "Is that all?" the bear said. The blue jay got angry and threw the acorn in the fire. It popped all over the place and there was acorn all over the ground. The bear swallowed it all down and got awfully sick. Some birds tried to sing for him but it did not help. Nothing helped. Finally the hummingbird said, "Lie down and open your mouth," and then the hummingbird zipped right through him. That's why the bear has such a big anus and can't hold his feces. (Y. p. 286.)

Second in emphasis to cautious intake is the prohibition of swearing, that is, verbal offense committed especially by reference to death and dead people; i.e. verbal elimination.

In accordance with the Yurok's tendency to rush their children along on the path of maturation, they have an interesting concept of regression. It is bad for the child, they say, to sleep in the afternoon, for there is an affinity between dusk and death. In its time the fetus was kept awake in the afternoon by the mother's rubbing of her abdomen. At dusk, children are hurriedly called into the house, because then they may see some "wise" people, i.e. members of the race that inhabited the earth before the Yurok took possession of it. The description of these "wise" people seems to mark them as a materialization of pregenitality, their attraction as a regressive tendency. They are adult at six months of age. They procreate orally and have no genitals. They do not know what it means to be "clean" and they never die. The child who seems a member of this race develops symptoms such as lack of appetite, nightmares, disobedience. He may waste away if he is not given treatment.

There are various forms of treatment. The parents themselves should stay out of it; maybe the grandmother next door will sing the proper songs. In severe cases, however, a psychotherapist is consulted. The author was able to interview the last of these women shaman. Her techniques embrace the psychosomatic, the bisexual and the ambivalent nature of neurosis. The shaman sucks two "pains" out of the child's body—one residing always above the child's navel (where it obstructs the nutritional tube) and its "mate" from wherever the child feels pain. Then follows the interpretation and the group therapy. The child is laid on the floor and his parents and relatives gather around in a circle. After elaborate rituals, the shaman has a vision and describes it. She will see, for example, a man who had made a vow of abstinence, nevertheless have intercourse with a woman. Or she will see an old woman sitting in the hills trying to "sorcerize" somebody. Whatever it is, one or the other of the child's relatives will get up and confess that he has committed that crime. The fact that this procedure is said to result in cures can be attributed to the shaman's intuitive skill in making the child's relatives confess to whatever secret guilt caused ambivalent tension in the home and anxiety in the child, both of which are thus ameliorated.

The very healing power of the shaman is derived from a potentially pathogenic set of events.

Long before F., the daughter and granddaughter of shamans, reached puberty, people had predicted that she probably would turn into a shaman too because "she slept so much", that is, had a neurotic inclination to regress. During her premenarche, her grandmother tested her by taking a "pain" out of her own mouth and trying to make F. swallow it. F. ran away from home. The following night, however, she had an anxiety dream in which an old woman threw a basket over her mouth in such a way that she swallowed its "yellow, black bloody, nasty" content. She woke up in extreme anxiety but kept this dream to herself because she realized that people would force her to become a shaman if they knew that her grandmother's suggestion had invaded her dream life. At breakfast, however, she gave herself away by vomiting, whereupon the community made her confess and in great excitement prepared her novitiate. She now had to learn to transform this involuntary vomiting of stomach content into the ability to swallow and to throw up "pains" without throwing up food with it—a mastery over the oral-nutritional tube which gives F. the power to cure people. Here the abhorred double-vector becomes beneficial.

Unlike F., the ordinary Yurok girl when menstruating the first time, is forced to "close up" all around. Silently sitting in the corner of her home with her back turned to the fire, she moves as little as possible. On leaving the house once a day, she does not look about. For four days or longer, she abstains from food. Then she takes her food to a spot where she can not hear any sound except the noise of the river. To the girl who has thus learned to guard her receptivity, her mother demonstrates the purpose of her inceptive organization by putting in front of her twenty sticks, calling ten of them sons, and ten, daughters.

F., however, acquired all the prerogatives forbidden to other women. She could sleep in the sweat house, pray for money, and smoke a pipe. She became as rich as any man and stronger in magic power. From F.'s and other shaman's dreams, the author concludes that F. was destined to become her mother's successor because she, alone among her sisters, early showed hysterical traits of "masculine protest" which are promoted to a plane of magic usefulness by the community. The author secured fragments of the case history of another woman who had fled her home just as F. had, when the career of a shaman was suggested to her. However, no inner pressure made her produce ("against her will") either a dream or the symptom of vomiting, the two involuntary affirmations of shamanism that alone convince the people of a shaman's calling. This woman had lifelong chronic indigestion and compulsively spoke of her interrupted novitiate until her death.

IX

The author discusses the relationship of such institutionalized infantile behavior as the Yurok's crying and bickering to the problem of tribal character and to neurosis. The Yurok is, of course, helpless only in his magic protestations, not in his activities. He builds snares and nets and accomplishes the technical feat of the fish dam. The author believes that the closing of the two gigantic jaws of the dam is analogous to the Sioux Sun Dance in two respects: it is the event of highest collective significance in the tribe's life; and it dramatizes the oral (biting) taboo. The Yurok finds it necessary afterwards to assure his trapped prey that no malice was intended. In fact he claims that he really cannot harm his prey. "I will," says the salmon—according to Yurok Platonism—"leave my scales on nets and they will turn into salmon, but I, myself, will go by and not be killed." It is as if this combination of crying, snaring and protesting innocence, represented a collective play with the greatest dangers of both ontogeny and phylogeny: the loss of the mother at the biting stage; the mythical banishment of the creator from the women of this world; and historically: the loss of salmon supply during bad years. There are further indications that the salmon (the food which refuses to enter the mouth of the world if you desire it too voraciously) is associated with nipple and penis, the too highly cathexed life-giving organs.

Toward his fellow men, however, the Yurok's receptivity loses all its helplessness. He claims, demands, whines, fusses, bickers, and alibis—as the author puts it, "like a jealous child who, now so touchingly helpless in the presence of the mother, uses an instant of her absence to turn on his sibling and to protest that this or that object—anything will do—is his". As for the ontogenetic basis of this behavior, we mentioned that a child who is weaned early will find himself in the company of a younger rival.

It obviously would take detailed studies to establish the Yurok's collective character, including the way in which a Yurok manages to be an individual. For it is only within the official character of a given people that a personological inquiry can begin. Each system, whether it emphasizes generosity or avarice, admits of additions and exemptions of individual avarice and generosity. To know a people's character one has to know their laws of conduct and the way they circumvent them.

The author believes that neurosis and culture, although using the same inventory of human potentialities, are systematically different phenomena. Sioux "sadism" does, of course, not keep a Sioux man from being a devoted lover and husband. As for the Yurok's "help-lessness":

Does it mean that the Yurok anywhere within his technology is more helpless, more paralyzed by sadness, than are members of a tribe which does not develop these "traits"? Certainly not; his institutionalized helplessness *eo ipso* is neither a trait nor a neurotic symptom. It is an infantile attitude which the culture chose to preserve and to put at the disposal of the individual, to be used by him and his fellow men in a limited area of existence. Such an institutionalized attitude neither spreads beyond its defined area nor makes impossible the development to full potency of its opposite: it is probable that the really successful Yurok was the one who could cry most heart-breakingly or bicker most convincingly in some situations and be full of fortitude in others, that is, the Yurok whose ego was strong enough to *synthesize orality and "sense"*. In comparison, the oral types whom we may be able to discern today in our culture and to whom we would be inclined to liken what we have said about the Yurok, are bewildered people who find themselves victims of an overgrown and insatiable potentiality without the corresponding homogeneous cultural reality. (Y. p. 295-296.)

In contrast, an oral neurosis is non-adjustive and tends to be all inclusive. Most important, it interferes with the development of genital primacy in the individual.

Among our neurotics this retentiveness is common enough: it interferes with psychosexual development and genital potency. But here again the comparison between the cultural and the neurotic character ends; for, on this level too, the strong Yurok is he who never risks, over sexual matters, his property or his luck in hunting or fishing, but who would still be man enough to use with unimpaired sexual potency opportunities without danger of commitment. The understanding between the sexes in these matters goes so far (or can go so far) that one informant defined a "nice girl" as one who always tells the boy beforehand when she is menstruating, thus saving him ritual trouble and subsequent loss of working time. (Y. p. 298.)

Wherever the emphasis of the ontogenetic trauma lies, every culture must insure that the majority of its members will reach a certain amount of genitality—enough to support a strong personal ego and to secure a group-ego; but not more than is compatible with group living.

This applies to other pregenital factors as well. The collective or official character structure of the Yurok shows all the traits which Freud and Abraham found to be of typical significance in patients with "anal fixations", namely compulsiveness, suspiciousness, retentiveness, etc. The author, however, was unable to find in Yurok childhood an emphasis on feces or on the anal zone that would fulfill the criteria of a collective "anal fixation". He feels that Yurok attitude toward property is alimentary in its incorporative aspects, and in its eliminative ones, rather concerns the total inside of the body with its mixture of excreta. This may be true for most primitives.

Anal character in our culture often appears to be a result of the impact on a retentive child of a certain type of maternal behavior in Western civilization, namely, a narcissistic and phobic overconcern with matters of elimination. This attitude helps to overdevelop retentive and eliminative potentialities and to fixate them in the anal zone; it creates the strongest social ambivalence in the child, and it remains an isolating factor in his social and sexual development. Forms of "individualism" in Western culture which represent a mere insistence on the privilege to sit in isolation on possessions can be suspected of representing just such an inroad of anality into cultural and political life. Otherwise it seems that homogeneous cultural life and anality contradict one another. (Y. p. 297.)

The ground work for the Yurok's genital attitudes is laid in the child's earlier conditioning which teaches him, to subordinate drive to economic considerations. Within such basic limits sex is viewed with leniency and humor. The fact that sex contact necessitates purification seems to be considered a duty or a nuisance, but does not reflect on sex as such or on individual women. There is no shame concerning the surface of the human body: it is its "inside" which, by implication, is covered when the young girl between menarche and marriage avoids bathing with others. Otherwise, everybody is free to bathe in the nude. But the girl knows that virtue, or shall we say an unblemished name, will gain her a husband who can pay well and that her status and that of her children and her children's children will depend on the amount her husband will offer to her father when asking for her. The boy, on the other hand, wishes to accumulate enough wealth to buy a worthwhile wife. If he were to make an unworthy girl pregnant, he would have to marry her. Above all, habitual deviant behavior is usually explained as a result of the delinquent's mother or grandmother not having been "paid for in full". This, it seems, means that the man in question was so eager to marry that he borrowed his wife on a down payment without being able to pay the installments; he thus proved that his ego was too weak to integrate sexual needs and economic virtues.

Exactly how genital the average genitality of any group can be said to be is debatable. The Sioux has an elaborate courtship during which, by restraint and the use of the love flute, he demonstrates to his girl that he has more than rape in mind. She, to be sure, brings a small knife along. Beyond this, intercourse in both tribes is mentioned by the men (of today!) as a primitive act of copulation without any aspiration to artfulness nor with any consciousness of a female orgasm. "After all," one Yurok said, "our women were bought." Since highly male societies restrict the verbal consciousness of women it probably would have been difficult under ancient circumstances to elicit data on female sex attitudes; at and during the time of the author's short trips, it was impossible.

As we saw, Sioux and Yurok children learned to associate both locomotor and genital modes with those of hunting and fishing. The Sioux, in his official sexuality, was more phallic-sadistic in that he pursued whatever roamed: game, enemy, woman. (Just as he could "count coup", i.e., gain prestige points by merely touching an enemy, a Sioux man could claim to have taken a girl's virtue by touching her vulva.) The Yurok was more phobic-compulsive in that, in his sexuality, he identified with his prey. He avoided being "snared" by the wrong woman or at the wrong time or place—*wrong* meaning any circumstances that would compromise his assets as an economic being. To this end he is said to have had intercourse in the open, outside the configuration of the living house, ostensibly in order to avoid offending the money in the house. The Yurok woman, in turn, took care not to be bought too cheaply. The snaring configuration occurs in one final item of the primal father story: having promised to be a good god, but venturing down the coast, he found the skate woman lying on the beach, invitingly spreading her legs.[4] ("The skatefish looks like a woman's inside.") He could not resist her. But as soon as he had inserted his penis, she held on to him with vagina and legs and abducted him. On the basis of an analogous equation (fish that looks like woman's inside = female genitals = woman) the author has tentatively assumed that the oblong salmon sent by the gods also represents the god's phallus and the god. In the fishdam ceremonials, then, all three are snared—without being harmed. Thus the symbolic meaning of catching the unwilling penis is added to that of holding on to the elusive nipple. This seems to enhance the enjoyment of the rejuvenation orgies for both sexes; for it gives reassurance that the incestuous and sadistic fantasies emphasized in the Yurok version of childhood dependence have not only not offended either the ontogenetic or the phylogenetic providers, but have been successfully applied to the common good for one more year. This permits the Yurok to accomplish a most precarious feat, namely, to eat their salmon and have it next year, too.

As these excerpts show, the author's data are largely data of verbal tradition, not of observation. They reflect what women remembered doing or saying to their children. There is no reason to doubt, however, that this selection, as far as it goes, is representative. To be sure, there is a great emphasis on feeding procedures; yet it may well be that in human groups who concentrate as homogeneous entities on a direct hand-to-mouth contact with one segment of nature, there is a communal and magic emphasis on first ontogenetic feeding problems.

In the primitive child's later childhood, as it fuses into community life, there probably is a diffusion of those pathogenit tensions that are typical for our each-family-for-itself training. It is in experiences connected with food that the primitive child is closest to his family, and especially to his mother, on whom falls the task in feeding him of

4.This may indicate that the Yurok position in intercourse was the same as the most usual one among Indians and whites today.

laying the basis for his attitude toward the world as a whole. Some consciousness of this mission which gives female functions and modes equality in cultural importance with those of men, may prevent the vast majority of primitive women from resenting their restricted participation in the more spectacular activities of men.

X

The instinctive mental hygiene measures of homogeneous cultures are impressive: parent-fixations are diffused in extended families; children are largely educated by other children, are kept in check by fear of ridicule rather than by the bite of guilt feelings, and are encouraged to be virtuous by the promise of tangible and universal prestige points. On the plains at least, no threat of violence or abandonment estranges parent and child, no talk of sinfulness, body and self. As we consider our means of child rearing in a planned democracy, it may pay to ponder over the polarity of child training:

> The Sioux baby is permitted to remain an individualist (for example, in the way he weans himself from his mother) while he builds an unequivocal trust in himself and in his surroundings. Then when strong in body and confident in himself, he is asked to bow to a tradition of unrelenting public opinion which focuses on his social behavior rather than on his bodily functions and their psychological concomitants. He is forced into a stern tradition which satisfies his social needs and conspires with him in projecting any possible source of sin and guilt into the supernatural. As long as he is able to conform, he can feel free. (S. p. 152-153).

In comparison,

> the dominating classes in the Anglo-Saxon world tend more and more to regulate early functions and impulses in childhood. They implant the never silent metronome into the impressionable baby to regulate his first experiences with his body and with the immediate physical surroundings. After the establishment of these safety devices, he is encouraged to become an individualist. He pursues masculine strivings but often compulsively remains within standardized careers which tend to substitute themselves for communal conscience.

However, as just demonstrated, child training is not an isolated field governed or governable by attitudes of malice or love of children, insight or ignorance; it is a part of the totality of a culture's economic and ideational striving. The systematic difference between "primitive" and "civilized" cultures almost forbids comparison of details. What follows are reflections with some bearing on the study of childhood by clinical psychoanalytic means.

As we have seen, primitive cultures are exclusive. Their image of man coincides with their consciousness of being a strong or "clean" Yurok or Sioux. We do not know how and how long they would have succeeded in remaining homogeneous if left alone. In civilization the image of man is expanding and is ever more inclusive. New syntheses of economic and emotional safety are sought in inclusive formations of new entities and new identities: regions, nations, classes, races, ideologies. These new entities, however, overlap, and anachronistic fears of extinction cause some areas to seek archaic safety in spasms of reactionary exclusion. The viciousness of the battlefields is matched in that of the wars of standards (including those of child training) and in the conflicts which individuals wage with themselves.

Primitive tribes have a direct relation to the sources and means of production. Their techniques are extensions of the human body, their magic is a projection of body concepts. Children in these groups participate in technical and in magic pursuits; body and environment, childhood and culture may be full of dangers, but they are all one world. The expansiveness of civilization, its stratification and specialization make it impossible for children to include in their ego synthesis more than a section or sections of their society. Machines, far from remaining an extension of the body, destine whole classes to be extensions of machinery; magic becomes secondary, serving intermediate links only; and childhood, in some classes, becomes a separate segment of life with its own folklore. Neuroses, we find, are unconscious attempts to adjust to the heterogeneous present with the magic means of a homogeneous past. But individual neuroses are only parts of collective ones. It may well be, for example, that such mechanical child training as western civilization has developed during the last few decades, harbors an unconscious magic attempt to master machines by becoming more like them, comparable to the Sioux' identification with the buffalo, the Yurok's with the river and the salmon.

XI

According to the author, clinical descriptions, i.e. the description of one or several successive segments of a historical process defines every item of human behavior according to at least three kinds of organization:

(1) The biological one, which reflects the nature of the human organism as a space-time organization of mammalian organ-systems (evolution, epigenesis, pregenitality),

(2) The social one, which reflects the fact that human organisms are organized into geographic-historical units,

(3) The ego-principle, reflecting the synthesis of experience and the resulting defensive and creative mastery (ego development).

None of these principles can "cause" a human event; but no human event is explained except by an investigation that pursues the Gestalten evoked by each principle in constant relativity to the two others.

In the psychoanalysis of the individual Freud has introduced this threefold investigation in the dynamic concepts of an id, a superego, and an ego.

What psychoanalysis has contributed to the knowledge of childhood, step by step, depended on the shifting foci of its theoretical attention. The id and its few basic drives was studied first. The initial focus of a science, however, threatens to impose its form on all further findings. Thus the next focus of study, namely the superego, which represents the first conceptualization of the influence of society on the individual, was primarily conceived of as an anti-id; it was said to be observable only when the id forced it to act. At best it behaved like the Victorian mother (quoted by Anna Freud) who sits in the parlor and periodically sends the nurse upstairs to tell the children not to do whatever it is they are doing. This mother never goes upstairs herself to tell the children what they *may* do—or even to do it with them. But this is what cultures, parents, neighborhoods do—and at least some of the ego's guiding ideals result from it. The ego, in turn, was at first conceived of as an ego both against the id and against the culture "with much emphasis on the poor little fellow's painful adjustment to the big bad environment" and with little emphasis on the fact that only a supporting society and a loving mother can make a functioning ego.

In his last writings Freud formulated the id and the superego in historical terms:

> During the whole of a man's life . . . the superego . . . represents the influence of his childhood, of the care and education given to him by his parents, of his dependence on them—of the childhood which is so greatly prolonged in human beings by a common family life. And in all this what is operating is not only the personal qualities of these parents but also everything that produced a determining effect upon themselves, the tastes and standards of the social class in which they live and the characteristics and traditions of the race from which they spring. Those who have a liking for generalizations and sharp distinctions may say that the external world, in which the individual finds himself exposed after being detached from his parents, represents the power of the present; that his id, with its inherited trends, represents the organic past; and that the superego, which later joins them, represents more than anything the cultural past, of which the child has to pass through, as it were, an after-experience during the few years of his early childhood. ("An Outline of Psycho-Analysis", *International Journal of Psycho-Analysis*, XXI, p. 82.)

We are now studying the relationship of the ego to the "power of the present", that is the experience of perpetual change from the immediate past to the anticipated future.

In her book *The Ego and the Mechanisms of Defense,* Anna Freud asks whether or not the ego invents its defenses all by itself. She comes to the conclusion that the form of defense depends on the id content to be warded off, but does not discuss the relationship of ego mechanisms to the historical present.[5]

Anna Freud reports a case of altruism by identification and projection. A patient seems to have renounced all earthly pleasure. But far from being a Puritan, she does not insist that everybody else renounce these pleasures too. On the contrary, wherever possible she helps other people, even rivals, to enjoy what she herself seems neither to demand nor to need. This is called a defense mechanism, although at times it must have approached a symptom, and around it a personality must have been built. Beyond asking what infantile drives made such a mechanism necessary, and indeed pleasurable, we could inquire: Why, and at what stage of the patient's life did this mechanism develop and who was its model? Was it the parent of the same or of the other sex? Was it an ancestor, a priest, a teacher, a neighbor? Within what kind of a communal environment was this mechanism developed and within what kind of culture change: In what sections of her environment and at what period of her life did this kind of altruism secure to the patient glory and a halo, or shame and defamation, or indifference?

The need for clinical reconstructions that include the correlation of critical psychosexual phases with contemporaneous social changes becomes especially apparent—but it is by no means restricted to— American patients of psychoanalysis. This, I assume, is one major reason for the fact that the discussion of "social factors" that were energetically sought by some European workers in the field, has become more systematic and decisive in this country. This change of focus—like preceding ones—is accompanied by apologies and apostasies, and this, for reasons intrinsic in the psychoanalytic movement, but not to be discussed here.

This dynamic country, by its very nature, subjects its inhabitants to more extreme contrasts and abrupt changes during a lifetime or a generation than is normally the case with other great nations. The national character is formed by what we hope will ultimately prove to be fruitful polarities: open roads of immigration and closed areas of settlement; free influences of immigration and jealous islands of tra-

5. See however, A. Freud and D. T. Burlingham, *Infants Without Families.* New York, 1944.

dition; outgoing internationalism and defiant isolationism; boisterous competition and self-effacing cooperation; and many others. Which of the resulting contradictory slogans has the greatest influence on the development of an individual ego, probably depends on the relationship of critical growth periods to the rate of change in the family history.

It was customary in some psychiatric circles in Europe to discuss what appeared to be a relative "ego weakness" in American patients. There are indications that in the depths of their hearts American neurotics, beyond seeking relief for guilt and inferiority feelings, desire to be cured of a basic vagueness and confusion in their identifications. Often they turn to psychoanalysis as a savior from the discrepancies of American life; abroad, they were willing to dissimulate their American identity for the sake of what promised to be a more comfortable one, made in "the old country".

The less neurotic American,[6] however, as long as he does not feel endangered by some too unexpected turn of events, paradoxically enough receives his very ego strength from a kind of proud refusal to settle on any form of group-ego too early, and too definitely. To be sure, he acknowledges some fundamental decencies and some—incredibly fleeting—common experiences on crossroads. Otherwise premature harmony disconcerts him; he is rather prepared for and willing to tackle discontinuities. In the meantime he lives by slogans which are, as it were, experimental crystallizations—a mode of life that can, of course, turn into perverse shiftiness.[7]

Such slogans as "let's get the hell out of here", or "let's stay no matter what happens"—to mention only two of the most sweeping ones —are in the sphere of ethos what rationalizations are in that of the intellect. Often outmoded, and without any pretense of logic, they are convincing enough to those involved to justify action whether within or just outside of the law insofar as it happens to be enforced. Slogans contain time and space perspectives as definite as those elaborated in the Sioux or Yurok systems—a collective ego time-space to which individual ego defenses are coordinated. But they change.

A cartoon in the *New Yorker* not long ago pictured an old lady who sat in her little garden before a little colonial house, knitting

6. His elusive nature is only now being defined by anthropologists. See Margaret Mead, *And Keep Your Powder Dry*, 1942, for an attempt at such definition and for a relevant bibliography.

7. What is popularly called an "ego" in this country, seems to be the defiant expression of the owner's conviction that he is somebody without being identified with anybody in particular.

furiously but otherwise ignoring enormous bulldozers excavating the ground a hundred feet deep around her small property, to make space for the foundations of skyscrapers. Many a patient from Eastern mansions, finds himself regressing to such an *ego-space,* with all the defense mechanisms of exclusiveness, whenever he is frightened by competition outside, or by unbridled impulses from within.

Or take a patient whose grandparents came West "where never is heard a discouraging word". The grandfather, a powerful and powerfully driven man seeks ever new and challenging engineering tasks in widely separated regions. When the initial challenge is met, he hands the task over to others, and moves on. His wife sees him only for an occasional impregnation. According to a typical family pattern, his sons cannot keep pace with him and are left as respectable settlers by the wayside; only his daughter is and looks like him. Her very masculine identification, however, does not permit her to take a husband equal to her strong father. She marries a weak man and settles down. She brings her boy up to be God-fearing and industrious. He becomes reckless and shifting at times, depressed at others: somewhat of a juvenile delinquent now, later, maybe, a more enjoyable Westerner, with alcoholic moods.

What his worried mother does not know is that she herself all through his childhood has belittled the sedentary father; has decried the lack of mobility, geographic and social, of her marital existence; has idealized the grandfather's exploits; but has also reacted with panicky punitiveness to any display of friskiness in the boy, which was apt to disturb the now well-defined neighborhood.

In the course of a psychoanalysis patients repeat in transferences and regressions not only infantile instinctual tensions and ego defenses, but also their abortive (and often unconscious) infantile ego-ideals. These are often based on conditions and slogans which prevailed at the period of the family's greatest ascendancy. Specific conflicts and resistances result: the patient, on the one hand, is afraid that the brittleness of his ideal identity will be uncovered; on the other, he wishes the psychoanalyst, no matter with what means or terminologies, to free him from the ambiguity of his background and to provide him with the deceptive continuity of a magic psychoanalytic world.

This, however, is not the social function of psychoanalysis.

The individual is not merely the sum-total of his childhood identifications. Children—perhaps more pronouncedly in a highly mobile society—are early aware of their parents' position in the community;

of their reactions to friends, servants, superiors; of their behavior in pleasant, pious, angry or alcoholized company; of Saturday nights in town and of mild enthusiasms and panics pervading neighborhoods, not to speak of lynchings and wars. If not impoverished too early by indifferent communities and selfish mothers, children early develop a nucleus of separate identity. Anxiety may cause them to sacrifice this individual awareness to blind identifications with parental persons. In the psychoanalytic treatment of adults this nucleus should be recovered. The patient, instead of blaming his parents (i.e. turning his positive over-identifications into negative ones), should learn to understand the social forces responsible for the deficiencies of his childhood.

In our clinical attempts to reconstruct the childhood of adult patients we have studied "id resistances" as derivatives of the infantile fear of being deprived of urgent satisfactions; we have studied "superego resistances" as representatives of the infantile fear of being overpowered by such needs. The change in ego-potential or both these fears during maturational and psychological crises is well known to us. We perceive of the ego as a central regulator which, closest to the history of the day, guards a measure of safety, satisfaction and identity. As we add to our knowledge and technique the understanding of resistances that originate in contemporary conflicts of ego-ideals, we cannot fail to make new and, in a sense, perpetual contributions to the study of childhood in a world characterized by expanding identifications and by great fears of losing hard-won identities.

TRANSFERENCE AND GROUP FORMATION IN CHILDREN AND ADOLESCENTS

By EDITH BUXBAUM, Ph.D. (New York)

I.

Statistical observations show that children under five years of age associate in groups of two to three for periods of from ten to forty minutes. A definite change is noticed in the size and stability of groups in the age between five and seven, when four to ten children can be associated for one to three hours. After age seven, the spontaneous interest in group formation seems to come to a standstill, and even decreases slightly, until the peak of group development is reached in pre-adolescence and adolescence. According to Thrasher, 51% of youth between eleven and seventeen; and according to Bühler, 67% of boys and 59% of girls between ten and fifteen, belong to groups. Although in young children the sex difference seems unimportant in this connection, it is observed that in adolescent boys and girls varying reactions occur in and to groups.[1]

Most observers take it for granted that the main purpose of the group is educational: it makes the child sociable. Ideas as to what constitutes sociability vary. Ronald Lippitt,[2] in his study of the effects of authoritarian, democratic, and laissez-faire leadership on the development of groups, finds that the democratic one offers optimal development of initiative and friendliness among the group members; the laissez-faire groups show the greatest development of knowledge; and the authoritarian leadership develops dependence and obedience toward the leader at the expense of intra-group relationships.

---

1. Cf. D. S. Thomas, "Some New Techniques for Studying Social Behavior", *Child Development Monograph*, I, 1929; Charlotte Bühler, "Social Behavior of Children" in Hutchinson, *Handbook of Child Psychology*, 1933, pp. 374-416; and Frederick M Thrasher, *The Gang*, Chicago, 1927. The percentage which Bühler finds in her investigations is high in comparison to Thrasher's. Bühler has mainly studied German groups; Thrasher's research is confined to Chicago. The difference in numbers may find its explanation in the different political set-ups in which these groups live.

2. R. Lippitt, "The Morale of Youth Groups", in *Civilian Morale*, edited by Goodwin Watson, 1942, p. 119 ff.

The approach in this paper is different. I am concerned with the question of whether there are any needs within the child which the group satisfies; or even whether there are any needs which the group satisfies better than any other relationship in the child's life. We should like to establish what role the group has in the emotional development of the child. Freud, in *Group Psychology and the Analysis of the Ego,* points out that libidinal factors are at work in the formation and preservation of groups, and that the libidinal needs are satisfied through member-member relationships as well as through member-leader relationships. He implies that the group plays a role in the development of the group member's ego as well as of his superego.[3]

A number of psychoanalytic investigations have followed upon Freud's ideas.[4] Zulliger, for example, shows how common guilt feelings tie groups of children together; and how common confessions to the teacher-leader release their guilt and increase their positive response to him. Redl describes ten types of group formation each with its own kind of leadership. He substitutes for the ill-famed expression "leader" the term "central person". The "central person" does not necessarily have to assume a leading or even an active part, but sometimes may act as a catalytic. He attracts, through definite qualities, children who have corresponding drives. Finally Redl discriminates three main types of groups: those in which the central person is (1) an object of identification; (2) an object of instinctual drives; and (3) plays the part of a support for the ego of the group member.

In surveying these observations which we consider representative we find that the group satisfies many emotional demands of the child, but that some individual relationship could satisfy the same demands. Possibly the group offers a greater choice of persons than every-day life does, but otherwise its function does not seem to be specific.

3. Freud's formula reads: "A primary group of this kind is a number of individuals who have substituted one and the same object for their ego-ideal and have consequently identified themselves with one another in their egos." *Group Psychology and the Analysis of the Ego,* International Psycho-Analytical Library No. 6, p. 80.

4. Siegfried Bernfeld, "Vom Gemeinschaftsleben der Jugend" ("Group Life in Youth") in G. Fuchs, *Ein Schülerverein* (*A Pupils' Association*), Beiträge zur Jugend-forschung (Quellenschriften für Seelische Entwicklung), Leipzig, Wien, Zurich, 1922; Edith Buxbaum, "Massenpsychologie und Schule" ("Mass Psychology and the School"), *Zeitschrift für Psychoanalytische Pädagogik,* X, 1936, p. 215; Fritz Redl, "Group Emotion and Leadership", *Psychiatry,* V, 1942, p. 573 ff; and Hans Zulliger, "Psychoanalyse und Führerschaft in der Schule" ("Psychoanalysis and Leadership in School"), *Imago,* XVI, 1930, p. 39 ff.

However, there are indications to the contrary: The gang, says Thrasher,[5]

"largely an adolescent phenomenon . . . occupies a period in the life of the boy between childhood when he is usually incorporated into a family structure, and marriage, when he is reincorporated into a family and other orderly relations of work, religion and pleasure . . . The gang appears to be an *interstitial group, a manifestation of readjustment between childhood and maturity.*"

Thrasher maintains that the group has a part to play in the life of adolescents which cannot be substituted by any other human individual relationship. This may serve to explain the tremendous increase of groups among them. As mentioned above, there is a similar period of increased group formation at the age between five and seven. These two peaks are significant; they indicate that there are certain needs within the child which force him into the group and which are independent of educational aims. Public school systems of all Western countries have made use of these needs by setting the beginning of schooling at age six or seven. In turning our attention to these peaks of group development in childhood and adolescence we hope to understand what are the needs for which child and adolescent seek satisfaction in the group more than in any other social setting.

II

Observation of two- and three-year-old children in nursery schools shows that in the beginning there is little contact between them. They do not notice each other. After some time, however, Billy notices John playing with a toy that seems interesting. Billy tries to get it from John, who will either surrender the toy without showing particular feeling, or will yell; or they will fight for it. The other solution to the dilemma is introduced by the teacher, who shows Billy and John how to play together with the desired toy. This little group of two, or perhaps three children is then able to play together as long as the toy holds their common interest. As soon as they feel tired, however, they will start fighting again.

This is the picture until about age four, when the group may contain three or four children, and the periods of playing together may increase to thirty or forty minutes. Becoming tired, one or another

5. F. M. Thrasher, op. cit., p. 37.

child may then be hostile toward the group, and the teacher is forced to interfere. She may either try to settle the fight and get the children to continue their play or change to another game; or she may find it better to let the group dissolve and let the children play alone for a while; or she may gather them around herself and tell stories or sing songs to them. Gradually they quiet down and are ready to return to their play with each other.

In the moment of tension when the children threaten each other with murder, or at least bloody noses, the presence of the teacher is required. The child is under a certain strain as long as he is on his own with the others. He knows that he does not feel altogether friendly towards them, and expects no more from them. Only in the presence of the teacher is he able to relax completely, by letting her take care of his security. At the same time, he expects her to control his own aggressive impulses against his playmates, instead of having to exercise control himself. She will see that nothing happens to him, that nobody attacks him, and that he, too, keeps peace. In this respect the teacher is temporarily accepted as a substitute for the mother.

Children who are strongly attached to their mothers are often almost unable to form any kind of relationship to either adults or children. Dicky, age five, was one of these. The time he spent in school was filled with waiting for his mother to come. He had not learned to dress or toilet himself. The teacher took over the mother's functions, with the result that Dicky would not let her get out of sight; yet he was constantly dissatisfied because mother's care was better than teacher's. At the slightest discomfort he would cry desperately for his mother. Gradually, however, Dicky did learn how to take care of himself, and no longer spent his time waiting for her. He took part in the activities with the other children. His relationship to the teacher became less anxious. Instead of crying, "Where is Mommy, I want my Mommy!" he would ask quietly, "Where is my teacher, where is my group?"

Adujstment to both teacher and group was not simply a matter of time for Dicky. His physical helplessness made it impossible for him to exist without his mother; there was no one whom he could trust sufficiently to take her place. She was the only one who knew what he needed, and he was painfully anxious without her. As long as the teacher offered herself as an unsatisfactory substitute, Dicky's anxiety only increased: he was then depending on two people instead of one. It was the newly-acquired independence, however, that detached him partially from the mother and opened up a new area of relationship for him. He became able to bestow affection on people without expecting them to take care of his immediate physical needs.

This process takes place so gradually and slowly in all individuals that we are generally not aware of it. Every skill that the child requires —his learning to grasp and hold, to move about and walk, to feed himself, to dress, and so on—all help him become independent of the person who has previously done these things for him. The physical independence is also expressed emotionally. The feelings of the child which were centered around the care-taking person out of a mere instinct of self-preservation, become free to be used elsewhere and in other ways. Freud's explanation of this phenomenon is that anaclitic object-choice is transformed into libidinal object-choice. The word "attachment" which we use in describing anaclitic relationships, preserves the original meaning of the physical adherence. It seems that the child is not just once detached from the umbilical cord. With every new development he withdraws further from the physical unity with his mother. Every such step reflects itself in an increase of object-libido.

This detachment is reinforced in the phallic phase of the child's development. While his oral and anal needs are satisfied by the mother to a certain degree, the sexual needs of the child are disregarded in the normal mother-child relationship of our society. The child is rejected in his genital demands by his mother and must find gratification elsewhere. Her complete rejection of his libidinal demands, together with the castration threat coming from the father, force the child to his last step in the process of physical withdrawal from the mother. There is no physical satisfaction which he can further derive from her. He is physically independent; his attachment to her is free of the anxiety for the gratification of immediate bodily needs.[6] Nevertheless the child's desire for physical affection persists basically, and he is not satisfied in this new kind of relationship. He

6. Freud, op. cit., p. 72 ff: "In his first phase which has usually come to an end by the time he is five years old, a child has found the first object for his love in one or the other of his parents, and all of his sexual instincts with their demand for satisfaction have been united in this object. The repression which then sets in compels him to renounce the greater number of these infantile sexual aims, and leaves behind a profound modification in his relation to his parents. The child still remains tied to his parents, but by instincts which must be described as being inhibited in their aim ("zielgehemmte"). The emotions which he feels henceforward towards these objects of his love are characterized as 'tender' It is well known that the earlier 'sensual' tendencies remain more or less strongly preserved in the unconscious, so that in a certain sense the whole of the original current continues to exist."

must reach out for other love-objects, and transfer part of his feelings to them.[7]

One of the objects which lends itself to his need may be the teacher. He expects the same kind of understanding from her as he has been used to getting from his mother. He is even more willing to accept it because he does not hold against her the grudge which he has against his mother for rejecting his libidinal demands, and for disappointing him. He forms a transference to the teacher, following the anaclitic type of object-choice.

His independence and comparative freedom from fear enable him to use his energies in exploring the world around him. He is now eager to learn. We realize that the time for the beginning of academic teaching has been chosen wisely. It would be rewarding to follow up the development of the child's interest and intelligence in connection with his growing independence from his primary objects and his predisposition to form transferences. This, however, is not the object of this paper.

The increase in object-libido manifests itself also in the greater sociability of the children. While the two- to four-year-old children form small groups for short periods, the size of the group, as well as the period of common satisfactory activity increases after the fourth year; the children associate in groups of eight to ten, and extend their common activities to two to three hours. Independent as far as his immediate physical needs are concerned, and emotionally secure through the transference that he has formed to the teacher, the child does not feel threatened any more by the other children, and can accept them better than before. Yet his feeling for the group is far more than an unwilling resignation. The children are tied together

7. The child who is ready to transfer his feelings from mother to another person and the child who is unable to do so each require a different approach in the analytic treatment. A three-year-old boy was treated for constipation. He stayed in the room with me and his mother. At first he reacted to my interpretations by turning to her and demanding, "Now you say it!" After a while he was satisfied to ask her, "Is it true?" When she confirmed my explanation, he accepted it. The young child, who is still completely dependent on his mother, cannot transfer his feelings to the analyst; he is also unable to form or reform his reactions independently of his mother. The analyst must therefore work with the mother in order to moderate her reactions or to get her cooperation in changing those of the child. When the child reaches the age of about five we can work with him directly; he is then sufficiently detached from mother and his object-libido is sufficiently developed for him to make a transference. We should reserve the name of psychoanalysis to the treatment of children who have reached this stage of development, and call what we do with the others education or child guidance. Frequently we have to work with and through the mother even with older children who, like Dicky (p. 354), are retarded in their development of independence and object-relationship. We must apply methods of guidance and education in order to get the child ready for psychoanalytic treatment.

through mutual identification. They get a feeling of safety in the group which contrasts with their previous feeling of being threatened by the rivalry-situation. At this stage group formation in a dynamic sense takes place. Freud's phylogenetic construct concerning the development of the group may here be quoted:[8]

"One can imagine only one possibility: the primal father had prevented his sons from satisfying their sexual tendencies directly; he forced them into abstinence and consequently into the emotional ties with him and with one another which could arise out of those of their tendencies that were inhibited in their sexual aim. He forced them, so to speak, into group psychology."

We find this imaginary "Urvater" represented in the child's castration fear, which is derived from the oedipus complex. It lends mother's rejection additional power through the threat of the father-rival and thereby makes it insurmountable. In the attempt to master this double pressure the child becomes more independent than he would wish to be. He reacts with the need to transfer his feelings from mother to other people, and is ready to be part of a group because it offers him something he cannot find elsewhere.

However, while we understand the child's readiness to form transferences and while we recognize that this transference is essential to his being part of the group, we have not yet answered a crucial question: In what does the gratification afforded by the group differ from that gratification which could be afforded by the individual relationship of two children outside the group?

III

We now turn our attention to the other great period of group formation, to adolescence, for additional clues. In adolescence the youngster's desire to be part of a group is imperative; when he cannot find a group in school he will try elsewhere, but he is determined to find it.

Adolescence is known for the violence as well as for the inconsistency of its emotions.

"Adolescents are excessively egoistic, regarding themselves as the center of the universe and the sole object of interest; and yet at no time in later life are they capable of so much self-sacrifice and devotion. They form the most passionate love-relations, only to break them off as abruptly as they began them. *On the one hand they throw themselves enthusiastically into the*

8. Freud, op. cit., p. 93.

*life of the community and, on the other, they have an overpowering longing
for solitude. They oscillate between blind submission to some self-chosen leader
and defiant rebellion against any and every authority.*[9] They are selfish and
materially-minded and at the same time full of lofty idealism. They are ascetic but
will suddenly plunge into instinctual indulgence of the most primitive character.
At times their behavior to other people is rough and inconsiderate, yet they
themselves are extremely touchy. Their moods veer between light-hearted
optimism and the blackest pessimism. Sometimes they will work with inde-
fatigable enthusiasm and at other times they are sluggish and apathetic."[10]

The emotional upheaval of adolescence colors their group life. Their
study reveals general principles as if seen through a magnifying glass.

We propose to distinguish two different types of groups among
adolescents. First, those with a leader whose authority is enforced
and upheld by his own overbearing power—be it physical strength or
psychological skill—or by an outside authority which may be state,
school, parent, or any organization. This corresponds to what Freud
classifies as an artificial group,[11] held together by external control.
The other type of group is that which forms itself spontaneously
around a central person (Redl). One member of the group is accepted
as leader for a certain time; he may be replaced by another member
after a short or long period.

The artificial group apparently gives the individual who joins it a
feeling of strength. This becomes most obvious in the "gang" when
the youngsters feel strong enough to defy the state's authority, as
well as the moral code.[12] But also the child in the non-delinquent
adolescent group, feeling protected and anonymous, becomes audacious
and revolutionary against the previously acknowledged authorities.
Yet he is not really independent. His new authorities are the leader
and the group. Nor is he a revolutionary in the political sense, aiming
for a change in a definite direction. The adolescent is a revolutionary
by emotion. To leave home, to break away from the family and its
traditions, to become independent, is the painful struggle he has to

9. My italics.
10. A. Freud, *The Ego and the Mechanism of Defense*, 1936, p. 149.
11. S. Freud, op. cit., p. 41: "artificial groups, requiring an external force to keep
them together".
12. Ibid., p. 28: "A group impresses the individual with a sense of unlimited power
and of insurmountable peril. For the moment it replaces the whole of human society,
which is the wielder of authority, whose punishments the individual fears, and for whose
sake he has submitted to so many inhibitions. It is clearly perilous for him to put himself in opposition to it, and it will be safer to follow the example of those around him
and perhaps even to 'hunt with the pack'. In obedience to the new authority he may
put his former 'conscience' out of action, and so surrender to the attraction of the
increased pleasure that is certainly obtained from the removal of inhibitions."

go through. The leader and the group who agree with his revolutionary tendencies help him in his struggle. But the leader no longer serves this purpose when he becomes entirely identified with the parental authorities: the adolescent then tries to break away from him.

The process of breaking away from the leader occurs regularly in this type of group. It can be observed in the classroom of the formal school. A group of children, deeply attached to the teacher or to the leader of their own age whom they love and worship, suddenly turns against him. The obvious reason may be a minor one, yet it seems to be the spark that causes an explosion of long-stored resentments.[13] The leader has turned from god into devil. His erstwhile followers may then turn into his enemies; they may either join another leader, or choose one among themselves and unite under his leadership against the former leader. The uniting factor now is their hatred toward him, just as it was their love for him before. The ideas and ideals which the leader represented, are now dismissed together with him.

As long as a leader is acknowledged, love for him prevails. Yet we know that he has to put all sorts of restrictions on the individuals in the group which ordinarily would be reacted to with ill-feelings, resentment, and hatred. Where are these reactions in the group? What has happened to them? They exist, but the group does not allow their expression. The child who criticizes the leader soon becomes an outsider and does not belong to the group any more. On the other hand, every single member of the group tends to feel rejected by the leader, is jealous of his companions and resents the fact that he is not allowed to brush them aside. These accumulated feelings find their expression when the dependence on the leader becomes more painful than rewarding—when a large number of the group suffer under the rejection of their positive feelings and demands. The teacher who understands the situation will give the children an opportunity to tell him what their objections are and will thus be able, with them, to revise their feelings toward himself. In so doing, he is giving up his authoritative position for the time being and identifies himself with the children in their criticism against himself. He lowers himself to their level, sides with their ego rather than represents their superego.[14]

By submitting to their criticisms he allows them to change roles with him: they are the judge of his actions as he used to be of theirs.

13. E. Buxbaum, "Massenpsychologie und Schule", op. cit.
14. See E. Kris, *Some Problems of War Propaganda*, 1943, ch. XII, p. 395, where democratic group formation is "linked to the birth of criticism" and described as "one in which identification in the superego is supplemented by ego identification".

He makes it possible for them to identify with him by encouraging them to take his place for a while. By this process their identification with him becomes greater than before; their negative feelings are resolved along with part of the transference. The teacher's position among the children is slightly changed, but he maintains his position as a leader. The teacher who is not able to cope with the criticism and the negative feelings loses this position. The group either dissolves or forms again under the leadership of the main critic.

If the teacher or leader is successful in overcoming the opposition of the group he may be sure that a similar crisis will arise again. If the youngsters succeed in breaking away from one group they will soon join another, and will eventually take up the fight there. The succession of joining a group and breaking away from it seems to be a standard feature of the adolescent group. The more rigid the leader is the more dramatic the break will be.

In the "spontaneous" group of children the leader does not retain his position for as long a period as he does in the "artificial" group. The children accept him for a certain time or for a certain purpose. After that another child assumes the position of leader. The change is performed without great upheaval; in fact, any child in the group can be leader for some time. He can play both parts alternately, the part of the leader and the part of the group-member. There are of course children who never try to take a leading part. They are mostly those who lend themselves to being bossed and who for individual reasons are unable to assume any part but that of dependence. They are very often children with a history of seduction, which they repeat in the group. They are unable to identify with the rest of the children.

The spontaneous groups exist mostly within the frame of the artificial group. The common leadership reflects itself in the individual groups: the small-group leaders imitate the big chief. They either support the common leader or build the nucleus of the opposition against him. The joining and breaking away from these small groups within the big one takes place constantly (though less spectacularly than it does in authoritarian groups), along with the change of leadership.

The repeated change between submission and opposition toward the leader, joining and leaving the group, alternating between being obedient member and active leader, shows a certain pattern. We recognize the swinging back and forth between activity and passivity.

It reminds us of the repetitive character of children's dramatic play.[15] Children repeat actively what they have been subjected to passively before. The greater the trauma they have suffered, the longer the play which reenacts it, persists.[16] The child who had been treated by the doctor, however unpleasant the experience may have been, begins to play doctor with a doll or with another child. Similarly, the child who becomes leader in a group enjoys treating his companions as he has been treated by the former leader. The child in the doctor-play with his playmates will also accept the part of the patient. In play he will put himself into the unpleasant situation which in reality he feared and resented, without minding it too much; he even enjoys it. We should have reason to be concerned if he wanted to take the role of the patient all the time; we should then suspect him of being thoroughly masochistic. If, however, he takes both parts alternately, we consider it as a rule of the game and wonder just what he gets out of it. Apparently he is satisfied to have the situation in hand. He is putting himself into this position instead of being forced into it as he was in reality. He can break it up whenever he pleases. The same is true for the child in his position as a member of the group. Submission to the rules of the group is self-imposed to a certain extent. If he does not agree with the group he can leave it by staying out, by choosing another group, or by becoming a leader himself. Even the most rigid groups offer a chance for these possibilities through sub-groups which develop within the big one. When the child chooses to be a member he voluntarily chooses the position of submission, obedience, and dependence. As a group member he repeats the dependence situation of home in the transference to the leader.

The adolescent turns against his parents in a desperate attempt to establish life of his own; he may even run away from home or be rude and contemptuous without apparent reason. The more he fights the more we know how attached he really is. In adolescence this breaking away from home is connected with the youngster's growing desire for sexual relationships, which cannot be satisfied in the family. He is left strictly alone with his desire, and has the choice of either giving it up and staying in the family or of looking for satisfaction elsewhere and leaving the family. As in the time of the phallic phase, he is being deserted by the family in his sexual needs. He tries to shift his attachment from his parents to a love-object outside the family. The leader

15. R. Waelder, "The Psychoanalytic Theory of Play", *Psychoanalytic Quarterly,* II, 1933.

16. S. Freud, *Beyond the Pleasure Principle,* International Psycho-Analytical Library No. 4, 1920.

and the members of the group present themselves as intermediaries: the child finds in them now love-objects which nevertheless repeat the family-situation to a certain degree. In this group, too, overt sexual relationships are forbidden. The group of two is not compatible with the general group conditions. The couple has no need for the group, the group no room for the couple. In fact, when sexual relationships enter the group, the group dissolves. The members who find a sexual partner outside, leave a group temporarily or completely.[17] Yet it seems to be easier to make the step into adult sex life from the group than from home. The child's fear of being left alone when he leaves the family proves unwarranted. He finds a new family. While in the original one it was forbidden to take the father's place he now discovers that it is possible to take the leader's place without being in any danger of punishment. Every time he breaks away from the leader or himself takes the leader's position he becomes more assured in his independence. When by entering upon sexual relations he takes the final step in identification with him, he gives up his dependence. The repeated experience of breaking away from the leader and of being allowed to assume his place, makes the adolescent less afraid to do in every respect what adults do, to be fully an adult himself.

IV.

We return to our question: what has the group to offer to the child? What needs within him does it meet? The two periods in which he tends to be part of a group are high points in his sexual development: the phallic phase, and the onset of adolescence. Both times "castration fear forces them into group-formation" (Freud).

To put it briefly: the childhood period of group-formation occurs at a time in which the child is forced to give up his physical dependence on his mother. His close relationship to her has been severed gradually by his achieving independence in mobility, expression, eating, and body care. He does not need his mother any more in order to survive. His relationship to her changes from an anaclitic one to one of object-libidinal character. The rejection of his sexual wishes leaves him frustrated, and drives him into transferring his feelings for her to other people. It is this readiness to form new relationships that brings him into the group. The increased need of adolescents for groups arises from similar sources. The growing

17. S. Bernfeld, "Vom Gemeinschaftsleben der Jugend", op. cit., and E. Buxbaum, "Massenpsychologie und Schule" op. cit.

sexual drive forces the adolescent to seek satisfaction which the family normally refuses to give. He therefore looks for it outside the family.

Whereas the young child finds in the group support for his new-found physical independence from mother, the adolescent finds reassurance for his moral independence from home. Both child and adolescent feel deserted, ousted from the protective atmosphere upon which they have used to rely and not yet sure enough to face the world alone. The group is a highly welcome shelter in the meantime. Fear of separation from mother and home is overcome by transfering allegiance to the group leader.

With young children, who gain constantly in independence through a widening range of activities, it can be expected that the development of boys and girls would be similar. It is different with the adolescent: striving for intellectual independence, he accepts, together with the group and the group leader, the ideas for which they stand; when he breaks with the leader he throws away the ideas. Thus, while the young child grows primarily in the sphere of the ego, the adolescent changes occur in the superego. We should therefore expect adolescent boys and girls to show a difference in their relation to groups, in line with the different development of their superego. We hope that further studies will bring more light on this question.

The adolescent's breaking away from the leader attracts the attention of the observer more than his submission. It seems, however, that both processes are of equal importance for his development. In breaking away from the leader he repeats his attempt to break away from home. Every break results in an increase in identification with the leader, which in turn makes him more independent. On the other hand, the periods of submission give him a chance to repeat actively experiences to which he had to submit passively before. But being able to choose such experience as well as to terminate it makes it pleasant and acceptable; and the adolescent is enabled to satisfy his passive tendencies. He learns that submission as well as attempts to take the leader's place do not result in punishment and castration. Dependence, as well as independence, are imposed upon the child by his parents. They are situations and relationships which are largely beyond his control. The group makes it possible for him to choose his place between indifference, membership, and leadership. While he is afraid to disagree with his parents for fear of losing their love he is courageous in the group because he feels strong in

the identification with his companions. He is supported in his
striving for independence as well as he is accepted when he finds it
more comfortable to submit. Instead of being forced to submit, he is
obedient because he chooses to be. Instead of being forced into independence by the traumatic process of rejection, he does the rejecting
on his own. His preconscious knowledge that his companions share
his desire to take the leader's place diminish his guilt feelings and
his castration fear to the extent that he is able to actually be the leader
himself. The allowed identification with the leader prepares and
encourages him to give up his position as a child and to behave in an
adult way outside of the group also. The swinging back and forth
between submission and revolt is most apparent in adolescent groups,
especially in those with an authoritarian type of leadership. We
see the same tendencies in groups of younger children—they have
plenty of opportunity to turn their passive experiences into active
ones in different forms of dramatic play—but their desire to obtain
final independence is less strong than their need for protection in
the group. The opportunity to submit and revolt alternately against
leadership and group is one of the characteristics which in particular
make the group indispensable for the adolescent.

It seems that the forcefulness of the group, put to use in everyday life to surmount obstacles that individuals cannot tackle alone,
is used by the child and the adolescent in order to fight obstacles
within himself. It helps him at the crucial point in his development,
in his physical and emotional breaking away from home. It serves
as a medium between the dependence of the child and the independence of the adult, as a "manifestation of readjustment between childhood and maturity" (Thrasher).[18]

18. This paper originated in some thoughts concerning the problem of mass-evacuation
of young children. Anna Freud's and Dorothy Burlingham's reports on the Hampstead
Children's Nursery have pointed out the dangerous effect which the separation of small
children from their mothers may have. When it is a matter of saving children from death
or injury there can be no doubt about what to do. We must remove them from areas of
danger just as the surgeon must operate in order to save a life, whether or not psychological difficulties will result. One may, however, be allowed to wish for the best possible conditions for children's evacuation. It seems that young children cannot be expected
to make any adjustment in groups before they are ready to form a transference to the
teacher. According to our theory and statistical material they are able to do so only after
their fourth year. Children younger than this should preferably stay with their mothers
or be boarded out in foster-homes, where a substitute mother can take care of one to
three children. When the child is ready to be part of a group we can expect that he
will stand the trauma of a longer separation from mother more easily. The same consideration should hold in the question of whether children should be sent away to
boarding schools or camps, where they would be separated from their mothers for long
periods.

V.

In observing groups of children we cannot help comparing them with the group-formations of adults. Freud has pointed out what libidinal factors are responsible for making people in groups behave differently from individuals. He emphasized that people in groups are apt to regress to infantile levels.

Looking at people who are easily inclined to join one group after another, we are struck by the similarity in their behavior to that of adolescents. They are entirely devoted to their leader, unable to be critical of him or his ideas; they are unable to face or to discuss reasonably criticism of their viewpoint which is, of course, that of the group to which they belong. When they are disappointed for one reason or another, they turn against the leader, the group, and the ideas for which it stands, and are most likely to become bitter enemies who form or join an opposing group. There are also individuals who stick to the leader or the group whatever development he or it may take. They are tied to both, and entirely helpless and hopeless without them.

It seems that the group, like other situations in life, revives old patterns to which the person responds according to his own fixations. We know that the neurotic lives to a varying degree in the shadow of his past. He has difficulties in seeing reality for what it is at the present moment. The group which the individual has joined to further a certain cause revives in him the old situation in which he found consolation and reassurance for his infantile anxieties. He regresses to the level at which he needed the group for his own purposes. The reason why he originally joined it becomes secondary.

It is obvious that education plays an important part in establishing the adult's relationship to the group. The more mature a person is, the more valuable his contribution to the group will be. The degree of maturity to which education will try to develop the children will, however, greatly depend on the degree of maturity which the society, whose servant education is, will find desirable in its future citizens.

THE PSYCHOLOGY OF GANG FORMATION AND THE TREATMENT OF JUVENILE DELINQUENTS[1]

By FRITZ REDL, Ph.D. (Detroit) [2]

This is not a clinical study of delinquent juveniles exposed to psychoanalytic treatment. On the other hand, it is not a sociological essay on "society and the individual" either. It might best de described as an attempt to make an analysis of the group psychological conditions under which delinquent traits are reinforced or counteracted, as the case may be. It is the assumption of the author that such a study, while it assumes its final meaning only after it is connected with specific clinical material, may be of stimulation value for the psychiatrist on his job.

Which Delinquents Are we Talking About?

While it is impossible to load this little paper with the task of establishing and defending a categorization of delinquent cases or a definition of delinquency, we should like to clarify the way in which the word is being used here, just so as to avoid major terminological misunderstandings. We think we can distinguish four fundamentally different types of delinquency among juveniles. These are:

Type I: Basically healthy individuals whose delinquent behavior is a natural defense against *wrong handling, a wrong setting* in which to live, or against *traumatic experiences* of certain types.

Type II: Basically non-delinquent youngsters who are drifting into delinquent behavior on the basis of some acute adolescent *growth confusion*.

Type III: Delinquencies which are really *"on a neurotic basis"*, by which we mean that the delinquent behavior in itself is part of a neurosis, or that it is developed in order to disguise one.

1. Read before the American Psychoanalytic Association, Philadelphia, May, 1944.
2. From the Department of Social Work and Public Affairs, Wayne University.

Type IV: "Genuine Delinquency"—by which we mean certain disturbances in the Impulse System of the individual, and/or malformations of ego, superego and ego ideal, in intensity or content.

It seems to me that type III has so far been the most successful domain of psychoanalytic treatment: where the delinquency of a juvenile is really only part of or a superstructure over a neurosis, it is logical to expect that it will clear up soon after this neurosis in itself has been removed. However, type IV seems to puzzle the psychoanalyst no end. Treatment often seems to go through phases encouraging good prognoses, in order to end up by sudden and unexpected relapses all along the line, in spite of an obviously positive transference to the analyst. It is this type I shall exclusively select for discussion today—needless to say that I refer to these types not in strict isolation from each other, but mainly in regard to emphasis and preponderance.

Group Psychological Support of Delinquent Traits

Too long have we indulged in stereotyping the "delinquent" along the lines of psychiatric romanticism. According to these theories the genuine delinquent is the "a-social" or "anti-social" individual, too egotistic and narcissistic to submit to the demands of "society", and bent on getting the gratification of his impulses against the limitations of society. The "lone wolf" against "the world" idea is still clearly traceable even in clinical descriptions of our time. There is no doubt that representatives of such types do exist, and this is not an attempt to deny them or to wave away their importance. However, at least as far as delinquent juveniles go, it seems to us that an entirely different type is much more frequent and less studied. This type comes closer to what Topping, Hewitt, and Jenkins[3] used to call the "pseudosocial"—though "pseudo-anti-social" would probably be a better term.

The confusion about this type rises out of a stereotyped use of the term "society"—talking of it as if it were a unified code of ethics to which "everybody adheres", while only the mean and befuddled delinquent doesn't see the light. Well, there is no such thing. Our delinquent youngsters do not live in a group psychological vacuum against "society". Society itself is not a simple and unified structure, but highly substratified into thousands of little subcultures, all of them vitally different from each other in essential items.

3. Ruth Topping, "The Treatment of the Pseudosocial Boy", *American Journal of Orthopsychiatry*, April, 1943. Richard L. Jenkins and Lester Hewitt, "Types of Personality Structure Encountered in Child Guidance Clinics", ibid., January, 1944.

What really happens with our delinquent juveniles could more adequately be described this way: He refuses to identify with exactly that substratification of society which the parents or the law-enforcing middle class represent. He rather identifies with the one or other sub-group, the group code of which is not as prohibitive of some of his vital gratifications as the other seems to be. This subgroup identification may happen in three ways:

1. *On a class-basis.* The delinquent juvenile in some cases makes an enthusiastic identification with "the tough way of life" versus the "sissy stuff" that school teachers and middle class church boards represent to him in the name of "the law".

2. *On a development basis.* This delinquent juvenile identifies heavily with the unwritten code of his *peer-culture,* versus the code of behavior represented by "the Adult"—which includes the adult of his own social stratum. Since many laws forbid the juvenile the same gratification that are not only permissible but openly bragged about by the adult of his own subcultural pattern, this in itself constitutes a simple source for "juvenile delinquency".

3. *On a neighborhood gang basis.* The third possibility is not only not contradictory to the first two, it is often nothing but a more concrete expression of either or both. In fact, sometimes this small "neighborhood gang" is nothing but the concrete way in which the youngster meets his "class culture" or his "adolescent peer code", as we mentioned them before. In other cases, however, it must be admitted that some such "gangs" add their own quirks of code deviations and assume a more specialized content.

It is true that conventionally, the word "gang" is usually limited to these smaller neighborhood groups mentioned under 3. For the purpose of this study, however, we shall ignore this fact and talk about "gang psychology" whenever either of the three group psychological ties is referred to. Without having a chance to justify such terminological deviation at this point, we can venture the following statement:

The larger number of the "genuine delinquent" type does not comprise "individuals against the group", but "members of group I against group II". In fact, we are ready to go even so far as to say: far from being the "strong personality that defies law and order", the genuine delinquent is deeply dependent upon *group psychological support* so as to be able to "defy law and order" and to "afford" his delinquency at all. The resistance we meet in our attempts to "treat" this delinquent, then, is not only due to the personal resistance any individual would develop in the course of a therapeutic procedure, the laws of which we know so well from the clinical picture of the neurotic. The forces that resist our efforts in the case of delinquent juveniles are richer than this: besides his "personal resistance" the delinquent juvenile is equipped with excellent "group psychological defenses" which he plays against our therapeutic attempts with tremendous force.

Needless to say that the nature of just these group psychological defenses must be of great interest to the therapist.

Just How Does "Gang Psychology" Do It?

The intricacies of the way in which group psychological elements hit the organism of the individual, and the process of group formation as well as leadership effect are too elaborate a story to be gone into here. At a previous occasion I have tried to discuss ten different bases for group psychological effect on individuals and I should like to summarize here some of the suggestions directly related to the topic before us.[4]

It seems to me that the operation of "gang psychology" supports the individual's delinquent trends especially in three basic ways:

1. The process of *"magical seduction"*.

   By this we mean that whatever delinquency-directed impulses are active within the individual member, they are "reinforced"—made more intensive and more daring—within the gang climate in two different ways:

   (a) Through the mere *visualization* of guilt—and fearless drive-satisfaction by other members of the group. The infectious value of the "bad example", which is hard to demonstrate in a few words, can best be remembered if we think of the increase in anxieties compulsive children experience when exposed to the display of reckless behavior in their less inhibited pals. The "increase" in defenses in such a moment is direct proof of an underlying increase in drive-upsurge.

   (b) Through the *"exculpation magic of the initiatory act"*. We mean by this mechanism the ability of the group leader or co-member to put existing inhibitions out of force by simply "doing things first" and thus bringing about unconscious exculpation.

   In both cases the individual has his "seduction" guaranteed, which is one direct service the gang renders to delinquency aspirants.

2. *Ego Support through organization of ways and means.*

   Our formula for the organizing function of the central person in gang formational processes reads thus:

   "The central person renders an important service to the ego of the potential group members. He does so by providing the means for the

44. "Group Emotion and Leadership", *Psychiatry*, V, 1942, 573 ff.

satisfaction of common undesirable drives and thus prevents guilt feelings, anxieties and conflicts which otherwise would be involved in that process for them."

Or, in other words: Johnny is ready guiltlessly to participate in a raid on a box car or candy store. However, he would feel too guilty to *plan* such a thing, too scared that something might go wrong. He can afford his delinquency if somebody else does the planning for him, and if somebody else will shoot the guard, if it should come to that.

Through this mechanism a wider range of delinquent satisfactions becomes possible than the individual superego of the delinquent could otherwise afford.

3. *Guilt-insurance through coverage by the group code.*

It cannot be expected that a delinquent juvenile has no trace of ego criticisms or conscience left. Therefore at least the one or other of his delinquent gratifications has to be bought at superego-expense. Those who are not only interested in occasional illegal satisfactions but are bent on developing good and thorough delinquent character traits so as to be morally tax-exempt ever hereafter, need the group psychological support especially badly. Gang psychology operates for them on the following basis: through their emotional tie to the group they eventually identify with the "group code"—which corresponds to what we could call superego in an individual. It is the residue of all values the group "stands for". This group code supplants the individual superego and puts it out of business—temporarily, first; on a retirement basis, later on. It is not true that delinquent youngsters do "not have any superego". They may have a very finicky one, indeed—only its content is filled with the group code which may be highly different from or even contradictory to the societal demands on the basis of which laws are written. Their conscience as well as their ego ideal is still in operation—but it functions only within the confine of the "group code".

On the basis of these three mechanisms, "gang psychology" enables the youngster to enjoy otherwise guilt-loaded or dangerous gratifications without the expense of guilt feeling and fear. It even offers him all the gratifications of "morality" at the same time: pride, moral indignation, the feeling of "being in the right" are still maintained, only they were carefully defined in terms of group code criteria.

Group Code Defenses

However, the production of identifications with the group code would not be enough. There is no doubt that it works very visibly as long as the group is "together". The question is what happens to all these group code identifications as soon as the individual steps out into "private life" or even into "group affiliations" of a different nature?

Can groups take a chance and just expect that the individual's group loyalty will be so strong that nobody else's value system will ever make a dent on their member?

The fact is—groups do not take such a chance. On the contrary, they all seem to be very highly concerned with this as their greatest danger: that the group code identification of individuals may be successfully attacked or may peter out in non-group-life. This is true of all groups, no matter what type. Thus the greatest fear of the "educator" is that the children so obediently identified with the good and the beautiful might be impressed by some dirty ragamuffin who does not believe in Emily Post and succeeds in undermining Johnny's virtue in no time. In the same way, however, the "tough" organizer of a delinquent gang takes good care that his clientele is imbued with thorough contempt against "sissy stuff teachers want you to believe in", lest they admire the "wrong" guy and fall in love with virtue overnight.

Therefore, groups have developed *special mechanisms* by which they inoculate their members against this danger. These mechanisms are not visible while the group is together. They can easily be studied, however, in retrospect, when we watch clashes between a group member and outgroup standards of a different code-content. To make it possible to describe these mechanisms of "group code defense" in short space, we shall introduce a few auxiliary concepts here.

We shall use the term *"outgroup"* for any other group but the one whose code we are talking about.

We shall call *"overgroup"* the larger organization of which the group we are talking about is a part.

We shall talk about *"code-dangerous outgroups"* and mean such groups whose code is basically hostile to the code of the group we are talking about.

The following seem to be the mechanisms of defense by which groups secure the post-group loyalty of their members against outside attack:

1. *Segregation and Individual Hatred.*

Some groups demand of their members that they avoid people who are not members of the same group psychological unit or that they hate those who belong to groups of a different kind. Such segregation demands and individual hatred are carefully practised and prepared when the group is together, and reinforced through the application of well-known devices long studied and well-described by the scientists who do research on propaganda. It is this mechanism through which even large group psychological units operate—political parties, religious bodies, racial and class structures. The success with which racial superiority theories can be maintained on the basis of such devices in a large part of the population is so well known through contemporary history that we can save ourselves details here.[5]

It should be added, though, that this is a very extreme technique applicable only under certain very specific conditions. Besides, only basically very insecure groups usually have to stoop to such primitive mechanisms.

2. *Depersonalizing Symbolization.*

By this artificially introduced term we refer to a rather complex process which can be described thus.

Some groups do not insist that their members keep away from non-members or from members of other groups. They do not need to be so fussy—they do a better job of inoculating their code loyalty to begin with. They allow their members to associate freely with anybody, to like or dislike people as they wish. However, the moment a person belongs to a code-dangerous outgroup, things are different: in that moment a beautifully prepared mechanism goes into action. People who belong to a code-dangerous outgroup are not to be considered as "people" any more, but only as symbolizing the value system of this outgroup which is to be rejected and fought. They rob these people of their weight as "persons", they demand that the group member consider them as just that much representation of the hostile unit.

This defense seems to be a very efficient device—people can afford to stick to their race prejudices, for example, and brag that "some of their best friends are Jews". They can do so without feeling disloyal to their antisemitic cause—for *in items that matter* they know that these "friends" will certainly lose their quality of personal relationship and will be treated by them as just so many representatives of the "code-dangerous outgroups". With this safety device in their pockets, they can be allowed to associate freely with whom they like, without any basic danger being involved to the code of their group.

3. *Tabu Against Code-dangerous Identification.*

The two previous mechanisms are not applicable universally enough either; therefore groups have developed a third one for last ditch defense: their members can have all the freedom of even entering libidinous ties with non-group members or even outgroup members, as long as they only remember this: you may *love* a member of the outgroup, but you must never "identify" with him, especially not where code-dangerous items are involved. This mechanism insures the tough businessman from allowing his socially inclined and beloved wife to have too much "influence" on his loyalty to his business associates . . . it also enables the member of a delinquent gang

5. See A. McLung Lee and N. Humphrey, *Race Riot,* The Dryden Press, 1943.

to become an efficient member of many other groups without really jeopardizing the code of his own. This mechanism can be studied beautifully by watching the behavior of some delinquency identified youngsters in a camp situation. Their development looks somewhat like this: they start with avoidance and suspicion of the adult group leader, since she is definitely an "adult" and outsider on that basis. After the adult is able to crash through this, they enter strong personal affectionate relationships with her. But the moment this adult acts as a "representative of the outgroup" (the world of adults), she is "depersonalized" and becomes nothing but a symbolic representative of the hostile code. Thus youngsters who have obviously "loved and adored" their counsellor will turn rudely against her whenever she meets them in such a role of outgroup representation. In cases where this can be broken down, the youngster is pushed against this last ditch stand: he accepts the adult as a friend, he also accepts her leadership and discipline. But the moment it comes to criticisms or discussions of certain code-dangerous items, like the matter of "stealing" or "delinquency"—the youngster withdraws any relationship he has previously developed, closes up like a clam, and refuses to identify with what the adult stands for.

In a nutshell, what we want to point out is this: Through the inoculative mechanism of gang psychology, delinquent juveniles act under the influence of their gang loyalties even when they operate in other groups or are in consultative isolation with an adult psychiatrist. They will protect their own identification with the delinquent group code by either avoiding or hating us as persons, or by treating us as though we represented a code-hostile outgroup, or they will feel safe in going far in love as well as identification with us, except in code-dangerous items.

Implication for Psychotherapy

If some of the previous observations are true, then it is obvious that they must have important bearing upon limitations as well as chances of psychiatric therapy with delinquent juveniles.

The prognosis for treatment of delinquents has been a hesitant one to begin with, and the odds against which the psychiatrist works have been expounded at great length and are so well known that we shall not endeavor to list them here again. The additions to which our group psychological observations challenge us are these:

I. *Group Psychological Barriers of Treatment.*

1. The psychiatrist who sees his patient in his private consultation room or at a guidance clinic—which means in group psychological isolation —is still "marked" by the fact that he is an obvious representative of an "outgroup". Thus he finds that his client, over and above whatever resistances he would have developed anyway on the basis of his case

history or through the treatment process, is constantly being furnished with *group psychologically produced defenses*. This is not only true of youngsters who are actually members of delinquent gangs. For the mobilization of defenses mentioned above it is sufficient that the youngster be identified with what is commonly referred to as a "tough guy philosophy" of life. These "group psychologically produced" defenses are not traceable without a thorough insight into the nature of the group climate of which the patient feels himself a part, and they offer strong resistance against techniques which are otherwise effective with the neurotic client.

2. The psychiatrist who works on the staff of an institution, or of an agency that is closely identified with one, is marked to begin with as a member not only of an outgroup, but of *the* hostile overgroup against which most of the gang code is directed in its most vicious heat. This situation is most glaringly exemplified in the grotesque situation we find in many court clinics or guidance clinics that try to serve out detention homes or punitive institutions for juvenile delinquents. In those cases youngsters are stored for weeks and months in a group psychological climate well known to be most delinquency-productive of all, and even more vicious in the defenses with which it furnishes its participants than the delinquent gang itself. Several times a week the youngster is taken out of this climate for an hour or a half, is exposed to the influence of a psychiatrist in interview contact and is from there sent back to a place where every wall oozes gang psychological defense.

The situation, while pretty universal, is just about as grotesque as if a hospital were to offer pharmacological treatment to pneumonia cases but would take good care that the air they breathe in between these applications is carefully emptied of oxygen. . . .

II. *Group Psychological Chances.*

If the Group Medium has such powers over individual resistance even beyond the immediate presence of the group, then this should encourage us in an attempt at harnessing those same powers into the service of therapy. The following opportunities seem to offer themselves as a possibility at this stage of the game:

1. *Supportive Group Climate.*

Instead of working in group psychological midair, special types of group climate might be created or initiated by the psychiatrist and his helpers, which would counteract the original "delinquent defenses" and at the same time provide for the normal group psychological needs growing youngsters have anyway. In saying this we mean more, of course, than the general advice of sending youngsters into the Boy Scouts or to the Y because "groups are good for them". We are thinking of an elaborate, near to pharmacologically-precise, prescription of just the type of group organization, climate and leadership that would fit treatment needs exactly. Our experiences in the "Detroit Group Project"—an agency created by the School for Social Work and Public Affairs for just such type of research—encourage us to think that such group psychological prescriptions could be worked out with some degree of accuracy right now.

2. *Group-Climatic Participation of the Therapist.*

In some cases we have been able to watch the disappearance of even heavy defenses of the group psychologically produced type, as soon as the psychiatrist did not operate in group psychological midair, but became part and parcel of the group life of the delinquent juvenile himself. By this we do not mean that he should join a delinquent gang, nor is it sufficient for him to be administratively on the "staff" of a group work agency or institution. We mean, however, that he should live in or close to the group psychological facilities created for the youngster's therapy, and that he be considered as "belonging" in terms of the member-psychology of the youngsters themselves. Especially in camp settings—preferably of the all-year-round type—it can easily be observed that some youngsters are ready to surrender group psychological resistances towards the person who is part of their group life. Thus the defenses the therapist has to work with are reduced to the individual minimum he would meet anyway. Whether the psychiatrist himself should be part of this group setting and to what degree, or to what extent cooperation with a group therapist can be worked out successfully, is not to be decided at this point.

Conclusions

1. Psychotherapy with delinquent juveniles, even if operating on the traditional interview basis, must not operate entirely in *"group psychological midair"*.

2. It is essential for the individual therapist to have as thorough a diagnostic picture of the *group psychological characteristics* of the climate the youngster lives in as of the individual dynamics of the case.

3. For certain types of cases—especially those with highly developed "tabu against code-dangerous identifications", it is advisable to undertake treatment in a setting which combines group therapy with the individual approach and in which the psychiatrist or his group therapeutic helper is part and parcel of the group in which the youngster lives.

4. It is desirable that group psychologically correct prescriptions be worked out by which *supportive treatment* in and through the group

can be added to the work of the psychiatrist within or outside of institutional situations. Places where youngsters are being stored must not only comply with the best that is known in practice educationally and clinically, but they must absolutely obey the laws of *group psychological antisepsis*. At this moment there is hardly a handful of such places in existence in the whole United States.

SURVEYS AND COMMENTS

GREGORY BATESON and MARGARET MEAD: BALINESE CHARACTER, A PHOTOGRAPHIC ANALYSIS [1]

Comments by BERTRAM D. LEWIN, M.D. (New York)

Balinese Character is an important book. With the lucidity and succinctness we are accustomed to expect of her, Miss Mead begins with a fifty-page account of the authors' observations of a year and a half in Bali. The book is "not about Balinese custom, but about the Balinese . . . as living persons, moving, standing, eating, sleeping, dancing, going into trance". A hundred large plates follow (about eight photographs to each plate) with the pictures arranged to bring out ontogenetic relationships. For example, one series of pictures consists of a little boy playing with his genital, another playing with a toy stuck between his legs, then a man dancing ceremonially with a lance held in the identical position; another series shows a little boy playing with a bird on a string, then men with fighting cocks. Bateson, to whom the photographs are mainly due, illuminates and clarifies them by legends that give added observations or relevant comments. He explains, for example, that the sling which the evil Witch carries in a certain popular play bears the same name as the sling in which a mother carries her baby. In order of arrangement, the plates parallel the subjects discussed in the preceding exposition, with many cross-references and mutual clarifications. The book is a descriptive atlas of many important Balinese experiences from birth through burial.

The wealth of observation and the stylistic economy of the presentation preclude an exhaustive summary of this book. Nor is this due only to quantity; the book is that type of scientific report which itself is so nearly a true statement that reading becomes observation. The following account is therefore not a resumé, but an extensive selection from among the facts which are nearest to the psychoanalyst's field of interest.

The birth of a Balinese child is a sort of Epiphany. Before he is born he is courteously addressed by the midwife and invited to appear. The baby is a god, its divinity persists for about eighteen months. (At other times, conversely, gods are treated as children.) Besides being a god, the baby is an autocosmic symbol—i.e., an object in the outside world identified as an extension of a given person's body. In this instance the baby is treated as "something midway between a toy and a puppet", to speak descriptively. He is carried about almost

---

[1] New York Academy of Sciences, 1942. Pp. xvi + 277.

continuously, passed from arm to arm in a crowd, flicked under the chin, tweaked at various places on his body. His penis is given occasional repeated tugs. He is the constant plaything of his mother, her friends, and of the children who act as his nursery maids. He is called "mouse", "caterpillar", "grub"; these small nibblers appear in paintings of corpses and "the woman who has refused to have children on earth is punished by having to suckle a caterpillar in hell"—perhaps in what an analyst would call self-retributive wish fulfillment. Toys are handled autocosmically by children. "When Balinese children are offered a mechanical mouse, or a doll, or a toy koala, they do not construct scenes with these toys. . . . They take one toy at a time, and handle it as part of their own body, if they are boys; or they treat the toy as a baby, or more occasionally as a hand, if they are girls."

Balinese children are carried on their mothers' left hip in or out of a sling. The baby's left arm is free, his right arm tucked in next to the breast. When the child reaches for something with the free arm, this arm is grasped and pulled back by the mother, who then pulls out the right arm. From this originates a great willingness to be passively molded, which is later exploited for example, by dancing teachers, who themselves practically dance, holding their charges before them and molding their minutest motions. This quality the authors call "waxy flexibility", though they do not explicitly equate it with clinical catalepsy.

Infant feeding is picturesque. The child is suckled and fed solid food practically from the start. The suckling phase is very prolonged; the child, carried for perhaps eighteen months, turns for a drink whenever he wishes. Solid food is first chewed by the mother, then pushed as a wad into the spluttering child's mouth. The action is rightly denominated an "attack on the mouth". There are numerous consequences of this double dietary system: the dichotomy persists later in life when "snacks" and liquid food are pleasurable, and regular meals and solid food painful, as many eating customs show. The mouth is protected in various ways; it is a psychologically sensitive zone. The eating of meals is accompanied by shame, the food for meals and feasts is pre-chopped, and at ceremonial feasts as much penalty is entailed by not taking one's share as by taking too much. There is a good deal of finger sucking and, later, fingering of the mouth throughout life.

Although the Balinese are not clean people, feces are regarded with disgust, while "urine is unimportant and the act of urination is performed very casually and without conspicuous modesty". Defecation indeed becomes a private function, performed in the secrecy of the outhouse and quite a fuss is made over a child's defecating in the wrong place. Before training is completed the apparently ubiquitous dogs gulp the feces, even while they are being extruded. In certain feasts for the lower spirits, where the eating is accompanied by shouting and revelry, with a certain amount of "rowdyism reminiscent of behavior in handling a corpse", offerings laid out on the ground for the spirits are actually eaten by the dogs. Scrambling for money thrown on the ground at funeral ceremonies suggests an analogy to the dog's scrambling for the scraps of food (and feces). The body is in some ways thought of as "a tube"; the parts of the body are given a certain amount of separate and independent life.

Fear is so early and general a reaction and so pervades Balinese behavior, that Margaret Mead considers it the basis for the general character formation. The child, it is emphasized, is not afraid *of* his mother but *with* her. Constantly in physical contact with her, he takes fright when she is afraid or when she deliberately frightens him by simulating fear.[2] Fear later is an enjoyable emotion, and actors conventionally portray it in dances. Fear may lead to a peculiar kind of sleep, a commonly observed manifestation in all age groups. The authors tell how Balinese employees, sent ahead by truck to set up camp, were overcome by the strangeness of the place and fell asleep at once. Photographs show two men falling asleep while being tried for theft.

Described and depicted is another Balinese peculiarity which resembles the "Tantalus situation". It consists in stimulating a child's emotional activity without permitting a climax. The child, flirted with or aggressively teased to a high pitch of affection or rage, is suddenly ignored. The adult goes into an absent-minded state of "awayness" and is completely heedless of the child, even though he is in a howling tantrum. Such stimulation is persistent; Balinese apparently spend a large part of their time petting or roughing children, with a good deal of tugging at little boys' penises. This tugging gets progressively rougher, till finally when the child is able to escape, he often backs away from any adult that makes a gesture in his direction.

Sibling rivalry is intense and overt. After the breast baby becomes the "knee baby", he tries violently to distract his mother and to act out his hatred and resentment of the new baby. He turns for consolation to the father, who plays with him, cuddles him, instructs him, and sometimes even suckles him a little. When the child is about four or five he is usually referred to as the third from the youngest—for that is then his usual position in the family. Regardless of whether he has younger siblings, however, his personality changes. He becomes seclusive, brooding and sullen; he withdraws into a detached state of "awayness" (which will be commented upon later in this review). About this age the larger social relations develop, the girls becoming child nurses, the boys helping their fathers in the fields.

Sibling rivalry is well understood by the Balinese. Figure 2 on plate 70 shows a native drawing of two brothers and their mother. The younger child is on a higher level and drinking, while the older brother is farther from the mother, kneeling and holding a dish of food. "The mother's face is turned toward the younger child and she holds a bowl in her hands." Unless there is some error, it also looks as if she were exposing her genital to the older

2. In describing this type of infantile fear Bateson and Mead apparently have publication priority over Freud and Burlingham (1). (Reference at end of paper.) Among the five types of fear shown by infants during the London air raids, their type four, fear through identification with the mother's fear, is of the same sort. "A child in the infant stage of one, two, three, and four years of age will shake and tremble with the anxiety of its mother, and this anxiety will impart itself the more thoroughly to the child the younger it is." The other four types of fear were the familiar "real anxiety", "fear of instinct", and "fear of conscience"; and a fifth type was the compulsive repetition of a frightening experience with loss of the love object.

Analysts and observers of children are nearer in method to Bateson and Mead than are those analysts who treat adults, as later instances will show. Apparently type four predominated in Bali, leaving a query as to the presence or absence of the other types.

brother. Two characters from a well-known folk drama are shown in a figure on plate 12: "I Tjoepak, the gross, boastful and cowardly elder brother, and I Gerantang, the refined and brave younger brother. . . . The picture shows I Gerantang . . . acting as a servant in washing I Tjoepak's hands, and the meal of sucking pig [a hint of the elder brother's feeling about the younger brother], on which I Tjoepak will gorge himself. In the story they go out to kill a demon (represented by a Witch mask). I Gerantang climbs down a rope into the demon's hole and kills the demon. I Tjoepak takes away the rope and goes home and claims the credit, leaving I Gerantang to starve in the hole . . ." He escapes, becomes a baby, is cared for by a fisherman's wife, and finally returns to expose I Tjoepak.

In the period of latency, girls take part in ceremonial dances and religious rituals; the boys play in gangs and are generally neglected by their elders. At some time between infancy and puberty children of both sexes have their teeth filed, as a *rite de passage*. "Courtship either for marriage or for a love affair, is a matter of glances and a few stolen words, and the romantic excitement steadily dies down after the first encounter. Once married, a Balinese husband finds that the girl he has married does indeed act like his mother—for she knows no other pattern of personal relationship—his brief unreal ardor cools and he counts himself lucky if he begets children." In the theater a favorite theme resembles the Leah and Rachel story; the hero has the unattractive sister palmed off on him. The courtship dances include the baby sling, the magic Witch's cloth, and in it the Witch (who is either very old and ugly or young and desirable) plays an obvious mother role.

The most extraordinary piece of drama, presented in this book with great vividness, is the Witch play, which contains "the definitive dramatic theme of the Balinese parent-child relations" and "not only expresses the residue in the adults of what they experienced as children, but is also watched by children and shapes their reading of the experiences to which they are subjected daily". The Witch is angry at a king, and trains her disciples—little boys and girls play their roles—to harass the land. The king sends an emissary to fight the Witch. He fails, retires from the stage, but reappears as a Dragon, and Dragon and Witch hold an altercation in ecclesiastical old Javanese. "Followers of the Dragon, armed with krisses, enter and approach the Witch ready to attack her. But she waves her magic cloth—the cloth baby sling—and after each attack they crouch down before her, magically cowed. Finally they rush upon her in pairs, stabbing ineffectively at the Witch who has become a limp bundle in their tense arms. She is uninvolved and offers no resistance, but one by one they fall on the ground in deep trance, some limp, some rigid. From this trance they are aroused by the Dragon who claps his jaw over them, or by his priest sprinkling his holy water. Now, able to move again but not returned to normal consciousness, they move about in a somnambulistic state, turning their daggers which were powerless against the Witch, against their own breasts, fixing them against a spot which is said to itch unbearably." The trance is a mixture of agony and ecstasy. "Some men actually fall backward onto the ground with an extreme backward bending of the trunk, and lie on the ground writhing in some sort of orgasmic climax."

The trance is said to occur in different proportions in different communities. In some villages everyone has had a trance, in others none; but every

Balinese has witnessed trance often. We are promised a special study called "Trance in Bali" by Jane Belo, who took part in the expedition. Balinese of all ages readily enter a trance, especially by means of a device which consists of two rods with a connecting string, to which the person holds. One rod is then pounded up and down rhythmically and the vibration transmitted through the string.

Balinese funerals are fascinatingly depicted in this book. They are rowdy affairs, the ceremonial prolonged and repetitive. The corpse or what is left of it or the simulacrum of it is buried over and over, with a variety of exhumations and cremations in gaudy funeral towers, including cremations and burials of its symbolical resurrections as "souls"—i.e., of puppets or animal representations. The mood of the funeral is excited and rowdy, with much tense boasting, laughing and joking. This same mood was referred to in the description of the feast for the lower spirits.

The above account is by no means exhaustive. Other reviewers, with other special interests, will no doubt be more impressed by other facts. Psychoanalysts will undoubtedly be more impressed and accessible to the tenor of Bateson's and Mead's thoughts than will a classical anthropologist. Their proof of the influence of infantile conflicts on the content of Balinese drama and art is very strong. On the other hand some of their explanations do not go far enough, and might be reconsidered here.

To begin with, a comment on the title of the book, *Balinese Character*, may be in order. The authors explain in the introduction that they find in Bali that "the ordinary adjustment of the individual approximates in form the sort of ·maladjustment which, in our own cultural setting, we call schizoid". The analyst would not dissent from this; the moody, inward, sensitive Balinese can be called schizoid. But he would caution against expecting too much from such a name-giving, and a certain amount of caution is warranted in regard to the concept of character, at least in psychiatry. Such terms as "schizoid character", "hysterical character", "obsessive character" and the like are purely descriptive; they are artefacts of psychiatric or psychoanalytic practice. A "schizoid" person is so called because he resembles in many particulars a schizophrenic; the idea has no special dynamic theoretical foundation, and due to its historic origin has one rather bad connotation. It tends to be considered a counter-term of "cycloid" and this antonymy leads into the innate character and constitution folklore of Kraepelin, Jung and Kretschmer.

Bateson and Mead must be absolved of any such counter-revolutionary intention. They state that the child's anxiety situations give substance to later character. This is a fruitful idea, makes sense to analysts, and brings to mind the work of Greenacre on "borderline personalities"(2). The best that analysts can do with the idea of character is still to think of it as a mixture or combination of sublimations and defense reactions, and in specifying these the usefulness of the general concept diminishes. As Ernest Jones pointed out in comparing the British and German methods of selecting army officers(3), it is better to assess the capacity for behavior than to enumerate the possession of specific qualities. Bateson and Mead notably do this, so that, regardless of any theory of character their observations are accessible to psychoanalytic critique.

The cannibal impulses are evident; not only in children, but in many fields of activity not directly connected with infant feeding. The newborn baby is a "god" till he gets big enough to trust to his own strength and no longer needs his "divinity" to protect him; for food is also a "god". So are corpses "gods". Feces, too, are apparently food, certainly to the scavenger dogs, and child training in bowel habits seems largely concerned in seeing that the feces should not be eaten. The number of times the Balinese change their minds about burying or not burying a corpse and the barbecue picnic atmosphere of the funeral suggests that they are in conflict as to whether to eat the corpse or not. Those who have analyzed patients with cremated relatives will appreciate the interpretation that cremation is "cooking". Viewing the range of cannibal impulses in Bali, regardless of their accessibility to consciousness, it is not strange that the mouth should be "attacked" so early and that the eating of solid food should be made painful and shameful. In cramming food into the spluttering mouths of tiny babies, the mothers appear to be vicariously attacking their own cannibal impulses.

Certain ideas brought out in other contexts are familiar to analysts as derivatives of cannibal impulses. Among these is the Balinese conception of the body as a tube, a version of the body-phallus equation, which is an oral fantasy(4, 5, 6, 7). Another is the idea that the body is constituted of separable parts that have each an independent life. This is related to what Bromberg and Schilder(8) have reported as the "dismemberment fantasy" of drug deliria, for which Malcove(9) discovered the correct interpretation in her study of children—that the dismemberment is a reminiscence of food being cut up.

As to such matters as the superego, nothing very definite can be inferred from the presented material. It is impossible to distinguish the type of anxiety that afflicts the Balinese at different ages. The presentation makes this all the more difficult by emphasizing the similarities rather than the differences between child and adult. It is here that the analyst will miss most those products of the psychoanalytic technique that enable him to judge the nature and strength of the defense mechanisms. However, when Bateson remarks that "the relationship between Balinese child nurse [herself a young child] and baby is still very far from being comparable to the relationships in which, in Western cultures, the image of an adult is introjected to form a personalized superego", his statement is quite plausible.

Nowhere in the little boy's direct behavior, as seen in this work, is there evidence of any hostility to his father or of any desire for genital congress with his mother. He is shown hating his mother and his siblings, and being sexually aroused and frustrated by her. As a man, we are told, he will be relatively impotent in marriage and disappointed in his wife or mistress. Far from hating his real father, he is found turning to him as a kind playmate and protector. The Dragon-father in the drama is a lovable puppy personality. The brother is the usual enemy. The teasing, narcissistic mother, who certainly resembles the mother of many Occidental schizophrenics, appears as the hated evil Witch. To judge by the public presentations in art and the drama, the Balinese accept the existence of hostility between siblings and between mother and child but do not know of sexual rivalry between father and son. This is the superficial interpretation.

To leave it at that and to say that the Balinese have no oedipus complex would be an error. The drama of the Witch and the Dragon seems not fully explained as a revenge on the bad mother by the good father for what she has done to the child. The young men approach the Witch with knives, and when they turn these against their own breasts, "play dead", and go into a trance, the Witch and Dragon keep up the fight. This suggests a "primal scene". Margaret Mead tells us that for a long while the child is held in contact with the mother, and is sometimes even in the same bed during delivery. A suspicion (which is capable of confirmation or rejection) arises that he is also there during parental sexual intercourse, and that this occurs while he is in the hypnagogic state that precedes sleep; or that in some other way sleep and erotic excitement combine. At the theater, we are told, the spectators identify themselves with the actors as they did with their mothers, "molding" their bodies accordingly. In fact, the facility with which adult feeling is communicated to babies is one of the author's surest observations. The usual method of sending children into a trance is to communicate to them through a string the rhythm of a stick, which a man pounds up and down against a bowl. This trance, like the erotic sleep of the men in the Witch drama, would be an equivalent of infantile masturbation, and repetitive of the erotic sleep during the primal scene. The curious fear-narcolepsy, which resembles clinical states reported in the first World War(10), may be interpreted as the same reaction with an altered (anxious) content. In short, we seem to have a "conversion symptom", "neurotic" sleep, which is a "genital" manifestation of the oedipus complex, a reminiscence of the primal scene.[3]

A contributory bit of evidence is supplied by the authors in their observation that at the age of two or three the child's behavior undergoes a marked change, "regardless of whether another younger child is born in the family . . . although being displaced from the mother's attention would hasten the change", and it is suggested that the coarseness of the elder-brother stereotype in art and the drama is related to this stage of childhood. "The child's habitual postures and facial expression change toward coarseness. The corners of the mouth become drawn in so that the lips protrude, as though the child were constantly on the verge of tears." Photographs show the children self-absorbed, brooding or sullen.

The convincing description and illustrations permit a "blind" diagnosis. These children have a "primal depression", as described by that great psychoanalytic clinician, Karl Abraham(6). He reports the "infantile prototype of the melancholic depressions" of one of his adult manic-depressive patients. The infantile depression occurred when the patient was five, during a period in which he was the involuntary and "tortured" witness of parental coitus. Abraham writes: "I should like to speak of a 'primal depression' (Urverstimmung) originating in the little boy's oedipus complex. The longing of the child to win over the mother as an ally against the father was strikingly evident. His disappointment at having his own tender approaches repulsed came to a climax in the very exciting impressions he received in the parents' bed-

---

3. Sleep as an infantile masturbation equivalent is mentioned in "Symposium on Neurotic Disturbances in Sleep" (11) with some reference to the role of the primal scene. For some of the oral implications of the hypnagogic states, see Isakower (12).

room. Terrifying vindictive plans fermented in him, but because of his emotional ambivalence, they were impractical and destined to hopelessness. . . . In later years the child repeatedly renewed his attempts to be successful in his object-love. Each failure in this direction caused a mental state which was a true replica of the primal depression." This passage is quoted to suggest a parallel with the Witch drama, and as a possible clue to the marital disappointment of Balinese men.

As to castration anxiety, Plate 17 includes invaluable pictures of little children learning to walk. The anxious little boy, unsure of his balance, holds on to his penis; the little girl clasps her hands in front of her abdomen. The little boy, presumably, is putting first things first and in his anxiety is reassuring himself that he still has his penis; while the girl reassures herself about what ever it is she thinks she has there. Walking seems to be an erotic experience, fear of falling is equated to fear of losing the penis. The erotized locomotion is doubtless the basis for future sublimated dancing pleasure, in which, as a later illustration shows, the boy having become a man boldly holds aloft a lance pivoted on his pelvis. Bateson and Mead suggest that the locomotor anxiety is related to a sort of primitive agoraphobia, which repeats the child's fear of going too far from the stick to which he is tethered while he is learning to walk. Later, fears are not assuaged by clasping the genital, but through magic. Analysts will be reminded by these observations of Abraham's paper on loco-motor anxiety(13), in which he too refers to the dancing of his patients as expressions of erotized locomotion, and attributes their fear of walking to an infantile erotization of that function and its repression under the influence of castration fear. Fenichel discusses the same phenomena in two papers(14).

The Balinese attach great importance to a child's walking as soon as possible, and to the prevention of crawling. Their objection to crawling and to "animality" brings to mind Freud's remarks about the assumption of the erect posture and its influence on the instinctual history of the human race. The erect posture interferes with the pleasure obtained from smelling and from using the mouth as a direct organ of prehension. In Bali, certainly, it prevents children from identifying themselves with the coprophagic dogs. The human contempt for dogs, Freud(15) tells us in this same connection, is due to the dogs' lack of inhibitions in respect to feces. In children, it is evident, in some way the pride in walking offsets the loss of the "zonal" animal pleasures.

Besides furnishing data which intercalate so nicely with analytic theory and experience, the book furnishes its readers a rare esthetic treat. Both in choice of words and in the selection of photographs for reproduction, the authors display an impeccable taste. They admirably solve the difficulty, to which they refer in their introduction, of transmitting to their readers an immediate sense of Balinese life.

BIBLIOGRAPHY

1. Freud, A. and Burlingham, D., *War and Children*, New York, 1943, p. 32.
2. Greenacre, P., "The Predisposition to Anxiety", *Psychoanalytic Quarterly*, X, 1941.
3. Jones, E., "Psychology of War", *Psychoanalytic Quarterly*, XIV, 1945.

BALINESE CHARACTER

387

4. Tausk, V., "On the Origin of the 'Influencing Machine' in Schizophrenia", *Psychoanalytic Quarterly*, II, 1933.
5. Ferenczi, S., "Gulliver Phantasies", *International Journal of Psycho-Analysis*, IX, 1928; and also "Disease- or Patho-neuroses", in *Further Contributions to the Theory and Technique of Psychoanalysis*, London, 1926.
6. Abraham, K., "Development of the Libido", in *Selected Papers*, London, 1927.
7. Lewin, B. D., "The Body as Phallus", *Psychoanalytic Quarterly*, II, 1933.
8. Bromberg, W. and Schilder, P., "Psychologic Considerations in Alcoholic Hallucinosis —Castration and Dismemberment Motives", *International Journal of Psycho-Analysis*, XIV, 1933.
9. Malcove, L., "Bodily Mutilation and Learning to Eat", *Psychoanalytic Quarterly*, II, 1933.
10. Winterstein, H., *Schlaf und Traum*, Berlin, 1932.
11. Symposium on Neurotic Disturbances of Sleep, *International Journal of Psycho-Analysis*, XXIII, 1942.
12. Isakower, O., "A Contribution to the Patho-Psychology of Phenomena Associated with Falling Asleep", *International Journal of Psycho-Analysis*, XIX, 1938.
13. Abraham, K., "A Constitutional Basis of Locomotor Anxiety", in *Selected Papers*, London, 1927.
14. Fenichel, O., "Über organlibidinöse Begleiterscheinungen der Triebabwehr", *Internationale Zeitschrift für Psychoanalyse*, XIV, 1928; and also "Remarks on the Common Phobias", *Psychoanalytic Quarterly*, XIII, 1944.
15. Freud, S., *Civilization and Its Discontents*, London, 1930.

EVACUATION OF CHILDREN IN WARTIME

A Survey of the Literature, with Bibliography.

By KATHERINE M. WOLF, Ph.D. (New York)

I. *Introduction.*

Modern warfare has confronted the authorities of the belligerent countries with a new problem. The bombing of large areas made the protection of civilians necessary(124).[1] Beside the construction of shelters, evacuation, i.e., the removal of civilians from areas in which bombing is probable to areas in which it is highly improbable, was considered the safest device. This scheme did not work out for the average adult (6) who was engaged either in an important war job or at least in some vocational activity essential to livelihood. The evacuation plan was therefore mainly carried out with children. So in Great Britain alone 734,883 children were evacuated(154). This constituted not only a technical problem from the viewpoint of transportation, schooling, physical health and sleeping accommodations, but a very specific psychological problem as well(17, 18, 41, 82, 83).

734,883 children were evacuated. At first glance this seems only a statistical figure, albeit a large one. For the psychologist, however, the figure loses its merely statistical character, since he realizes that it means that in a few days almost three-quarters of a million children were separated from their parents in so relatively small an island as Great Britain. History has here made a cruel psychological experiment on a large scale.

Unfortunately the literature on evacuation, though voluminous, as shown by the bibliography, is not wholly satisfactory by the psychologist's standards. Moreover it is far from homogenous and it is therefore difficult to evaluate the results in any uniform fashion.

II. *Methodological Problems in the Literature.*

The methodological difficulties in the literature on evacuation are of kinds.

---

1. Numbers in parentheses refer to the bibliography.

1. The statistics compiled vary in degree of reliability due to the emergency situation in which they were collected. There is almost no way of determining the level of reliability of any individual study of this kind.

2. From the methodological point of view many of the studies on evacuation lack the necessary comparable material on children in peace time. For instance, when John(118) says that 44% of the children were maladjusted after bombing and evacuation, we need to know how large a percentage of this group was maladjusted before.

3. A great number of articles on evacuation give neither statistical proof nor any observational material verifying their conclusions. It would be satisfying to have some charts, tables, or at least quotations by Coromina(65) when she asserts that children separated from their parents show no neurotic symptoms whereas those evacuated with their parents show very definite symptoms.

4. Other papers again do not mention the age of their subjects or at least not the age distribution in the group observed. This is especially regrettable in the case of the very interesting papers by Alcock(2, 71).

5. Although the date of publication usually gives a hint as to the time in which the special research on evacuation was carried out, a more exact statement of the date would be desirable. As Valentine(217) points out, the results depend to a great extent on whether they were collected in the beginning, or at a later period of evacuation.

6. The method by which the different authors gather their material varies enormously. To quote just three examples: Burt(46-50) studies the behavior of children by direct observation. The same group of children had been observed before evacuation. Isaacs(114) collects all her material indirectly with the exception of a small percentage that was directly observed at the Child Guidance Clinic. She deduced the data used in the Cambridge Survey from reports of the "friendly visitor" (a kind of social worker), from the teacher who knew the children in London and came to Cambridge with them, and from an essay by the children entitled: "What I like and what I miss in Cambridge". Vernon(218) bases her conclusions on specific interviews with girls before evacuation, interviews about their schoolwork, their leisure occupations and their ideas about careers.

7. The quantitative aspect of the material in the literature is equally lacking in homogeneity. It varies from well under a hundred cases to many thousands.

III. *The Influence of the Evacuation Situation on the Child's Mental Equilibrium.*

In describing the influence of the evacuation situation on the child's behavior we shall introduce a distinction, unfortunately not clearly made in most of these articles. We shall try to differentiate between the formation of neurosis in children and the child's adaptation or maladaptation to his foster home.

We believe that such differentiation is important. Adaptation and mal-adaptation is a circumscribed problem that begins and ends in the area in which it takes place. Neurosis formation transcends the limits of the foster home environment as a psychological situation and extends over the child's whole life.

To keep the enumeration from becoming too complicated we forego an-other distinction. We shall not at first make any distinction between positive and negative modifications of the child's behavior. So in a first part of our discussion we describe the factors favoring or inhibiting the child's adaptation to the foster home and, considering these factors, state how many children suc-ceeded in making a positive adaptation. Later we shall see how the child's general behavior was modified, and then describe how many children acquired a neurosis, and what kind. We shall also describe how the children's behavior in general came to be positively influenced by evacuation.

The results obtained from the different authors on these questions are extremely contradictory. There is almost no point on which they completely agree. This is partly due to the above mentioned differences of method, but partly it is probably also due to the psychologically complex character of the evacuation situation.

A. Adaptation to the Billet.

All papers agree that successful adaptation to the billet is surprisingly high. There are few figures on this point except in Isaacs book(114), who reports that 46 of 689 children were not able to adapt themselves. 26 of these cases could be explained by the children's behavior difficulties, 10 by difficulties in the foster homes. 2 of the 26 children were really unplaceable; 3 of the 10 foster homes could not be used. There is no such agreement on the factors that favored adaptation. Whereas Isaacs maintains that a continuation of contact with the parents through constant visits favors adaptation, Burt em-phasizes that repeated visits of parents have a harmful influence on adapta-tion to the billet(46). Davidson and Slade's figures(70) tend to support Isaac's view, but their statistical significance is doubtful according to the authors. Burt stresses the importance of similar social levels of parents and foster parents. Isaacs can find no statistical support for this thesis in her material. Davidson and Slade state that age has no bearing on the adaptation of the children to their foster homes, whereas Isaacs proves that only 3.3% of the children under thirteen years of age were maladjusted, compared to a group of 18.5% of children of more than thirteen years. Again Isaacs makes the very plausible conclusion that children who changed their billet frequently were not so well adapted as children who were left in the same billet. But Davidson and Slade in evaluating their material on this point could not find any such positive correlation between changes of billeting and maladap-tation. Another fact on which Isaacs and Davidson and Slade disagree is the influence of siblings in the same foster home. Isaacs maintains that the presence of siblings makes adaptation easier, Davidson and Slade do not encounter this positive influence. The only factor to which Davidson and Slade concede a definitely positive influence on adaptation to billeting is intel-ligence. Yet Isaacs sees no correlation whatsoever on this point, and John(118) shows that intelligent children demonstrate twice as many maladaptations as unintelligent ones.

There are only a few statements about this adaptation problem that have been accepted without question, but only, we believe, because they occur as the single statement of one author. To this group belongs Isaacs' claim that maladaptation is likely to occur when the foster parents are more than sixty years old, as well as Burt's statements(46) that older boys adapt better to homes having a male influence and that excitable children should be billeted either alone or with stable children.

In view of their many other disagreements on the subject of factors favorable to adaptation, these few mildly positive statements are the more interesting, especially when taken in context with Isaacs' detailed analysis(114) of 46 cases of billeting in which no adaptation could be achieved.

These children were observed and described thoroughly by both a psychologist and a psychiatrist.

They were given a psychological examination including the Stanford revision of the Binet-Simon test, the Merrill Palmer, the Healy picture completion I and II, and the Oakley form board. Their attitude towards both the examiner and the test was observed. Afterward the children were interviewed by a psychiatrist. From the adapted children a control group of 40 children comparable in point of age and various other factors was chosen. They all went through the same procedure and although these two groups did not show any statistically relevant difference in intelligence, they differed distinctively in regard to their mental health. The psychiatrist working with Isaacs classified the mentally sick children into six groups(51); (1) anxious, (2) withdrawn, (3) jealous and quarrelsome, (4) active and aggressive, (5) manic depressive, and (6) delinquent. In each of these groups three degrees of mental sickness were distinguished: (a) those showing slight symptoms, (b) those showing a clear picture of specific mental disease, and (c) those showing a picture of mental disease so grave as to need immediate psychiatric treatment.

If one compares the adjusted and the maladjusted groups in regard to their mental health, one finds that in the adjusted group 24 were normal, 9 slightly and 7 strongly or very strongly disturbed. In the maladjusted group only 7 were normal, 10 slightly, and 29 strongly or very strongly disturbed.

The character of the disturbances in the two groups is not the same. The sick children of the maladjusted group belong mostly to the jealous quarrelsome, active-aggressive, or manic depressive types. The sick of the adjusted group are either anxious or withdrawn.

To round out the description Isaacs distinguishes two personality types among the normal children: the outgoing, friendly, active type and the quiet, passive type. She finds that the majority of the healthy adjusted children belong to the first and the healthy maladjusted children to the second group. From this she draws the conclusion that mental health is very important for adaptation to a billet. If the children are outgoing and friendly it helps their adaptation and when children are mentally ill they can still adapt if they belong to the anxious or withdrawn type.   If these children are billeted in quiet conventional homes where they are left alone, no real problems of adaptation are likely to arise.   The most difficult group for placement are the active aggressive boys and the corresponding jealous and quarrelsome girls. Their chance of adapting is very slight though sometimes in very free and unconventional homes adaptation does succeed.

B.   The influence of billeting on the child's general behavior.

Evacuated children had to adapt to more than a new foster home since they changed from city to country life.   They had to give up their usual leisure occupations.   They were separated from their friends.   Although none of these influences has the same importance as the essential one, changing one's home, they surely contributed to the psychological picture.   Some high-lights on this adaptation problem are given by the different authors on evacuation.   There is the interesting observation that the London children did not mix with the Cambridge children, but nevertheless acquired a Cambridge accent (Isaacs: Teacher's report)(114). Or Vernon's statement contradicting this, that evacuated children replaced their home friends by new friendships in the reception area(218).

On the whole descriptions of changes in the behavior of children in reception areas are on a superficial level.   There are some allusions to an improvement in manners, in self-discipline, in attachment to school, to greater independence and self-reliance.   This last statement cannot be general-ized since other authors state that evacuated childrn are afraid of taking jobs that would mean another separation from their parents.

By far more interesting than the so-called positive influence of evacua-tion on the child's mental status are the accounts of the negative changes, whether they are merely negative variations of normal behavior, or those variations that must be recognized as neurosis formation.

Neurosis formation induced by evacuation can be considered neither a developmental neurosis nor a traumatic neurosis in the strict sense of the word.   The best illustration of the strange type of neurosis formation precipi-tated by evacuation can be found in the second part of Freud and Burlingham's *War and Children*(87): Children under the strain of separation develop habits which express an emotional attitude toward the situation, but which then lose their direct expressional value and gradually become symptoms in themselves.   An instance of such a transformation is the tic that poor little Patrick, aged three years and two months, developed.   He did not want to cry but instead constantly assured himself, by nodding his head, that his mother would come to get him.

All authors agree that the effects of bombing and of evacuation must be distinguished from each other psychologically.   There are even a few authors (Pritchert, Rosenzweig, Alcock and others)(124, 170) who maintain that while separation leads to psychosomatic or psychoneurotic disorders, bombing leads to unmanageable behavior and aggressivity.

The majority of authors find that evacuation has a greater influence on the mental habits of the child than bombing. Thus Burbury(45) shows that in 52% of evacuated children a formation of neurotic symptoms or an exacerbation of their already present symptoms can be found, while only 20% of the bombed children showed such a negative influence on their adaptation to reality. Yet Coromina(65) finds no neurotic symptoms in evacuated children, but slight ones in children exposed to air-raids; and Bowley(37) maintains that he could observe eight times as many symptoms in children exposed to air-raids, as in children subjected to evacuation.

On the important question of what is the percentage of neuroses created by evacuation we find neither homogenous material nor agreement among the authors. The findings range all the way from Coromina's assertion(65) that no neuroses are created by evacuation, through Bodman's paper(32, 33) claiming neurotic symptoms found in 61% of the children, to Boyd's assertion(38) that evacuation improves their mental and physical health(7). This material is not only not homogenous, but it is frequently uninformative on the two following points. On one hand it says nothing about the time elapsing between the immediate evacuation shock and the date the survey was conducted(217), and on the other, we learn nothing about the incidence of neurosis in the children prior to evacuation(51).

That the first is important is shown by the above quoted article of Bodman(32, 33) who finds a behavior disturbance in 61% of the children observed immediately after evacuation, and only 11% in those studied seven months later. The relative value of statements that mention the incidence of neuroses only after evacuation is clarified by Burt's articles(46-50). He finds 25% of evacuated children to be neurotic, but 17% of these had been neurotic before. By eliminating all papers whose methods seem lacking in carefulness, as well as those whose material seems too scanty, we would probably be safe in saying that the percentage of neurotic disorders in evacuated children was between 25 and 44% (Bodman and Dunsdon, 34). Again, by considering only those differences that seem well confirmed, we may assume that one-third of these children either acquired or suffered an aggravation of their neurosis due to evacuation alone. This would amount to saying that 8 to 15% of the children had acquired a neurotic behavior or had their condition aggravated by evacuation.

The specific factors that influenced this neurosis creation are again discussed in a completely contradictory fashion. We single out one factor, because we believe it to be of the greatest theoretic importance. This is the child's age. It would certainly throw some light on the question of the formation of a traumatic neurosis, (or on that of a neurosis of a similar structure such as the separation neurosis happens to be) if we knew in which age group this neurosis can most easily be evoked. Kris(122) claims convincingly that Burt's results(49) on this point prove the greater readiness of the ages critical for libidinal development, such as the oedipal phase or puberty, in forming a neurotic response to a difficult situation. Unfortunately these data of Burt do not stand uncontradicted. Burt finds the peaks of neurotic response to war effects in the age groups between two and five years and in the age groups between fourteen and sixteen. While the latter phenomenon is corroborated by Isaacs no evidence for the former can be found in her material. Partial corroboration is to be found in Bodman's article(32, 33). But on the other hand he maintains that symptom formation and symptom persistence is greatest from one year on, which is in opposition to Burt, who finds that the occurrence of neurotic symptoms in children younger than two years is negligible. Bowley(37) asserts that the age group between two and five adapts best, that the climax of psychoneurotic symptoms are found between five and seven, and the gravest psychosomatic symptoms between eleven and fourteen. Alcock(3, 71), in complete contradiction to Burt, discovered the maximum of neurosis formation in school children, 89% of all the children she observed. Only 7% of the children developing a neurosis were in the age group from two to five years. We will try to show the divergencies among the authors by a table in which the vertical column gives the ages and the horizontal column states the maximum and minimum of neurosis formation.

Age	Maximum according to	Minimum according to
1- 2	Bodman(32, 33)	Burt(49)
2- 5	Burt(49)	Alcock(3, 71)
5- 7	Bowley(37)	Isaacs (Tottenham group, 114)
7- 9	Alcock(3, 71)	Isaacs (Islington group, 114)
9-11	Keir (girls, 120)	Burt(49)
11-13	Keir (boys, 120)	Burt(49)
13-15	Burt(49), Isaacs(114)	————

After reading this table one is not astonished that Davidson and Slade(70) find that neurosis formation has no correlation with age. The sole fact emerging as relatively uncontradicted is that adolescents develop an evacuation neurosis more frequently than do children.

The question of "Neurosenwahl" favored by separation is one in which there is more agreement among different authors than there is on the question of neurosis formation. As far as the fact is mentioned at all by such authors as Isaacs(114), Burt(46-50), Vernon(218) and others, evacuation always leads to a lack of concentration. It is an interesting subsidiary point to this statement that Vernon finds that a large percentage of adolescent girls who before evacuation had planned to study, afterwards gave up this decision. Another neurotic disturbance frequently mentioned in the reports is the occurrence of enuresis(103). Probably its frequent mention arises from the fact that it is the symptom that gave overt trouble to the foster parents and therefore was always brought up in any discussion at evacuation centers. But in addition it also seems to represent one of the most commonly observed syndromes in reaction to evacuation. We need not go so far as Gill(36), who found 80% of all evacuated children to be bedwetters, since his survey was made immediately after evacuation had started. But even Isaacs' statement (114) that 48% of all children who came to the Cambridge Child Guidance Clinic were enuretic is impressive. It is still more impressive when we learn from Burt(46) that in the case of enuresis there was not only an increase of 33% but an increase of 50% compared to the occurrence of this symptom in peace time. Alcock(3) and all her coworkers, as well as John(118) also emphasize the frequency of enuresis. Beside the relative agreement on the occurrence of enuresis, the only other relative agreement is to be found in regard to anxiety states(16, 45, 118, 218, 219), which are noted by almost every author dealing with evacuation. But this category is one of the lowest in percentage with Isaacs(114), whereas it is one of the highest with Burt(46).

In America a great deal has been written about war and delinquency (100, 101, 224). It would be interesting to learn something of the role of evacuation in influencing the delinquency of children in whom war has produced insecurity and aggressive behavior(21). Indeed the American Outpost in Great Britain(4) states that delinquency has been increased 41% through evacuation. Cook(64) characterizes as alarming the increase he has observed. On the other hand, the Child Guidance Council(194) seems to expose both these statements as unreliable, since the increase in delinquency during the war is in actuality only part of a general increase in delinquency that has been occurring during the last ten years. Bell(26), who agrees with the criticism of the Child Guidance Council, adds an interesting point. In the United States the peak of delinquency occurs at eighteen years of age while in Great Britain it is at thirteen. In the face of this difference and in spite of all assertions to the contrary it still would seem plausible to infer that evacuation does have some negative influence on the moral behavior of children.

More light is shed on this problem by Bodman and Dunsdon(34), who claim a delinquency increase of 44% but who relate that a group of children with I.Q.'s below 85 shows an increase of delinquency of 74% whereas in the group with I.Q.'s above 85 the delinquency shows a decrease of 23% during the war.

IV. Conclusions and Summary.

This material in spite of its lack of homogeneity shows two striking results.

1. The percentage of neurosis formation caused by evacuation is relatively low considering the deep trauma which we would have expected separation from parents to constitute.

2. Enuresis stands out as the dominant symptom of the syndrome evacuation neurosis.

Both of these results seem partially understandable (we do not even attempt a complete explanation or interpretation) through the clues we have to the kind of mechanism employed by the child in coping with the fact of his separation from his parents. The child's dealing with this experience seems to depend on whether his prior relationship to his parents was stable or one of conflict.

A stable relationship seems to be responsible for the relatively high rate of successful adaptation to the billeting situation. The adaptive mechanism in this case consists in a modification of the images of the parents which takes place throughout the whole experience of evacuation. There are only two books that illuminate this point. These are Freud and Burlingham's *War and Children*(87) and the *Cambridge Survey* edited by Isaacs(114).

These two books are to a large extent incomparable. The children on which Isaacs bases her report almost all were more than four years old, in foster homes in the reception area of Cambridge. Freud and Burlingham collected their material from the observation of pre-school age children in a nursery. It is therefore the more interesting that the same fact can be derived from both books, although Isaacs does not explicitly mention it: the fact is that evacuated children had an extremely vague memory of their homes. The image of their parents acquired a shadowy, uncertain character that lends itself readily to various psychological mechanisms such as displacement, condensation, etc.

Even when Freud and Burlingham relate that the memory pictures of little evacuated children are very vague (citing instances) we must realize that the rudimentary character of the child's memory does not suffice to explain this phenomenon. We know that from the end of his first year the infant has acquired an enduring image of his parents. But every attempt to explain the vague picture of parents on the basis of an adequate development of memory fails when we examine the material Isaacs(114) presents in the essays of the children ("What I like and what I miss in Cambridge"). Although the great majority of children mention their parents as one of the items missed, the mentioning is done with a conventional and unemotional attitude. When children go beyond this conventional utterance, they become surprisingly vague and confused for their age level and for their intelligence.

An example is that of an intelligent girl of seven:

"I miss my doll Pram and mummy and Daddy and granma and bathing her at night, and putting to bed and putting cums down her throat, and bits of fish and dressing her in the morning and put her plates in. And cleaning her hair and nursing her."

Even by reading this attentively one cannot discover whether she is speaking of her doll or of her grandmother. Certainly the parents are merely the stage hands in the drama "Home".

Or another example, a boy of thirteen, who impresses observers and teachers by his intelligence, starts his report with the sentence: "Most of all I miss my parents." This remark, similar to the stock replies of many other children, nevertheless seems to have more true emotional value, and so would seem a case disproving our thesis. Yet on closer knowledge of the facts, we learn that this boy's mother died when he was a little child, and that since then he has lived alone with his father.

It seems that evacuation produces a process in the child's mental apparatus that in turn adapts this apparatus to a separation from the parents for an indefinite period. The child suspends his relationship to his parents for this given time. This creates a vagueness in his image of his home and probably produces a disturbance of his perceptive and imaginative processes in general. It expresses itself in a lack of concentration which is an almost uniform characteristic of evacuated children. This arrangement seems to make adaptation to evacuation fairly successful and explains the low incidence of neurosis formation in children who did not show neurotic symptoms prior to evacuation.

However, the literature seems to indicate that this mechanism of suspension is limited to those cases in which the child's relationship to his parents had been a stable one. Where there was conflict, the conflict is so exacerbated that the child is compelled to act it out in the foster home environment.

For instance, a thirteen-year-old girl whose father had died when she was little and whose mother has deserted her, was brought up in an institution without showing any particular behavior problems. Immediately after billeting, however, she reported that her foster parents were starving her and that her foster father had assaulted her. Neither of these accusations turned out to be true.

The pattern this example demonstrates might be formulated in more general terms as follows: Though a conflict had once existed in this child's relationship to her parents it was of a kind that did not express itself in terms of neurotic symptoms (probably because of the specific libidinal situation in the institution). When evacuation came, however, and by its traumatic character impelled the child to regress to this period of conflict the mitigating or modifying factors that had been present when the conflict was first experienced were absent in the billet. Consequently the latent neurosis became manifest. Such manifestation may have the specific form of the example given above. In the majority of cases, however, the child probably shows a much more generalized reaction to his own anxiety and aggression. It conforms closely to our knowledge of children's neuroses to hear that enuresis in this situation is the most frequent neurotic symptom.

In summary let us say: The child interpreted his role as a wartime guest very literally. He was only a guest, but a guest at a party, which was not of his choosing. Therefore he did not want to think too clearly of his losses. The child preferred to be a "War Time Guest" rather than a "Borrowed Child". In preserving his home somewhere in his mind, and in not allowing the new home to become a rival, the normal child from a normal home could adapt to the situation. But it is probably too much to be a guest with a stone in one's stomach.

BIBLIOGRAPHY

1. *A Children's Charter in Wartime.* Published by the Children's Bureau, Committee on Children in Wartime.
2. Alcock, A. T.: War Strain in Children. *Brit. Med. J.,* 1, 1941, 124.
3. Alcock, A. T.: The Bombed Child and the Rorschach test. *Brit. Med. J.,* 2, 1941, 787.
4. *American Outpost in Great Britain.* Aldwyck House, London, November, 1941.
5. Anderson, E. W.: Psychiatric Syndromes Following Blast. *J. Men. Sci.,* LXXXVIII, No. 371, 228.
6. Anon.: Evacuation of Mothers and Young Children. *Brit. Med. J.,* 1, 1940, 488.
7. Anon.: Medical Examination and Evacuation. *Brit. Med. J.,* 1, 1940, 1000.
8. Anon.: Evacuation of Children from London, *Brit. Med. J.,* 1, 1940, 921.
9. Anon.: War Strain in Evacuated Children. *Brit. Med. J.,* 1, 1941, 128.
10. Anon.: Medico Social Problems of Evacuation. *Brit. Med. J.,* 1, 1940, 660.
11. Anon.: The Young Visitors, *Lancet,* 1, 1940, 133.
12. Anon.: Transplanted Children. *Lancet,* 1, 1941, 118.
13. Anon.: Town-Country. *Lancet,* 2, 1941, 609.
14. Anon.: War Strain in Children. *Lancet,* 1, 1941, 121.
15. Anon.: Community Actions for Children in War Time. *U.S.A. Child Bureau Publications,* No. 295, 1943, 9.
16. *Anxiety and its Control.* Guide for Civilian Defense Personnel. Reactions of People under Stress. Training Schedule No. 1. Prepared by the Military Mobilization Committee of the American Psychiatric Association.

17. Association of Architects, Surveyors and Technical Assistants. Evacuation Committee: *Evacuation in Practice. A Study of a Rural Reception Area*. No. 123, 1939, Duplic., 28.
18. Association of Architects, Surveyors and Technical Assistants. Evacuation Committee: *—Evacuation—The Under Fives*. 1940, No. 127, Duplic., 34. The A.A.S.T.A., 57, New End, London, N.W. 3, in collaboration with the A.A. School Rural Planning Group.
19. Astbury, B. E.: *Letters from an English Social Worker in Wartime*. Published by the Family Welfare Association of America. 27.
20. Astbury, B. E.: Interviewing after Air Raids. *Family*, XXIV, 1943, 128.
21. Bagot, J. H.: Juvenile Delinquency (App. 1, Delinquency during War-Time), London, Cape, 1937.
22. Baruch, D. W.: *You, your Children and War*. New York, Appleton Century, 1942, pp. 12+234.
23. Baruch, D. W.: Helping Children for War. *Marriage and Family Living*, 1943, No. 5, 49.
24. Beals, F. L.: Wartime Problems of Children. *Hygeia*, 22, 1944, 268.
25. Beals, F. L.: Wartime Problems of Children. *Hygeia*, 22, 1944, 296.
26. Bell, M.: Delinquency in Wartime England. *Probation*, XX, 1942, No. 4, 97.
27. Bell, M.: Delinquency in Wartime England. *Probation*, XX, 1942, No. 4, 111.
28. Bender, L. & Frosh, J.: Children's Reaction to the War. *Amer. J. Orthopsychiat.*, 12, 1942, 571.
29. Beverly, B. I.: The Reactions of Children and Youth to Wartime. *J. Pediat.*, 20, 1942, 665.
30. Beverly, B. I.: Effect of War upon the Minds of Children. *Amer. J. for Pub. Health*, 33, 1943, 793.
31. Bibring, M.: Child Guidance during Crisis. *Somas*, 69.
32. Bodman, F. H.: War Conditions and the Mental Health of the Child. *Brit. Med. J.*, 2, 1941, 486.
33. Bodman, F. H.: Effects of Air Raids on Children. *Brit. Med. J.*, 2, 1941, Nov. 11.
34. Bodman, F. H. & Dunsdon, M. I.: Juvenile Delinquency in Wartime. Report from the British Child Guidance Clinic. *Lancet*, 2, 1941, 572.
35. Body, A. H.: *Children in Flight*. Some Pictures of Evacuation. Foreword, Earl De La War. London, University of London Press, 1940, pp. 95.
36. Bottome, P.: *London Pride*. New York, Little, Brown & Co., 1941.
37. Bowley, A. H.: Child Guidance Surveys in Wartime. *Ment. Health*, July 1940, 176.
38. Boyd, W.: The Effects of Evacuation on the Children. *Brit. J. Educ. Psychol.*, 11, 1941, 120.
39. Brander, T.: Kinderpsychiatrische Beobachtungen während des Krieges in Finnland. 1939-1940. *Zeitschr. f. Kinderpsychiat.*, 7, 1941, 177.
40. Brander, T.: Psychiatric Observations among Finnish Children during the Russo-Finnish War. 1939-1940. *Nervous Child*, IV, 2, 1943, 313.
41. British Psychological Society: *Shelter and Evacuation Problems*. Papers read at the meeting of the Brit. Psychol. Soc., July 26, 1941.
42. Brothwood, W. C. W.: Experience of Evacuation in a Country Reception Area. *Public Health*, LIII, 1940, 6, 125.
43. Bulletins from Britain, No. 84: *Children in Wartime*: The Under Fives.
44. Burlingham, D.: see Freud & Burlingham.
45. Burbury, W. M.: Effects of Evacuation and of Air Raids on City Children. *Brit. Med. J.*, 2, 1941, 660.
46. Burt, C.: The Incidence of Neurotic Symptoms among Evacuated School Children. *Brit. J. Educ. Psychol.*, 10, 1940, 8.
47. Burt, C.: War Neuroses in Soldiers, Civilians, and Children. (roneo'd summary for private circulation). London, Psychol. Lab. Univ. Coll., November, 1939.
48. Burt, C.: The Billeting of Evacuated Children. *Brit. J. Educ. Psychol.*, 11, 1941, 85.
49. Burt, C.: Under Fives in Total War. December 20, 1941. Printed for circulation to members of the British Psychological Society.
50. Burt, C.: War Neurosis in British Children. *Nervous Child*, II, 4, 1943, 324.
51. Burt, C. & Simmins, C. A.: Critical Notice of the Cambridge Evacuation Survey. *Brit. J. Educ. Psychol.* 12, 1942, 71.
52 Castendyck, E.: Refugee Children in Europe. *Social Service Review*, 13, 1939, 587.

53. Chess, S.: War Ideologies of Children. In Gerard, M. W. and others: Psychology of Preadolescent Children in Wartime. *Amer. J. Orthopsychiat.*, 13. 1943.
54. *Children in a Democracy*. General Report adopted by the White House Conference on Children in a Democracy. January, 1940.
55. *Children in Wartime*. Child Study Association, New York.
56. *Children in Wartime*. Committee for the Care of Young Children in Wartime, Supt. of Documents, Washington, D. C.
57. Clifton, E.: Some Psychological Effects of the War. *Family*, XXIV, 1943, 123.
58. Coghill, H. de J.: The Effect of War on the Behavior of Children. *Virg. Med. Mon.*, 69, 1942, 1929.
59. Committee of Neuropsychiatric Societies, N. Y.: *Monthly Abstracts*, Jan.-Oct. 1944.
60. Committee on Psychological Problems of Children in War Time. *Growing up in a World at War; Emotional Problems of Children in Wartime*. Chicago, Institute for Psychoanalysis, 1942, 25.
61. Community Projects for Child Welfare. Bulletin published by the National Citizen's Committee of White House Conference on *Children in a Democracy*. See: 54.
62. Conference on Emergency Problems of Children and Youth. *Committee on Child Development of National Research Council*. November, 1941.
63. Conover, H. F.: *Children and War: A selected List of References*. Washington, D. C., Library of Congress, 1942, 21.
64. Cook, P. H.: Evacuation Problems in Britain. Trans. Kans. Acad. Sci., 44, 1941, 343.
65. Coromina, J.: Repercussions of the War on Children as Observed during the Spanish War. *Nervous Child*, II, 4, 1943.
66. Cosens, M. E.: Evacuation, a Social Revolution. *Social Work*, I, 3, 1940, 165.
67. Crosthwaite, A. A.: French Evacuation. *Social Work*, I, 5, 1940, 298.
68. *Cultivating the Roots of Democracy*. Published by National Association for Nursery Education, University of Iowa, Iowa City, Lt.
69. Davis, A. E.: Clinical Experience with Children in Wartime. *Social Service Review*, 17, 1943, 170.
70. Davidson, M. A. & Slade, J. M.: Results of a Survey of Senior School Evacuees. *Brit. J. Educ. Psychol.*, 10, 1940, 179.
71. De La War, Earl & Others (Rickman J., Isaacs S., Bowlby J., Winnicott D. W., Thomas L., Yates S. L., Milner M., Alcock A. T.) *Children in War Time*. London, New Education Fellowship, Latimer House, 1940, 80.
72. Democratic Education. Suggestions for Education and National Defense. *Progressive Education Association*, September, 1940.
73. Despert, J. L.: School Children in War Time. *J. Educ. Sociology*, 16, 1942, 219.
74. Despert, J. L.: *Preliminary Report on Children's Reaction to the War, Including a Critical Survey of the Literature*. N. Y., Cornell Univ., Medical College, 1942.
75. Dunsdon, M. I.: A Psychologist's Contribution to Air-Raid Problems. *Mental Health*, 2, 1941, 37.
76. *Education for Victory*. An Official Biweekly of the United States Office of Education, Federal Security Agency. Washington, D. C.
77. *Education for Civilian Defense Pamphlets*. Issued jointly by the N. Y. State Council of Defense and the State Depts. of Education, Health, Labor, Mental Hygiene, Social Welfare. Albany, 1942. (Three Pamphlets.)
78. Education Problems of Evacuation, by One who Has dealt with them. *J. of Educ.*, 71, 844, 1939, 699.
79. Elliot, M. M.: The Effect of War and Civil Defense on Children; The British Experience. *Social Service Review*, 1942, 16, 1.
80. Elliot, M. M.: Civil Defense Measures for Protection of Children. *United States Department of Labor Publications*, No. 279, 1942, 186.
81. *Embassy of U.S.S.R.: Information Bulletin*. (48, 51, 57, 59, 70, 83) 1942.
82. Evacuation from the Reception End, by One who was there. *J. of Educ.*, 71, 843, 1939, 653.
83. Evans, Capt. F.: Evacuation and its Problems. *Quarterly Review*, 543, 1940, 50.
84. Fox, E.: Emergency Hostels for Difficult Children. *Ment. Health*, 1, 1940, No. 4, 97.
85. Freud, A. & Burlingham, D. T.: *Monthly Reports* on Hampstead Nurseries. Released by Foster Parents' Plan for War Children.
86. Freud, A. & Burlingham, D. T.: *Young Children in War Time*. Allen & Unwin, London, 1942.
87. Freud, A. & Burlingham, D. T.: *War and Children*. Intern. Univ. Press, N. Y., 1943.

88. Freud, A. & Burlingham, D. T.: *Infants without Families*. International University Press, New York, 1944.
89. Fries, M. E.: National and International Difficulties. *Amer. J. Orthopsychiat.* XI, 1941, 3.
90. Gardner, G. E.: The Family in a World at War. *Ment. Hygiene*, 26, 1, 1942, 50.
91. Gardner, G. E.: Child Behavior in a World at War. *Ment. Hygiene*, 27, 3, 1943, 353.
92. Gastwirth, P. & Silberblatt, J.: Reactions of Junior High School Children to the War. *High Points*, 25, 1943, 59.
93. Geleerd, E. R.: Psychiatric Care of Children in War Time. *Amer. J. Orthopsychiat.*, 12, 1942, 587.
94. Gentile, F. M.: The Effects of the War upon the Family and its Members. *Psychiatry*, 6, Feb. 1943, 37.
95. Gerard, M. W. & others: Psychology of Pre-adolescent Children in War Time. *Amer. J. Orthopsychiat*, 13, 1943, 493.
96. Gill, S. E.: Nocturnal Enuresis; Experience with Evacuated Children. *Brit. Med. J.*, 2, 1940, 99.
97. Gillepsie, R. D.: *Psychological Effects of War on Citizen and Soldier*. New York, Norton, 1942.
98. Glover, E.: Notes on the Psychological Effect of War Conditions on the Civilian Population. Part III: The Blitz. *International J. of Psycho-Analysis*, XXIII, 1, 1942, 17.
99. Glover, J. A.: Epidemological Aspects of Evacuation. *Brit. Med. J.*, 1940, 629.
100. Glueck, E. T.: The Morals of Youth in War Time. *Ment. Health*, XXVI, 2, 1942, 210.
101. Glueck, S.: Effects of the War on Juvenile Delinquency and Crime in England. *Crime News and Feature Service*, Bulletin of the Society for the Prevention of Crime, February, 1942.
102. Goldman, G. S.: Notes for Air Raid Wardens Concerning Civilian Morale and Panic. Prepared for the *Emergency Committee of Neuropsychiatric Societies in New York City*, May, 1942.
103. Gordon, I.: Allergy, Enuresis, and Stammering. *Brit. Med. J.*, 1, 1942, 357.
104. Greenberg, S., Editor: *The Family in a World at War*. By twenty outstanding experts. Child Study Association, New York.
105. Hadfield, I. A.: War Neurosis. *Brit. Med. J.*, 1, 1942, 281.
106. Harms, E.: The American Child on his Front of this War. *Nervous Child*, II, 4, 1943.
107. Henshaw, E. M.: Some Psychological Difficulties of Evacuation. *Ment. Health*, I, 1940, 5.
108. Henshaw, E. M. & Howarth, H. E.: Observed Effects of War Time Conditions on Children. *Ment. Health*, II, 4, 1941, 93.
109. Hendry, C. E.: Boys in War Time. *Scouting for Facts*, No. 4, 1942, 16.
110. Henriques, I. Q.: Evacuation and Welfare. *Social Work*, I, 4, 1940, 235.
111. Hutchinson, D.: Orphans, Fact and Fiction. *Nervous Child*, II. 1943, 48.
112. Isaacs, S.: Children of Great Britain in Wartime. *Child Study*, Winter 1941-1942.
113. Isaacs, S.: Cambridge Evacuation Survey. *The Fortnightly*, June, 1940, 619.
114. Isaacs, S., Editor, with the cooperation of Brown, S. C., and Thoules R. H.: *The Cambridge Evacuation Survey*, a Wartime Study in Social Welfare and Education. (Written by Bathurst, G., Brown S. C., Bowlby J., Bullen G. A., Fairbarn N., Isaacs S., Mercer N. S., Rooff M., Thoules R. H.). Methuen & Co., London, 1941.
115. Jensen R. A.: Children's Psychosomatic Complaints and the War. *Lancet*, 64, May 1944, 161.
116. Jersild, A. T.: Children and the War. *Teach. Coll. Rec.*, No. 44, 1942, 7.
117. Jersild, T. T. & Meigs, M. F.: Children and War. *Psychol. Bull.* No. 40, 1943, 541.
118. John, E. M.: A Study of the Effects of Evacuation and Air Raids on Children of Pre-school Age. *Brit. J. Educ. Psychol.*, 11, 1941, 173.
119. Jones, H. E. & Jones, M. C.: Attitudes of Youth towards War and Peace. *Calif. J. Sec. Educ.*, 16, 1941, 427.
120. Keir, G.: Special Evacuation Difficulties of the Residential School Child. *Ment. Health*, III, 1, 1942, 1.
121. Kenna, J. C.: *Educational and Psychological Problems of Evacuation*. An Analysis of Experience in England. Melbourne, Australia, Australian Council for Educational Research, 1942, 54.

122. Kris, E.: Danger and Morale. *Amer. J. Orthopsychiat.*, Vol. 14, No. 1, 1944, 147.
123. Lampard, M. E.: Vermious Evacuees. *Brit. Med. J.*, 1, 1940, 656.
124. League of Nations Health Organization: *Medico-Social Questions Arising out of the Movements of Civil Populations.* Report of the Emergency Subcommittee of the Health Committee. Geneva, 1940, Ch. 1448(1), pp. 7.
125. League of Nations Health Organization: *Medical and Health Question Connected with Evacuations.* Chronicle of the Health Organization. II, 1, 1.
126. Lerner, E. & Murphy, L. B.: Further Report of Committee for Information on Children in War Time. *J. Soc. Psychol.*, 34, 1943, 321.
127. *Letter to the London Times.* March 12, 1941.
128. Leslie, I. M.: Some Problems of a Hostel in a Reception Area. *Social Work,* I, 5, 1940, 307.
129. Lewis, A.: *Report on the Incidence of Neurosis in England under War Conditions.*
130. Lewis, A.: *Report on the Incidence of Neurosis in England under War Conditions. Lancet.* 2, 1942, 175.
131. Lindsay, K.: The Problem of Youth. A Challenge to Social Responsibility. Feb. 28, 1940.
132. Lissen, L. R.: Some Problems in a Reception Area. *J. Educ.*, 71, 845, 1939, p. 742.
133. Liverpool University, Social Science Department: *Preliminary Report on the Problems of Evacuation.* London, Hodder & Stoughton, 1939.
134. Liverpool University, Social Science Department: *Our War Time Guests.* A Psychological Approach to Evacuation. London, Hodder & Stoughton, 1940.
135. McDonald, M. W.: Impact of War on Children and Youth—Intensification of Emotional Problems. *Amer. J. of Public Health,* 33, 1943.' 336.
136. McClure, A.: Effect of Air Raids on School Children. *Brit. J. Educ. Psychol.*, 13, 1943.
137. Manheim, H.: *Social Aspects of Crime in England between the Wars.* London, Allen & Unwin, 1940.
138. Manheim, H.: Crime in War-Time England. *Ann. Amer. Acad. of Pol. and Soc. Sci.* 3547 Walnut Street, Philadelphia, Pa., Sept. 1941, 128.
139. Massobservations: *War Begins at Home.* London, Chatto & Windus, 1940.
140. Mead, M.: We Need not Mar our Children. *N. Y. Times Magazine,* Feb. 15, 1942.
141. Mental Hygiene: *Ally of Victory.* Annual Report 1941-42, National Committee of Mental Hygiene.
142. Mercier, M. H.: The Suffering of French Children. *Nervous Child,* II, 1943, 308.
143. Mercier, M. H. & Despert,, J. L.: Psychological Effects of the War on French Children. *Psychosom. Med.*, 5, July 1943, 266.
144. Miller, D. C.: Youth and National Morale. *J. Educ. Sociol.*, 15, 1941, 17.
145. Mira, E.: Psychiatric Experiences in Spanish War. *Brit. Med. J.*, 1, 1939, 1217.
146. Mons, W. E. R.: Air Raids and the Child. *Brit. Med. J.*, 2, 1941, 625.
147. *Moral Implications of Child Development.* The Committee on National Morale.
148. *Morale in War Time.* An Outline for Defense Speakers, prepared by the N. Y. City Committee on Mental Hygiene of the State Charities Aid Association. April 1942.
149. Morgan, L.: Blitz Children at System Court, Gloucestershire. *News Chronicle,* March 17, 1941.
150. Murphy, L. B.: The Young Child's Experience in War Time. In Gerard, M. W. and others: Psychology of Pre-Adolescent Children in War Time. *Amer. J. Orthopsychiat.*, 13, 1943.
151. *Needs of Young People in Time of War.* Scottish Scheme for Mobilizing the Resources of Youth Organizations. Dec. 12, 1939.
152. New York State Association for Nursery Education Bulletins.
153. Neustatter, W. L.: Some Psychiatric Aspects of Total War. *Diseases of the Nervous System.* III. 3, 1942.
154. Notes in Parliament: *Brit. Med. J.*, 1, 1940, 197.
155. Notes in Parliament: *Brit. Med. J.*, 1, 1940, 283.
156. Notes in Parliament: *Brit. Med. J.*, 1, 1940, 675.
157. Notes in Parliament: *Brit. Med. J.*, 2, 1940, 282.
158. Notes in Parliament: *Brit. Med. J.*, 2, 1940, 420.
159. *Nursery Schools for Children in Reception Areas.* Board of Education Cir. 1495; Ministry of Health Cir. 1936; London, H. M. St. O. 1940.
160. Odlum, D. M.: The Teacher and the Evacuated Child. *Pub. Nat. Counc. for Ment. Hyg. of G. B.*

161. Odlum,, D. M.: The Teacher's Role in Air Raids. *Teacher's World and School Mistress*, England, June 14, 1939.
162. Odlum, D. M.: Notes for those in Charge of Air Raid Shelters. *Pub. Nat. Counc. for Ment. Hyg. of G. B.*
163. Owen, A. D. K.: The Great Evacuation. *Political Quarterly*, 11, 1940, 30.
164. Padley, R. & Cole, M.: *Evacuation Survey*: A Report to the Fabian Society. Routledge, London, 1940.
165. Paul, L.: How the Evacuation Went. Problems in the Reception Areas *The Schoolmaster and Women Teachers' Chronicle*, CXXXVI, 1579, 1939, 330.
166. Pegge, G.: Psychiatric Casualties in London. *Brit. Med. J.*, 2, 1940, 553.
167. Peller, L. E.: Eating in Groups in Wartime. *Ment. Hygiene*, New York, 27, 1943, 188.
168. Plaut, P.: Refugee Children in England. *Ment. Health*, I, 2, 1940.
169. Prescott, D. A.: Wartime Morale Problems of Public Schools. *Understanding the Child, a Magazine for Teachers*. X, 4, 1942.
170. Pritcherd, R. & Rosenzweig, S.: The Effects of War Stress upon Childhood and Youth. *J. Abnorm, and Soc. Psychol.*, 37, 1942, 329.
171. Proceedings of the White House Conference on *Children in a Democracy*. Children's Bureau, U.S.A. Dept. of Labor, Public. No. 266, 1940.
172. Pygot, F.: Conditions of Evacuated School Children. *Brit. Med. J.*, 1, 1940, 587.
173. Répond, A.: Problèmes actuels d'hygiène mentale et de la psychiatrie infantile en Angleterre. *Gesundheit und Wohlfahrt*. 1942.
174. *Reports of the Psychologist*, London County Council, 1913-30.
175. Rickman, J.: Panic and Air Raid Precautions. *Lancet*, 1, 1938.
176. Ring, F. A.: Some Reflections on Evacuation. *J. of Educ.*, 71, 845, 1939, 747.
177. Robson, W. A.: Evacuation, Town Planning, and the War. *Political Quarterly*, XI, 1, 1940, 45.
178. Ross, H.: *Child Guidance during Crisis*. Amer. Orthopsychiat. Assoc. Meeting, Feb. 1942.
179. Ross, H.: Emotional Forces of Children as Influenced by Current Events. In Gerard and others; Psychology of Pre-Adolescent Children in War Time. *Amer. J. Orthopsychiat.*, 13, 1943.
180. Schooling in an Emergency. *Board of Education Cir.* 1474, London, H. M. St. O., August, 1939.
181. Schreiber, M.: Junior Talks about the War. *High Points*, 24, No. 7. 1942, 23.
182. S. C. M.: *Children under Fire*. Longman Green, 1943.
183. Seipt, J. S.: *The Wartime Adjustment of the Exceptional Child*. Proc. Inst. Except. Child. Woods Schools 8, 1942, 50.
184. Secondary Schoolmaster: Evacuation As I See It. *J. of Educ.*, 71, 845, 1939, 745.
185. *Selfdiscipline in Wartime*. Published by the Mass. Dept. of Mental Health and the Mass. Society for Mental Health, 1942.
186. Shakespeare, G. M. P., (Committee under Chairmanship of—): *Report on Conditions in Reception Areas*. 1941, London, H. M. St. O., 18.
187. Sheldon & Evans: Townchildren in the Country. *Lancet*. 1940, 94.
188. Sheviakov, G. V.: War and Adolescents. *J. Psychol.*, 14, 1942, 161.
189. Shirley, M. & Poyntz, L.: The Influence of Separation from the Mother on Children's Emotional Responses. *J. Psychol.*, 1942, 251.
190. Simney, T. S.: *Our War Time Guests*. Opportunity or Menace. See: Liverpool University.
191. Smith, A. K.: Child Welfare in the Defense of Some British Dominions. *The Children's Bureau*, U.S.A. Dept. of Labor. Oct. 1941, 98.
192. Smith, R. M.: Children in War Time. *Diseases of Children*, 64, 1942, 497.
193. Solomon, J. C.: Reaction of Children to Blackouts. *Amer. J. Orthopsychiat.*, 12, 1942, 62.
194. Staff of British Child Guidance Council: Juvenile Delinquency and the War. *Ment. Health*, July 1941.
195. Stalker, H.: Panic States in Civilians. *Brit. Med. J.*, 1, 1940.
196. Steet, R. F.: *Children in a World of Conflict*. Boston, Christofer Publishing House, 1941.
197. Stewart, M. S.: America's Children. *Public Affairs Pamphlet* No. 47.
198. Straker, A. & Thouless, R. H.: Preliminary Results of Cambridge Survey of Evacuated Children. *Brit. J. Educ. Psychol.*, 12, 1942, 71.

199. Strachey, J. S. L.: *Borrowed Children,* a Popular Account of some Evacuation Problems and their Remedies.   New York, The Commonwealth Fund, 1940, pp. XIV+199.
200. Strachey, J. S. L.: *These Two Strange Years.* Letters from England. October 1939—September 1941.   New York, Commonwealth Fund, 1942.
201. Sullivan, H. S.: Psychiatry and the National Defense. *Psychiatry,* IV, 2, 1941, 201.
202. Sundquist, J. L.: *British Cities at War. Chicago,* Public Administration Service 1941
203. Sutherland, J. D.: One Hundred Cases of War Neuroses. *Brit. Med. J.,* 2, 1941, 366.
204. Tangye, C. H. W.: Some Observations on the Effect of Evacuation upon Mentally Defective Children. *Ment. Health,* 2, 1941, 75.
205. Tchukovsky, K.: *Children at War.* Typewritten reprint issued by Embassy of U.S.S.R. (Quoted by Despert, see: 74).
206. *The Education of Evacuated School Children in Time of War.*   Board of Education Circ. 1469, London, H. M. St. O. May, 1939.
207. *The Government Evacuation Scheme.* Ministry of Health Evacuation Memo. No. 4, London, H. M. St. O.
208. *The Government Evacuation Scheme.* Ministry of Health Circ. 1965. London, H. M. St. O., February, 1940.
209. *The Schools in War Time.* (Issued by the Ministry of Information in Behalf of the Board of Education). Published by H. M. St. O., 1941.
210. *They Still Draw Pictures.* A Collection of Sixty Drawings Made by Spanish Children during the War. Introduction by Aldous Huxley. New York, 1938.
211. Thom, D. A.: The Psychiatric Aspects of Civilian Morale as Related to Children. *Ment. Hygiene,* 25, 1941, 529.
212. Thomas, R.: Children in War Time: Foster Parents. *Bulletin from Britain,* No. 77.
213. *Times: Educational Supplement. Cambridge Survey of Evacuees.* January 27, 1940, 27.
214. *Times: Educational Supplement.* ibid. February 3, 1940, 92.
215. Towle, C.: The Effect of the War upon Children. *Social Service Review,* 17, 1943, 44.
216. Trotter, W.: Panic and its Consequences. *Brit. Med. J.* 1, 1940, 270.
217. Valentine, C. W.: Editorial Note on Evacuation Investigations. *Brit. J. Educ. Psychol.,* 11, 1941, 127.
218. Vernon, M. D.: A Study of Some Effects of Evacuation on Adolescent Girls. *Brit. J. Educ. Psychol.,* 10, 1940, 114.
219. Vernon, P. E.: Psychological Effects of Air Raids. *J. Abnorm. and Soc. Psychol.,* 36, 1941.
220. Wagner, C. W.: The Specific Nature of Temperament Traits and a Suggested Report Form. *Brit. J. Educ. Psychol,* 1939.
221. Wagner, G.: Evacuation. *Social Welfare,* IV, 6, 1940, 98.
222. White, W. L.: *Journey for Margaret.* New York, Harcourt, Brace & Co. 1941.
223. Williams, H. D.: Behavior Problems of Children in War Time. *Nervous Child,* II, 4, 1943, 376.
224. Winsore, M.: Delinquency in War Time. In Gerard, M. W. and others: Psychology of Pre-Adolescent Children in War Time. *Amer. J. Orthopsychiat.,* 13, 1943.
225. Wishik, S. M.: Your Child's Morale in War Time. *Radio Talk,* January 9, 1942. *Station WNYC.*
226. Wolman, I. J.: The Child in War. *Amer. J. Med. Sci.,* 205, 1943.
227. Youth in Britain in War Time. February 4, 1942, *British Press Service.*
228. *Youth in War Time.* December 16, 1941.
229. Zachry, C. B.: Research in Child and Youth as Defense Effort. *Amer. Orthopsychiat. Assoc. Meeting.* February 1942.

MARGARET E. FRIES' RESEARCH IN PROBLEMS OF INFANCY AND CHILDHOOD

A Survey

By LILLIAN MALCOVE, M.D. (New York)

While still a practising pediatrician, in 1928, Margaret E. Fries became interested in the mental hygiene aspects of child development. She began a project within the structure of Well Baby Clinic of the New York Infirmary for Women and Children. For the study she selected from the "larger" clinic group forty-five babies in whom the possibility of feeble-mindedness had been ruled out. Their ages ranged from six weeks to eighteen months. As the study progressed, newborn infants were added to the group. The therapeutic aim was to make the word "well baby" more "meaningful" by "adding mental hygiene to physical hygiene". The investigatory aim was to study the genetic aspects of integrated development. Fries thought that the modern tendency to shorten the period of infancy through early habit-training affected deleteriously the formation of character traits and produced symptom-atologies. Consequently she planned to investigate, in empirical fashion, the life experiences of the child within his milieu, in order to find out what factors influenced the development of character traits and symptomatologies. She took into consideration the fact that the child functions physically, emotionally, and intellectually in a social environment; thus the organization of the group formed to study the child consisted of a psychiatrist, a pediatrician, a social worker, and a psychologist.

Not long after the project was begun, Fries supplemented her pediatric skills with a training in mental hygiene and psychoanalysis, including child analysis. The structure of the group she then worked with, which included social workers and volunteer nurses, was similar to that of the already established child guidance clinics, but it differed in two main aspects. Its function was primarily preventive, and its method was the study of the child in his environment, from birth to adolescence. The development of the child, of his character traits and symptomatologies, were observed currently, and in their earliest appearances. Furthermore, this development was studied in relation to the existing influences and events in the child's life. The differentiation in development as related to differences in experiences were compared and evaluated.

The author originally began her study with the premise that there were three main contributing etiological factors in the child's psychic development: constitution, habit-training, and parental emotional stability.

The method selected to investigate the role of these three factors was to obtain as much pertinent data as possible about the child and his environment. This was done during the monthly clinic visits, and in the home visits, to promote optimal development. Later a play group was formed in order to continue the observations of the child when he had outgrown his infancy. Incidentally, this play group served the practical purpose of giving the mothers an added incentive to come to the clinic, and of providing therapeutic and/or recreational facilities for the child. Since the author assumed that early bowel and bladder training was harmful, the educational program was instituted at once to direct the mothers to coincide the time of bowel and bladder training with the physical (sitting up), psychological, and neuro-muscular optimal readiness in the infant; weaning time was determined by these factors in the child, and also by the psychological readiness in the mother. This therapeutic interest exacted a price from the scientific study: it eliminated the possibility of having a true control group of infants exposed to an early habit-training regime. As an alternative the author used the less intensively studied cases as a control group. She was aware of the fact that she did not have a true control group in the scientific sense of the word; nevertheless there were still quite valid and definitive observations that could be made on those cases in which the mothers, compelled by their own anxieties and compulsions, carried out their own methods of early training despite clinical efforts to reeducate them. Some study of early training of the infants of the first group who were under eighteen months old when the project was started was also possible.

Naturally these situations did not provide the ideal one for observing the effects of early habit-training in an otherwise satisfactory mother-child relationship. Only such a study could truly evaluate the specific effects of early training.

The written communications of the research work have, from 1935 to-date, appeared periodically in Pediatric, Obstetric, and Orthopsychiatric Journals. The presentations differed in form and emphasis, depending on the journals and on the stage of the research work. Although the titles varied, they expressed a common denominator: a study of the factors that determine normal and abnormal development. For the sake of simplicity and expediency main trends of all the reports will be discussed as one communication.

A plan was outlined at the start for obtaining direct data on the child through observations and examinations plus indirect anamnestic data of the child and all the adults in his environment. Monthly or more frequent contacts were recorded, and in six-monthly intervals summaries were made. Movies of important mother-child situations (like nursing) and of the Moro test, supplemented the written record. Three well-edited films with constructive guides are now available to the public at the New York University Film Library. The study of the child and the adults in his immediate milieu was extended, as the work progressed, to include, in the case of the child, the period of adolescence, and in the case of the mother, the period of pregnancy and puerperium. Observers were present during the entire time of labor, and daily full observations were made of the mother and infant in the ten-day lying-in period. To this data were added observations made of the children in the play group in their relation to other children, to teachers, to materials, and to their mothers and fathers.

A picture of the child as a physical, emotional, intellectual and socio-logical being within his specific environment was verbally drawn in the exten-sive and detailed summary form of eight-and-a-half printed pages. In this summary one can see the carefully gathered data on the original three etio-logical factors, within the larger picture of the child's total behavior and his relationship to his total environment and to its component parts. The study of the half-yearly psychological summaries does present an inclusive develop-mental life picture of the child. The method of the study in its basic structure is a sound one. In dealing with the data the author made allowance for the unavoidable inaccuracies due to parents' evasions, deceptions, and unreliability of memory. My general criticism is in regard to the voluminousness of the summaries, which detracts from their clarity and, to an extent, from their use-fulness. I feel that the author's conscientiousness exceeds her discrimination in the selection of pertinent categories. Another general handicap is the fact that without differentiation, factual data such as physical history, development, and progress, are recorded side by side with subjective interpretive findings such as "Disposition", "Identification", "Courage", "Object Relations", etc. This lends an unevenness to the values of the different parts of the summary. A more specific criticism applies to the inadequate organization of some parts of the outline form dealing with the emotional aspects of the child. To mention two examples: under one caption of "Behavior" there is a mixture of concepts, such as "Disposition", "Independence", "Courage", and "Miscellaneous"; of the Defenses, only "Reaction-Formation" is recorded. Then there is the questionable use of captions referable to the four libidinal phases: "Oral Symp-toms", "Anal Organic Symptoms", "Phallic Symptoms", "Genital Organic Symptoms", and "Genital Psychological Symptoms". These are not explained anywhere, and the subheadings of "What", "Began", "When", "Treatment", "Stopped", "Relapses", "Parents' Attention", and "Child's Reaction", only enhance the cryptic nature of this part of the summary. Keeping in mind the fact that much of this data is covered by the social workers and volunteer nurses who in their earlier years were probably not analytically trained and who were later trained in varying degrees, one wonders about the inevitable degree of error. This same (libidinal phase) classification is used in the his-tory of the mother, and it would seem to be even less reliable there without a psychoanalytic precision study. The reason for the use of this classification, one can infer, is that the author wished to observe the effect of a mother who has a predominance of traits derived from certain libidinal phases of develop-ment, on a child in his libidinal phase of development corresponding to the mother's. This seems to me to be very difficult for a study short of an analytic observation of both mother and child.[1]

The methodological process in the chronological periodic interviews and examinations, in the consecutive reports of psychiatric or analytic therapy with the child and/or the mother, and in the six-monthly summaries, was desig-nated by Fries as a "going forward" or "synthetic" approach. A "few" of the cases in the group were studied "intensively". From the repeated references to one particular case in different papers we can assume that intensive study meant psychoanalytic therapy and/or short periods of analysis,

1. The charts have since been discarded for a more dynamic and analytic approach to the material.

as in the case of one young child. It is not stated how many cases were thus studied. The microscopic pictures were then compared with the macroscopic ones. The physical and psychological examinations and the historical data were thorough in all of the cases. The project was most short-handed in psychiatrists, which probably accounts for the relatively small number of intensively studied cases. Psychological developmental tests (Gesell) were not given but intelligence tests were, in all cases.

The work in the project was therapeutically successful in proportion to the limited facilities. It was observed that "superficial psychotherapy" was often effectual. Pathological aspects of the mother-child relationship were definitely modified by the treatment. Methods of persuasion, suggestion and education failed in proportion to the degree of the mother's neurosis and her pathological involvement in her child. Analysis was found to be indicated in some instances. Direct psychiatric work with the very young child was helpful despite the failure to effect a change in the mother's neurotic behavior. The optimal time for therapy was found to be, for the mother, the period of pregnancy, and for the child, the period of infancy.

The results of the research aspects of the project were also successful from the point of view of forming the initial premise that psychic development depended on constitution, child-training, and parental emotional stability. The study of the "constitution" consisted of extensive and thorough medical and psychological examinations of the child at regular frequent intervals. Specific study was directed toward estimation of the infant's motoric responses within the range of normalcy. Fries utilized an extended form of the Moro test: her test consisted in dropping a padded weight near the child; and when the child was three months, using the weight without the pad.[1] The infant's responses were observed and recorded by written descriptions and by movies. The tests were done daily in the first ten days and then at periodic intervals until the age of five months, when the adult form of Startle Response took over. It was noted that this change coincided with the child's ability to hold up his head when sitting. After a great many responses, which varied in degree, intensity, and duration, were observed, they were classified into three groups with gradations between them: Active, Moderately Active, and Quiet. In addition to the testing of Startle Responses, observations were made of the infant's general motor activity and of his activity in nursing, sleeping, etc. This was also done daily for the first ten days, and later, periodically. The combination of the Startle Response and the general motor activity, which had a high correlation, constituted the Activity Pattern of the infant. It was noted that these variations in motoric responses probably persist throughout life: this is being further investigated. In the first five to ten days, eliminating the traumatic effect of the birth process, the total body response was observed to be "dependent upon the excitability of the neuro-muscular system. One can speculate that perhaps part of the excitability of the neuro-muscular system is congenital by result of inheritance, intra-uterine life, or birth itself; while part of the excitability is determined by temporary body changes, such as illness, growth, emotional state, etc." Therefore the Congenital Activity Type and what constitutes the Activity Pattern are identical only for the short period of the

---

1. This was later described as the Weight x Height Stimulus Test.

first five to ten days. The duration of the Congenital Activity Type is not fixed. What is certain about it is its brevity. Insofar as the Activity Pattern is seen to be environmentally determined it is modifiable. It was observed that environmental modifications tended to shift the Pattern from either extreme toward the mid-line, whereas destructive environmental influences tended to shift it further in the direction of the extremes; the Quiet response became quieter and the Active response more active. The effect of an emotionally stable mother satisfactorily related to her child influenced the response by keeping the Pattern the same or shifting it toward the mid-line; and the effect of the emotionally unstable mother who was pathologically related to her infant was to shift the response toward the extremes. This part of the study, which provided an estimation of the *kind* of motor response the infant was born with, could furthermore foresee the *tendency* in the direction of the response as it falls under the influence of physical and environmental factors. As such, it is of considerable importance both as a diagnostic tool in the repertoire of infant behavior tests and as an aid in preventive therapy. It provides us with the earliest picture of the functioning of the Infant Ego Apparatus. According to Fries all three types are normal. The child with the Moderately Active response has the greatest advantage; and if post-maturity without organic pathology is also present there is additional advantage in starting life.

From this material the author concluded that the character of the response, combined with the picture of the infant's response to frustration, as shown in the Oral Test, gives the form and the basic pattern generally indicative of the method an individual will later use in the "adult editions" of the Activity Pattern in dealing with obstacles and deprivations, and in meeting new situations. Within degrees of variation in a known direction, the "type" then persists throughout life, except in the psychopathologies, where the response can change; as for example, an active child can become a quiet child as a result of repression. The therapeutic value lies in the fact that the needs of infants with different types of responses differ. The quiet child who tends to withdraw under stress needs more than an average amount of stimulation, patience, and reassurance. Such an infant has to be introduced gradually to changes and to new situations. The active child fares particularly badly under restraint, which stimulates aggressiveness and other traits, like stubbornness and rebelliousness. Since the Activity Pattern expresses itself in involuntary as well as voluntary muscles, the effect of the Pattern on respiration, cardio-vascular and gastro-intestinal activity should be of particular interest to the pediatrician. The author's original statement that "constitution" is an unchangeable factor is true to a quite limited extent, since shifting of the Pattern is a true change, and is possible. However, the fact that "constitution" is a contributing factor is proved true.

Another test worked out by Fries and already referred to, the Oral Test, consists of Presentation, Removal and Restoration of the nipple. The results are instructive and helpful in diagnosis; they supplement the findings of the Activity Pattern study, with which they have a high correlation. The Active child becomes very active and may even have a Startle Response to the Removal of the nipple, and may take a short time to quiet down before sucking on the restored nipple. The Quiet child tends to withdraw in the face of thwarting and needs help to suck again on the restored nipple. The Moderately Active child is more responsive to the Removal of the nipple and more resourceful in his attempt to regain it; and the acceptance of the nipple in the Restoration is more active. In later papers, still unpublished, the author has worked out in various degrees of completion, "Oral" tests adapted to the older child. Mainly these gauge the response to new situations and to frustrations. There is one test for the one-and-a-half to five-year-old child, and two for the five- to eleven-year-old. These tests are less accurate than the original one since in the years beyond infancy it is very difficult to get so universal an object of gratification as the mother's breast to the infant, or so universal a basic need as sucking. There are also other complicating circumstances of the test situation, such as the relationship to the examiner, the mood of the moment, etc., which make for inaccuracies. Nevertheless the tests ought to be useful for diagnosis and prognosis, and as an aid in determining "integrative development", which is their main purpose.

A word about one aspect of the prophylactic work, which took the form of "predictions". At the end of the ten-day lying-in period, when the study to-date was completed, Fries analyzed her data and made "predictions", which consisted of foreseeing difficulties or smoothness in development. Although it at first seemed that these predictions depended on the factors "constitution" and "parental emotional stability", it was later found that the former contained too many unpredictables, such as intellectual endowment, endocrine functions, and birth process disturbances. Consequently the predictions were seen to be based primarily on the picture of the family history. Even so, they were found to be valuable and in many instances highly accurate.

The second factor, the role of habit-training, was studied thoroughly. That it influenced behavior was proved beyond doubt. The original thesis about the importance of timing of training was modified for it seemed to be only one of the situations in the mother-child relationship. In the original group, which included children up to eighteen months of age, some of whom had been subjected to early training, it was observed that babies were trained in a shorter time when the training began after six months.

It can be assumed that early training is very likely to have ill effects on emotional development, because the attempts to condition a neuro-muscular system to voluntary control before it has attained a state of physical maturity imposes a task on the infant before he is equipped to meet it. Untoward results are to be expected. What these results are in specific behavior has not yet been tabulated and set in conclusive terms. So far, the findings show clearly the direction of general behavior tendencies as either more active, aggressive and stubborn, or more passive and withdrawn. Less clearly is seen what traits or symptomatologies might derive from early or late weaning or from early, inconsistent or late training of the vegetative functions. It is possible that the abundant clinical data in the author's possession which have not as yet been published might give us these answers. In studying causation, the author observed consistently the existence of multiple determination in the formation of traits and symptoms. Also stressed was the interrelationship of physical, mental, emotional and sociological factors. This is doubtless true. Nevertheless, it is conceivable that eventually more specific cause-effect data may be forthcoming. As an example of what is meant by more specific findings, I refer to a study by Despert of young children in the Payne Whitney Nursery.[3] Despert found that early training produced an over-organized and compulsive personality.   Though the number of children in her early-trained group was very small, still her finding deserves further study.

Assuming multiple determination of behavior, and assuming that these determinants derive from many sources, as Fries has shown, it still seems possible to pursue the study of characterological formations and of particular problems relative to character development, as for instance, the development of ego functions. It would seem that the observation of relatively normal children, from infancy on, should provide an opportunity to study this problem analytically as well as developmentally. One aspect of such a study might be the Defenses, from their first appearances and throughout their vicissitudes, in the course of the psychological developmental stages. The only Defense recorded in the summary is Reaction-Formation; there is no reference to Denial, Repression, Projection, Isolation, etc. in the summary which is the completed study. Other important ego functions that need investigation are the development of ego mastery and the sense of reality, which includes the manifestations of the adaption to reality. Important, too, would be the study of the constellations in which there is retention in varying degrees within normalcy (normalcy to be established first), of earlier forms of thinking; this retention would probably be found to be related to Defense mechanisms. These are just a few of the problems that belong less to the laboratory of the analytic treatment situation and more to a research laboratory committee conducted by analysts in conjunction with psychologists, pediatricians, and social workers—a set-up such as, or similar to, the one of Fries.

A statement not yet verified about conditioning factors in psychopathologies was made by the author about schizophrenia. She believes that the candidate for schizophrenia is the infant who is from birth below or just average physically and in Central Nervous System maturation; who has an excessively hypo-Activity Pattern; who responds with quiet withdrawal to the Oral Test; who has feeding difficulties early in life; and who is exposed to severe deprivations or has a mother with a schizoid personality.

One practical aspect of the study on child-training is the author's expressed conviction that the pediatrician has a profound responsibility for the child's psychic as well as his physical health. His contribution lies primarily in the realm of habit-training, for which he needs knowledge of child psychology in order to guide the mother with psychiatric as well as medical wisdom. We know from experience that those pediatricians who have been able to assimilate into their pediatric framework the added tools of child psychology have shown us that it is a goal not only "devoutly to be wished" but an actual possibility. Furthermore, since 1930 several different kinds of pediatric-psychiatric clinical set-ups have been established and are now functioning with noteworthy success. The recent developments in the author's research work have been in the direction of organizing "an Integrated Health Plan" with a "Central Training Clinic" within a hospital, starting in the "Prenatal Clinic".   This "Central Training

3. J. L. Despert, "Urinary Control and Enuresis", *Psychosomatic Medicine,* VI, 4, 1944, p. 304.

Clinic" is based on the original project plan and the branch set-ups in the community are subsidiary to the main clinic. Among the goals of this plan, which includes treatment and research, is the one of training professional personnel in allied fields, particularly pediatricians. The need for this is unquestionable. In her original group Fries found that the infants under eighteen months who showed psychological deviations also suffered from physical deviations in most instances. This fact further emphasizes the need of a psychiatric pediatrician for the period of infancy.

The third etiological factor, the contribution of "parental emotional stability" to the child's psychic development, was demonstrated particularly well in the report of the development of a child from birth to the age of four, and in the full report of a complete case. Although the father and other members of the family were given due attention, it was found that of greatest importance to the child's development was his relationship to his mother— a fact now axiomatic. The author illustrated, in particular, that the way in which a mother affects the child's behavior depends, in broader categories of behavior form, on the child's Activity Pattern, which correlated with the Oral Test response. No conclusions were presented on specificity of symptom or character trait development, though the material for such study may well be available in the records of the cases. What was presented was the multiplicity of causation and the interrelation of the many existing factors. Fries discussed the close and subtle interaction of mother and child in the light of innate differences in children. The possibilities of different effects on mothers of very quiet or very active children is an often-missed fact, and is important prognostically as well as therapeutically. Fries believes that just as the child's integrated development depends on the mother who is his total environment, so does the mother's integrated development depend on the child. The latter is an exaggeration. The way in which the child utilizes the mother's contribution to his gratification contributes to the mother's emotional state and the mother is, to be sure, deeply affected. However, at her stage of development it is doubtful whether her integration is dependent on the relation to the child, as the author contends.

We can see from the foregoing review that the research work of Fries has accomplished the big task of creating a method of study and of pursuing to final verification the existence of three definite causative influences on child behavior. A number of additional problems have grown out of the study. Some of these have been ably pursued as the effect of different cultures and different sociological conditions on development. Of the three films referred to, one is on "Family Life of the Navaho Indians"; it has an eighteen-page guide which is in itself a paper of interest, and very informative. The study of the respective values of deep and superficial therapy has had considerable thought and work but is not yet completed. Some of the subjects mentioned in the communications, those that are still part of plans for the future, include "A Simultaneous and Comparative Study of Normal and Pathological Development", a study to see if patterns up to six months persist after six months, a study of the extent to which patterns established by six months can be modified, the "Significance of the Mother's Attitude to Foetal Movements", the "Study of Criteria for Normal Psychic Development at Different Age Levels", and others I may have overlooked. From this point on, it is hoped that the author will be in a position to present papers on individual research topics, and not feel obliged to present a picture of her project as a whole, as has been done heretofore in her communications on her research project.

The author's research work has not outweighed her interest in disseminating her findings to as large an audience as possible so that they could be applied practically. This has been done for the lay public by radio talks, films, pamphlets, newspaper and magazine articles. For the professional groups, articles have been published for nurses, dentists, obstetricians, pediatricians, and for the psychiatrically oriented allied professions in the Orthopsychiatric Journal. The widest extension of the mental hygiene interest in the child has culminated in the Integrated Health Program Plan, which the author has already presented in the Orthopsychiatric Journal and *Nervous Child*. The Plan, as it is now visualized, brings the child into the center of the community's active interest from the time of his embryonic stage of existence. Every person and institution that contributes toward his functioning and his total integrated development is brought into the scope of the Plan and the role of each is defined and to the fullest extent possible aided and abetted. The individual parts of the community are related to each other and to the central focus, the child, with the aim of integrating the community functions and mobilizing its potentialities of functioning for the child. In this Plan the primary aim of insuring and preserving the total health of man is carried out in the balance of the three aims of the Program, Treatment, Research, and Training of Personnel, to function effectively and cooperatively.

BIBLIOGRAPHY

I *Technical Papers*

1. "Behavior Problems in Children under Three Years of Age", *Archives of Pediatrics*, November, 1928, 653-663
2. "The Teaching of Mental Hygiene in Medical Schools", *Transactions of the Second International Pediatric Congress, Acta Paediatrica*, XI, 1930, 506-508.
3. "A Well-Integrated Personality", *School and Home*, XVI, November, 1934.
4. "The Formation of Character as Observed in the Well Baby Clinic", *American Journal of Diseases of Children*, 49, January, 1935, 28-42. (With Katherine Brokaw and V. F. Murray.)
5. "Interrelationship of Physical, Mental and Emotional Life of a Child from Birth to Four Years of Age", *American Journal of Diseases of Children*, 49, June, 1935, 1546-1563.
6. "The Study of the Emotional Development of Children", *Medical Woman's Journal*, August, 1936.
7. "The Value of a Playgroup in a Child Development Study", *Mental Hygiene*, XXI, January, 1937, 106-116.
8. "Factors in Character Development, Neuroses, Psychoses and Delinquency", *American Journal of Orthopsychiatry*, VII, April, 1937, 142-181.
9. "Play Technique in the Analysis of Young Children", *Psychoanalytic Review*, 24, July, 1937, 233-245.)
10. "Interrelated Factors in Development (A Study of Pregnancy, Labor, Delivery, Lying-in Period and Childhood)", *American Journal of Orthopsychiatry*, VIII, October, 1938, 726-752. (With Beatrice Lewi.)
11. "Psychiatry in Dentistry for Children", *Journal of the New Jersey State Dental Society*, April, 1941.
12. "Mental Hygiene in Pregnancy, Delivery and the Puerperium", *Mental Hygiene*, XXV, April, 1941, 221-236.

13. "Psychogenetic Implications in the Care of Obstetrical Patients", *The Trained Nurse and Hospital Review*, CVII, July, 1941.
14. "National and International Difficulties", *American Journal of Orthopsychiatry*, XI, July, 1941, 562-773. (With Paul J. Woolf.)
15. "Psychosomatic Relationships Between Mother and Infant", *Psychosomatic Medicine*, VI, April, 1944.
16. "Importance of Continuous Collaboration of All Agencies in Dynamic Handling of Each Child", *Nervous Child*, 3, 1944, 258-267.

II. *Publications for the Lay Public*

17. "All About Your Baby", *The Modern Homemaker*, McCall's, Dayton, Ohio, 1936.
18. "Baby's First Ten Days", *McCall's*, 1936.
19. "Anticipating Parenthood", *Extension Service New Jersey State College of Agriculture, Rutgers University*, 24, July, 1937.
20. "Your Baby and How to Train Him", *McCall's*, January, 1938.
21. "The Value of Play for a Child Development Study", *Understanding your Child*, II, June, 1938.
22. "Some Psychological Factors in the Physical Health of Children", *Child Study*, XVI, October, 1938.
23. "How Brave Can Parents Be?", *Parents' Magazine*, December, 1942.
24. "Democracy Begins in the Home", *New York Times Magazine*, August 29, 1943. (With Paul J. Woolf.)

III. *Films (available in the Film Library of New York University)*

1. Guide to Film I: "Some Basic Differences in the Newborn".
2. Guide to Film III: "Psychological Implications of Behavior During the Clinic Visit".
3. Guide to Film IV: "Family Life of the Navaho Indian".

MARGARET A. RIBBLE: THE RIGHTS OF INFANTS [1]

Comments by LAWRENCE S. KUBIE, M.D. (New York)

This little book is a healthy and stimulating challenge to every pediatrician, pediatrics nurse, and educator. Its spirit and its purpose is profoundly right. Its emphasis on the importance of the emotional factors in child care from the very moment of birth is sorely needed as a corrective to an era in which every mother and nurse has been encouraged to attempt to turn an infant into a clockwork mechanism, an era in which the only goal of child care seems to be to reduce trouble to a minimum, irrespective of what this costs the child's psychological development. Nothing could be more wholesome than the challenging picture this book presents to any young mother as to what constitutes the essence of mothering and what that mothering means to the emotional development of the child. No mother who reads it with an open mind and heart can ever again indulge in unashamed boasts as to how quickly after the baby's birth she scrambled back to her career.

The book is further stimulating to those who are interested in possibilities of improving the organization of infants' nurseries, because it opens up many avenues of speculation as to ways in which the infant can be assisted in the transition from intra-uterine to postnatal life.

On the other hand when one turns to the detailed physiological data which the author adduces to support her thesis, one is troubled. Sometimes the physiology is naive. Often it is dogmatic when it ought to be tentative. Thus the prenatal and early postnatal concentration of the blood with respect to red blood cells is precisely what occurs in adults who are accustomed to living at high altitudes; but this does not imply, as the author seems to think, either a relative or absolute anoxemia. Nor does the short inspiration and the prolonged expiration nor shallow and rapid breathing of the newborn indicate an inevitable anoxemia. In fact the whole picture of the relationship of sucking and respiration to anoxic states, though interesting and provocative, is hardly the open and shut affair that the author describes. It is true of course that the central nuclei which control all of these functions are situated in close proximity to one another; and that a close interrelationship exists between them is highly probable. However the particular type of interdependence of one on the other which the author describes, making the sucking process and the learning of sucking almost a panacea to all of the infant's struggles, may

[1] Columbia University Press, New York, 1943, pp. 118.

415

well turn out to be a partial truth and something of an over-simplification. This reviewer feels further that her concept of stuporous states in infants, and her concept of different types of sleep and partial sleep also are matters that require more precise definition, and clearer evidence, before they can be strictly evaluated.

It is somewhat puzzling therefore that from an argument, which both physiologically and psychologically must be characterized as naive, the author arrives at conclusions which in the main one must support with enthusiasm. This may be because the physiological and psychological arguments, despite their limitation, are in essence sound. Or alternatively, or in addition, it may be because the conclusions reached are derived from simple, pragmatic, honest clinical observation and feeling; and that their substantiation by psychological and physiological reasoning is in the nature of elaborate partially-scientific rationalizations. To the reviewer it does not seem to be particularly important to resolve this quandary in this review. It is far more important to stress the great potentialities for good that are inherent in the author's basic thesis.

EDOUARD PICHON: LE DEVELOPEMENT PSYCHOLOGIQUE DE L'ENFANT ET DE L'ADOLESCENT[1]

Comments by KATHERINE M. WOLF, Ph.D. (New York)

Pichon's book is planned as a text book for child psychologists, child psychiatrists, consulting psychologists, social workers; in short, for all who deal with the child's development and its abnormalities. As such it shows the usual organization of a text book on child psychiatry. It deals with the general approach to the child, with the methods of mental diagnosis such as interviews and tests. It enumerates mental syndromes known in child pathology, be they somatic, as in idiocy and imbecility, or purely psychological, as in enuresis and pavor nocturnus. Finally it deals with educational principles and with therapy. All these parts are not original. They can be found in any American handbook on child psychiatry. Carl Rogers' *The Clinical Treatment of the Problem Child*,[2] for example, gives all the information Pichon offers on the subject, and much more—it is based on a greater clinical material and incorporates more literature.

However, one portion of Pichon's book, the largest part, can legitimately claim originality; it gives an account of the child's development from birth to maturity. The originality lies not in a lot of new material but in the attempt, for the first time as far as we know, to give a picture of human development based on the findings of psychoanalysis and, at the same time, of experimental child psychology. Our review is limited to a report of this section of the book, and shows how Pichon attempts this synthesis.

He does so by a method of presentation that seems at first sight extremely plausible and natural. He views the child's development from two aspects, the emotional and the intellectual: the first, by means of psychoanalysis, the second, by means of experimental child psychology.

His description of the child's emotional development follows in the main rather closely the account that Freud has given in the *Three Contributions to the Theory of Sex* and that Anna Freud has elaborated in her books. As does psychoanalysis, Pichon divides the development during the first five years into three phases, the oral, the anal, and the phallic, which are succes-

1 (The Psychological Development of the Child and the Adolescent), Masson & Cie., Paris, 1936. Pp. 374.

2. Houghton Mifflin, New York, 1939.

sively determined by the erogenous zones, the mouth, the anus, and the genitals. Pichon considers the oedipal complex the climax of this emotional development in early childhood. He describes the formation of a superego as a result of the oedipal situation. He believes that the oedipal phase is followed by the latency period, the period in which the manifest sexual drives of the child seem to disappear, to reappear during puberty. He admits the libidinal character of sucking, of playing with the excrements, of masturbation, and considers the role of all these phenomena in the course of normal development.

There are, however, a few points on which Pichon disagrees with psychoanalysis. He argues against any identification of libido and sexuality and proposes to replace this identification by a new one that would characterize the libidinal drives as "hedonistic" ones, that is to say, drives seeking pleasure.

Beside a few minor differences in Pichon's description of emotional development from their description in psychoanalysis, there is another very important one. He does not accept the merely descriptive attitude of psychoanalysis which makes no moral evaluation. His view on the contrary is that emotional development tends to improve the human being. During the time of his development the human being becomes progressively able to renounce the egotistic pleasure of being loved in favor of the altruistic joy of loving. This love becomes at the same time increasingly independent of the original drive. "A healthy person is not a person whose drives are free, but who is free from drives." At birth man is a selfish animal, ready to devour his environment. The adult is "human", which means ready to sacrifice himself for his environment. He has become a "moral" person.

It goes without saying that this description of emotional development does not stop at puberty. On the contrary, the real achievement of development comes after puberty when the young man or woman finally succeeds in subordinating his or her different libidinal drives to a love that directs itself to one person, a person of the other sex, and "eternalizes" the drive in the social form of marriage.

Pichon's description of intellectual development also starts at birth. Here he does not pursue one line of thought consistently, but uses successively three different schools of genetic psychology in order to describe the child's intellectual development. In rough outline it would be correct to say that Pichon follows Wallon's book *L'enfant turbulent* in giving his picture of the first year of life. His description of the second and third years is based on his own studies. Piaget is used as a guide to show the trends of intellectual development from the fourth or fifth year on.

With Wallon, Pichon assumes that during his first year the baby learns to master the world by means of his muscular and sensory apparatus. He learns to react to and to distinguish between stimuli, be they optic, acoustic or tactile. He learns to enlarge his horizon by changing his body posture, by lifting his head, by sitting up, by standing, and by walking. At the beginning of this development the child is incapable of mastering his environment. Therefore he reacts to any stimulation as does any person who cannot master the situation, namely, with an emotional outburst. Pichon accepts Wallon's first stage of human development, the "Emotional Stage", and interprets it as the catastrophe reaction of an organism that cannot yet adapt to reality. He refuses, however, to associate these findings with any complicated theory about the development of the nervous system as Wallon does. The second phase of human development according to Wallon, the "Sensory Stage", is also accepted by Pichon. He sees in it the gradual adaptation of the organism to its environment by means of its sense organs and its muscular apparatus. Again he refuses to share Wallon's neurological explanation of this course of development.

This mastery of the infant's world by means of perceptual and motor reactions is achieved as soon as the child starts walking and grasping objects of his surrounding. This is at the end of the first year or at the beginning of the second.

But just at the moment when this development approaches its goal, the human being undergoes a new development in mastering the world, this time on another level. The sensory-motor level is replaced by the verbal one. The infant has become a child.

Although verbal development has its precursors in the first year of life, as in the baby's crying and babbling, the development of language has not yet begun during this period. Pichon cites evidence that the babbling of a child cannot be considered as language in any strict sense of the term. The selection of sounds that are like utterances have nothing to do with the phonetic units of any living language. The child babbles sounds that do not exist in his maternal tongue. He merely selects sounds according to his own acoustic and motoric pleasure; and babbles those that he prefers to hear and to produce.

Real language and its development start when the child utters something that the parents consider the child's "first words". In common with all psychologists dealing with the development of language, Pichon emphasizes that the term "word" is incorrect for this first linguistic effort of the child. The child's first language efforts result in single words that have the function of phrases and that bear a close relationship to the exclamations of adults. Pichon calls this first stage in speech development the stage of "enunciation" and shows that this enunciation serves to express the child's feelings, wishes, desires, and needs, but not to represent any objective fact. It lasts from one year to approximately a year-and-a-half.

This stage of extreme subjectivity is replaced by a phase of extreme objectivity. The child in his next phase describes everything as though it were independent of himself and of his emotional situation. "I" and "You" have become objects of the outside world that are described by names as are any other objects.

The final development of language is achieved when a new subjective element has been added to the child's language. Between the second and the third year the child becomes able to use the first and second person pronouns. This means that he has discovered that there are in the objective world of which he is speaking two points of reference, the speaker and the listener. The child has discovered "I" and "You", not in the first elementary usage that was characteristic of the stage of enunciation, but in the more complex usage that Pichon calls an attribute of "introspective conscience". The child does not only experience the "I" and "You" as a reality. This reality has become a specific object of his thinking.

This introspective conscience appearing in the last stage of verbal development, demonstrates itself in rudimentary forms only. A child of four or five is still unable to perform the mental operations involving real introspection.

This is shown clearly by the studies of Piaget, as Pichon demonstrates. It would lead us too far and be irrelevant to the theme of this review to discuss all the points in which Pichon disagrees with Piaget. Therefore we will limit ourselves to an enumeration of those in which Pichon agrees with Piaget and will describe the end of the intellectual development in Pichon's presentation of Piaget's theory.

The thought processes of the child between the fifth and eighth years is characterized by two features. Piaget calls them "syncretism" and "realism". Pichon prefers the words "globalism" and "absolutism".

The child of this age is not yet able to analyze any situation into its component parts. He always conceives any social and intellectual situation as a whole and therefore cannot speak of it otherwise than as a whole. It is clear that such envisaging of a situation excludes any causal explanation of it as well as any possibility of recognizing similar elements occurring in a different situation. It also excludes the capacity to describe a situation to another person in terms that would enable that person to understand it. Pichon uses this global attitude of the child towards the world as a basis for demonstrating a law that appears to him of utmost importance to anyone describing human development. He calls this law "the law of addition of possibilities" and shows that the globalism of thinking is not lost when we become adults but still has a function in our mental life. Artistic and personal thinking would be impossible were the adult always to analyze the content of his thoughts.

The second feature of the child's thinking is its "absolutism". The child having not yet developed a real faculty of introspection cannot distinguish between psychic reality and objective reality. Whatever he perceives has equal existence, whether it be a dream or a fantasy produced by the child himself, a prohibition or command pronounced by the parents, a figure invented by a poet, a picture created by an artist, or a table and a chair in the room. Piaget calls this thinking "realistic" because it believes in the reality of any psychic creation. Pichon calls it absolutistic because it neglects any relation to the person who has created it.

Only after eight years and very gradually does the child overcome this globalism and absolutism and become able to think analytically and relatively.

During this whole evolution one trend is obvious in every stage of intellectual development. Mastery of the world has been achieved in the first stage by means of the sensory-motor apparatus, in the second by means of language, in the third by means of thought. This changing of medium has a definite direction. The medium progressively loses its concreteness. It becomes more and more abstract. As the emotional development replaces instincts by morality, the intellectual development increasingly detaches the human being from the concrete situation and leads him to autonomous mastery of the world by means of thought. Pichon gives the latency period a characteristic name. He calls it the stage of "decarnalization", literally, the stage which breaks any links to the flesh. This literal translation coresponds exactly to what he wishes to point out. In his theory the latency period is the period of "real" development of the human being: in which the emotions lose their associations with the basic drives and thought loses its close relation to sensation and motor reactions.

One could evaluate or better criticize Pichon's book along several different lines. For example one could collect all the points in which he supplies actually incorrect information, such as his statement that the baby smiles during the first month and recognizes his parents in the course of the second or third, or his pedagogical advice which recommends toilet training in the first half of the first year and forbids the study of foreign languages throughout almost the whole of one's life. One could demonstrate that such incorrect statements are based partly on inadequate personal observations and partly on a strange scotomization of any literature not French. The index of Pichon's book on child psychology does not even mention the names of Gesell, Pratt, Shirley, McGraw, C. Bühler, Lewin, and others. We could also mention how disturbing we have found Pichon's tendency to change all the terms used by other psychologists.

It seems to us more fruitful, however, to ask whether Pichon succeeds in his attempt to synthesize psychoanalysis and experimental child psychology. .

It is the unavoidable consequence of his presentation that we have had to give his views on psychoanalysis and on experimental child psychology separately and almost without relation to each other. He presents the development of the emotions and the development of the intellect as though they were separate. He tries to establish a fragile bridge between these two realms of development; he assigns one exclusively to the field of genetic psychology and the other to psychoanalysis. He does this by means of a law which he asserts rules development. He calls it "the law of appetition". Any intellectual development is always preceded by an analogous emotional development.

Pichon's book makes any connection between these two types of development, any interaction between emotion and intellect, almost negligible. Nor does he make any reference to the mutual relation between the achievements of psychoanalysis and experimental child psychology. We believe that the basis of this failure to give a real synthesis lies in the fact that Pichon has not clearly understood and formulated the essential difference between these two schools of psychology. Instead of recognizing that they both deal with the same subject, namely, the development of the human being, and that they describe the same object by two different methods (one by direct observation and experiments and the other by reconstruction, interpretation, observation and explanation), he seems to believe that these two schools of psychology are each clearly limited to a specific field of human development, the one to the emotions and the other to the intellect.

This error is astonishing. Any one who has studied psychoanalysis knows that it explains the development of human beings as a whole and refrains from atomistic focusing on any one specific problem. A thorough student of the books of Wallon and Piaget must recognize that it is the aim of these authors in using their specific methods to trace the development of the human mind as a whole. Pichon has studied analysis, and practised it. His quotations show clearly that he has not only read Wallon and Piaget, but that he has tried to digest them. So his erroneous statement in regard to their fields of interest cannot be based on a lack of information. There must therefore be another reason for such misconception.

An author misinterprets other authors either because he does not know them sufficiently, or because they do not agree with his views. We may suppose the latter to be true in Pichon's case regarding psychoanalysis as well as in reference to the theories of Wallon and Piaget.

Psychoanalysis as well as both these special approaches of experimental child psychology attempts to describe human development as subject to certain laws that are in conformity with other laws of science. Pichon, however, thinks of this development as an achievement, subject to norms comparable to the norms of esthetics, ethics, or jurisprudence. Both psychoanalysis and experimental child psychology seek causal explanations of the history of man's becoming human, though in methodically different fields. Whereas psychoanalysis establishes a causal genetic unity throughout the whole development in relation to the conscious and unconscious contents and the mechanisms of the human mind, Wallon and Piaget try to demonstrate that the forms in which the human ego operates are equally subject to causal and genetic laws. The genetic continuity of content of mental processes can only be recognized by the method of psychoanalysis, while its formal development should be the subject of direct observation.

The moment one replaces this causal aim of psychology, common to experimental child psychology and psychoanalysis, by a finalistic or normative one, the relation between psychoanalysis and experimental child psychology changes its character. Their limitations are no longer determined by the limitations of their methods in finding causal relationships. Their value is determined exclusively by the test of how far they are able to support a finalistic point of view. Thus psychoanalysis, almost by accident, lends itself better to demonstrating that the child stigmatized by all possible perversions finally becomes the adult capable of monogamy, while experimental psychology demonstrates that the infant who cannot distinguish sound from light becomes the adult capable of solving scientific problems. We say "almost by accident" because we believe that neither does psychoanalysis set out to prove the one, nor experimental psychology the other.

This criticism would have taken too much space and would be as negativistic as others we eliminated in the beginning, had it only been able to show that Pichon is wrong and that he did not succeed in making an adequate synthesis of psychoanalysis and experimental child psychology. But in these considerations we believe there are two points of more general importance.

The first is that a synthesis of psychoanalysis and experimental child psychology would be successful if it could combine these two different methods to describe the one common object, the developing human being. The second is that neither psychoanalysis nor experimental child psychology can be arbitrarily interpreted for the sake of achieving that synthesis, nor even for the sake of applying the knowledge of either or both. It cannot be a question of personal taste, whether one is finalistic or causalistic; in subscribing either to psychoanalysis or to the genetic psychology of Wallon and Piaget, one is subscribing to their causalistic attitude. Not to do so is more than to disagree on minor points; it is to miss their main objective.

It is because Pichon's book attempts a synthesis of psychoanalysis and genetic psychology and because it shows a mistake typical of the kind that frustrates such an effort that we believe it is worth reading and worth careful thought.